OXFORD MEDICAL PUBLICATIONS

Modern Obstetrics
in General Practice

OXFORD GENERAL PRACTICE SERIES

Editorial Board

G. H. FOWLER, J. A. M. GRAY,
J. C. HASLER, A.-L. KINMONTH,
D. C. MORRELL

1. Paediatric problems in general practice
   M. Modell and R. H. Boyd
2. Geriatric problems in general practice
   G. K. Wilcock, J. A. M. Gray, and P. M. M. Pritchard
3. Preventive medicine in general practice
   edited by J. A. M. Gray and G. H. Fowler
5. Locomotor disability in general practice
   edited by M. I. V. Jayson and R. Million
6. The consultation: an approach to learning and teaching
   *D. Pendleton, T. P. C. Schofield, P. H. L. Tate, and
   P. B. Havelock*
7. Continuing care: the management of chronic disease
   edited by J. C. Hasler and T. P. C. Schofield
8. Management in general practice
   P. M. M. Pritchard, K. B. Low, and M. Whalen
9. Modern obstetrics in general practice
   edited by G. N. Marsh
10. Terminal care at home
    edited by R. Spilling
11. Rheumatology for GPs
    H. L. F. Currey and S. Hull
12. Women's problems in general practice
    Second edition
    edited by Ann McPherson

Modern Obstetrics in General Practice

Oxford General Practice Series 9

Edited by

G. N. MARSH, MD, FRCGP, MCFPC,
DCH, DObst, RCOG

General Practitioner, Stockton-on-Tees, Cleveland

OXFORD   NEW YORK   TOKYO
OXFORD UNIVERSITY PRESS

Oxford University Press, Walton Street, Oxford OX2 6DP

Oxford New York Toronto
Delhi Bombay Calcutta Madras Karachi
Petaling Jaya Singapore Hong Kong Tokyo
Nairobi Dar es Salaam Cape Town
Melbourne Auckland

and associated companies in
Beirut Berlin Ibadan Nicosia

Oxford is a trade mark of Oxford University Press

First published 1985
Reprinted 1987

British Library Cataloguing in Publication Data
Modern obstetrics in general practice.—(Oxford
general practice series; 9)
1. Gynaecology   2. Obstetrics
I. Marsh, G. N.
618   RG101

ISBN 0–19–261419–3

Library of Congress Cataloging in Publication Data
Modern obstetrics in general practice.
(Oxford general practice series; 9) (Oxford
medical publications)
Includes bibliographies and index.
1. Obstetrics.   2. Family medicine.   I. Marsh, G. N.
(Geoffrey Norman)   II. Series: Oxford general practice
series; no. 9.   III. Series: Oxford medical publications.
[DNLM: 1. Family Practice.   2. Obstetrics.   3. Pregnancy
W1 OX55 no. 9/WQ 200 M689]
RG524.M68 1985   618.2   85–4944

ISBN 0–19–261419–3

Printed in Great Britain
at the University Printing House, Oxford
by David Stanford
Printer to the University

Acknowledgements

I express my sincere thanks to all the following people:

Dr John Hasler—for initially suggesting the idea of this book to me, and encouraging me thereafter.

Dr Michael Bull—for his several contributions and his sensible guidance.

All the contributors—for many, many hours of hard work in the preparation of their chapters.

Kathleen McFarlane—for typing the text many times and generally assembling the book.

The staff of Oxford University Press.

My partners and trainees—for so much goodwill and for looking after my patients, during my time spent editing.

My patients for having taught me so much about pleasurable and even joyous obstetrics.

And finally my wife and family—for tolerating me sunk deeply in my armchair, not speaking, and not even wandering down the garden to look at my 'old roses'.

Contents

Section C: Intranatal care

Section D: Postpartum care

Contributors

Ms Catherine Boyd
Formerly Research Officer, Maternity Alliance, London

Dr M. J. V. Bull
General practitioner, Oxford

Dr S. R. Burne
General practitioner, Oxford

Ms. Hilary Cashman
A patient of Norton Medical Centre, Stockton-on-Tees

Professor G. Chamberlain
Professor of Obstetrics and Gynaecology,
St George's Hospital Medical School, London

Ms Chloe Fisher
Community midwife, Oxford

Mr Keith A. Godfrey
First Assistant in the Department of Obstetrics and Gynaecology,
University of Newcastle

Dr Marion H. Hall
Consultant Obstetrician and Gynaecologist, Aberdeen Teaching Hospitals

Mr K. B. Lim
Senior registrar in Obstetrics and Gynaecology, Hammersmith Hospital,
London

Professor D. F. Hawkins
Professor of Obstetric Therapeutics,
Institute of Obstetrics and Gynaecology, Hammersmith Hospital, London

Dr G. N. Marsh
General practitioner, Stockton-on-Tees

Dr M. McKendrick
General practitioner, Hexham, Northumberland

Dr A. H. Melhuish
General practitioner, Henley-on-Thames

Professor D. C. Morrell
Professor of General Practice, St Thomas's Hospital Medical School,
London

Dr R. G. Newcombe
Lecturer in Medical Statistics, University of Wales College of Medicine, Cardiff

Dr B. M. N. Pitt
Consultant Psychiatrist, St. Bartholomew's Hospital London

Dr B. A. Sides
General practitioner, Worsley, Salford

Mr Malcolm Stewart
Senior Research Assistant, St George's Hospital Medical School, London

Professor G. M. Stirrat
Professor of Obstetrics and Gynaecology, University of Bristol Medical School

Mrs Marjorie Tew
Research Statistician, University of Nottingham Medical School

Ms Sandy Tinson
Health visitor, Abingdon, Oxford

Ms Jean Towler
Director of Nursing Services (Midwifery), Manchester

Ms Rhiannon Walters
Researcher and commentator on modern obstetrics; mother of twins, London

Dr L. I. Zander
Senior Lecturer, Department of General Practice,
St Thomas's Hospital Medical School, London

Introduction

G. N. Marsh

The existence of this book bears witness to the rapid development of general practice in the 1960s and 1970s which has now reached the stage at which the clinical content of the work done can be reassessed and re-evaluated. Hence this is a book on obstetrics, yet edited by a general practitioner, and in which several of the chapters and sections have been written by general practitioners. By incorporating those chapters with others from specialists in relevant fields—obstetrics, statistics, sociology, midwifery etc.—a book has developed which describes what is special and peculiar to obstetrics within the setting of general practice. Thus emerges the 'specialty' of general practitioner obstetrics (Marsh 1982).

Between 1971 and 1981 the number of general practitioners increased by 15 per cent to 22,304 in Great Britain and the average list size fell by 10 per cent to approximately 2200 patients per doctor, creating the potential for improvement in general practitioner care resulting from smaller numbers of patients. Health centres containing good facilities in which to work numbered 270 in 1971 and 1000 in 1981. The proportion of general practioners working in a health centre rose from 8 to 15 per cent. An even larger proportion of general practioners now work in modern group-practice centres. By 1981 over 80 per cent of midwives, district nurses, and health visitors were attached to general practices. These rapid changes in the structure and personnel should have rebounded to the benefit of all types of clinical care within general practice, but especially to obstetrics with its considerable orientation on team work.

Paradoxically though, during the last two decades and coinciding with these improvements there has occurred a fading of interest by general practitioners in obstetrics, rather than the reverse. Major policy decisions were taken resulting in almost all deliveries taking place in hospital. In addition general practitioners realized that intranatal care was becoming increasingly technological, mechanized, and beyond their scope. With the Caesarean section rate rising towards 30 per cent in the United States, the universal use of monitors being proposed, epidural anaesthesia becoming more common, and the percentage of forceps deliveries increasing steadily it seemed impossible for 'just a general practitioner' to remain involved in the intranatal scene (Francome and Carson 1983). Birth was not only being 'medicalized', but 'surgicalized'. Concomitant with these changes, specialists were being held responsible for the results of their care. Perinatal mortality rates were being increasingly focused from region to area and even to district.

Realizing the importance of good antenatal care and feeling that it may have shortcomings in the general practice setting many specialists tried to undertake antenatal care too. Having lost the intranatal conclusion of their antenatal endeavours general practitioners saw less point in doing antenatal care and were accordingly prepared to let specialists take over. Increasingly, however, the specialists themselves were unable to provide enough staff or hours for the sheer volume of antenatal and postnatal care required. Much of what they did provide was seen to be inappropriate, or inadequate, or even inhumane by many women. Not only did the sheer volume of care overwhelm them, but specialists became increasingly weary of huge clinics of perfectly normal women performing for the most part a perfectly normal physiological function. They found that their highly specialized pathology-orientated training rendered much of what they were doing extremely boring. It is not surprising, therefore, that junior staff began to carry out a large amount of hospital antenatal clinic care.

Throughout the last two decades the number of complaints to organizations such as the Patients' Association and the Association for the Improvement of Maternity Services has been very high. The Patients' Association receives complaints across the whole medical spectrum yet 90 per cent of them were about obstetric care (Robinson 1974). Increasingly, women were demanding to be treated as women and not patients and protesting that having a baby should surely for the great majority of them be a physiological function. Many women with authoritative and well-thought-through views were writing to newspapers and women's magazines. Surveys and studies carried out showed that the thousands of anecdotes of dissatisfaction were increasingly amounting to statistically significant data (BBC TV 1981; Boyd Sellers 1982; Garcia 1982). Women wanted more emphasis on the behavioural aspects of having a baby and also wanted to participate in the discussions on some of the modern surgical techniques—episiotomy, induction, the use of monitors—and whether they are as necessary as they were becoming prevalent (*Lancet* editorial 1980).

An interestingly recurrent finding in the lay comments about obstetric care was that the general practitioner involvement elicited greater satisfaction than any other aspects (Lowthian 1981). Both general practitioner and midwife got good marks. These comments were substantiated by various media studies on television and film as well as in an authoritative lay literature (BBC TV 1979; Cartwright 1979; Oakley 1982; Rothman 1982; Spastics Society 1979).

At the same time and encouraged by the groundswell of support from women, general practitioners themselves were beginning to realize that the antenatal and postnatal period of a woman's life was very central to their role as family doctors. The psychological rapport that can develop during the antenatal period is of enormous significance in the family doctor/ patient relationship.

Two major reports—one written jointly from the Royal College of Obstetricians and Gynaecologists and the Royal College of General Practitioners and one solely from the Royal College of Obstetricians and Gynaecologists—both concluded that specialist antenatal and postnatal care should on the whole be concentrated on high-risk patients with obstetric problems and the vast majority of care could and should be done by community-based primary health care teams in the setting of general practice. (Royal College of Obstetrics and Gynaecology and Royal College of General Practitioners, 1982; Royal College of Obstetrics and Gynaecology Working Party 1982). Thus all general practitioners need to update and reassess their antenatal, puerperal, and postnatal care. There are obvious problems associated with intranatal care—one of the major ones being access to delivery facilities—but both reports recommended greater use of existing general practitioner facilities and that all specialist units should provide facilities for general practitioners to look after their own women in labour. Without the enthusiasm from these reports it is doubtful whether I would have agreed to edit this book.

So a small but significant proportion of general practitioners with access to intranatal care facilities need to consider its modern implications, and provide a viable and even competing alternative to care of normal patients by specialists. When concerned with intranatal care the general practitioner emphasis must be on 'normalizing' obstetrics where possible and most importantly responding to the woman's requests and suggestions. He must feel more satisfaction from the normal delivery than he would from one ending in forceps. It is this style of care for which women are asking and it is the general practitioner who can provide it. This does not preclude specialists doing so, but the general practitioner can offer the great advantage of continuity of care. But general practitioner obstetric intranatal care must above all be safe; Chapter 8 amasses the considerable evidence that it is. Klein has shown in Oxford that general practitioners manage normal cases better than their specialist colleagues (Klein *et al.* 1983). The conventional wisdom amongst general practitioners that this was so has now been substantiated statistically.

THE PRIMARY HEALTH CARE TEAM

Primary health care teams now exist increasingly in towns, cities, suburbs, and even in country areas. The teams are community set and community orientated (Marsh 1976). There is great potential for good obstetric care in their multidisciplinary approach. Obstetric care being a team affair, this book is written by team members and it moves from preconception to postnatal care and includes care of the newborn. This team approach is, in part, what is special about this book. Indeed other specialties could adopt this style. Psychiatry, paediatrics, and geriatrics would be particularly appropriate. It is important to remember that the team works despite the fact that some members of that team are independent professionals in their own right. That status does not preclude working in a team with others. In particular the changing character of the general practitioner/midwife relationship is explored in the book and attention is directed particularly to whether general practitioner and midwife are both needed for a normal pregnancy, delivery, and puerperium. It goes without saying that the book concludes that they are. In passing, it is worthy of note that there are a large number of women contributors, something for which I deliberately aimed. It is a sad commentary that the proportion of female specialists in obstetrics and gynaecology is extremely low and falling and lower than in many other specialities. By the same token elections for the Council of the Royal College of Obstetricians and Gynaecologists usually result in only one or two women being elected out of approximately 30 people.

The consumer contribution to the book is drawn from personal experience and then related to women in general (Chapter 1). It is further substantiated by much of the recent 'women's literature'. It emphasizes that despite the many participants in the care patients want a continuum of interest by a doctor whom they know.

WHO SHOULD READ THIS BOOK?

This book is not in any way a traditional textbook of obstetrics. Accordingly it is not for medical students unless they know that they intend to enter general practice. It is very much for the general practitioner beginning to do obstetrics, and even more relevant to the general practitioner who has been practising for a few years. Both groups are probably equally dismayed by the technological teaching and practice to which they have been exposed or become accustomed and which may well be daunting rather than encouraging them to continue in obstetric practice. It will be of similar benefit to those general practitioners who were trained in the 1950s and early 1960s before the era of a scientific approach to obstetrics and before the introduction of technology. This book describes what a good general practitioner should be doing in the 1980s and the data on which that is based.

It will of course be essential reading for anyone taking the DRCOG examination more particularly as the exam evolves from being a mere assessment of the performance of an SHO in a specialist obstetric unit, as it currently is, to an exam more relevant to future practice. Anyone wishing to score high marks in the MRCOG or wishing to become a consultant fully aware of the potential and practice of good general practitioner obstetrics will need to read it too. Although this is not a textbook each author has tried to provide a comprehensive list of references.

The final chapter describes a system of obstetric care which is not only safe, but also modern and personally fulfilling to all the participants and especially to the mother and baby. It is eminently applicable in the field of general practice. Having read this book all general practitioners should go to their surgeries bent on making changes in their antenatal and postnatal care. The fortuitous few with intranatal care facilities available should feel far more confident, and enthused to expand this component of their work.

REFERENCES

BBC 2 (1979). 'Will the baby be alright?' *Man alive* programme. Film of antenatal care at Norton Medical Centre.

BBC TV (1981). *That's Life* programme, February.

Boyd, C. and Sellers, L. (1982). *The British way of birth*. Pan, London.

Cartwright, A. (1979). *The dignity of labour?* Tavistock Publications, London.

Francome, C. and Carson, D. (1983). Can we avoid a caesarian crisis? *Occasional Paper No. 8*. Middlesex Polytechnic.

Garcia, J. (1982). Women's views of antenatal care. In *Effectiveness and satisfaction in antenatal care* (eds M. Enkin and I. Chalmers) *Clinics in developmental medicine nos 81/82*. London: Spastics International Medical Publications/William Heinemann Medical Books, pp. 81–91.

Klein M., Lloyd, I. Redman, C. Bull, M. and Turnbull, A. C. (1983). A comparison of low-risk pregnant women booked for delivery in two systems of care: shared care (consultant) and integrated general practice unit. II: Labour and delivery management and neonatal outcome. *Br. J. Obst. and Gynaecol.*, **90**, 125–8.

Lancet Editorial June 14 (1980).

Lowthian, R. (ed.) (1981). Antenatal clinics. A survey of 2000 readers. *Mother magazine*, July and November IPC Magazines, London.

Marsh, G. N. (1976). *Team care in general practice*. Croom Helm, London.

Marsh, G. N. (1982). The specialty of GP obstetrics. *Lancet* **1**, 669–72 and correspondence.

Oakley, A. (1982). *From here to maternity*. Penguin, Harmondsworth.

Robinson, J. (1974). *Consumer attitude to maternity care*. Oxford Consumer. May.

Rothman, B. K. (1982) *In Labour: Women and Power in the Birth-place*. Junction Books.

Royal College of Obstetricians and Gynaecologists and the Royal College of General Practitioners (1982). Report by a Joint Working Party on Training for obstetrics and gynaecology for general practitioners.

Royal College of Obstetricians and Gynaecologists (1982) *Report by working party on antenatal and intrapartum care*.

Spastics Society (1979). Film: *Feeling special* (the antenatal care at Norton Medical Centre).

Section A

1 The case for general practitioner obstetrics: the women's view

Hilary Cashman

My first child was born in January 1983, when I was 30 years old. A year or so later the euphoria surrounding that birth has still not been dispelled; and I offer here my own roughly researched blueprint for a safe, active, and happy birth, since this is unhappily a rarer event than it should be.

I had been interested in the subjects of pregnancy, birth, and women's fertility in general for some years, as an area in which women's choices seemed to be unnecessarily curtailed and the power and prestige of the medical profession used sometimes oppressively. There exists a kind of folklore about birth; almost every woman can quote a dozen or so cases from among her own friends or family of premature inductions, hiccuping fetal monitors, analgesia not given when wanted or given when not wanted, unnecessary episiotomies, delayed or incompetent perineal repairs and subsequent depression. Some doctors would dismiss this as anecdotal evidence; if so, it must be one of the most widespread anecdotes around!

Rumblings of discontent about such treatment have been heard for years, surfacing first among articulate middle-class women who were better equipped than most to seek alternatives (such as Michel Odent's clinic at Pithiviers) or press for a better deal within the NHS system. Most women, however, still had to put up with whatever treatment they were given, and be told that they were lucky to end up with a healthy baby and should not complain.

By the early 1980s things were beginning to change; the consumer movement in childbirth began to blossom and broaden out. There were several reasons for this but the primary one was probably mass media coverage of the issues. In 1981 and 1982 BBC television showed a film about Michel Odent's clinic, in which viewers saw women giving birth without drugs, in whatever position suited them, in quiet and calm surroundings. In 1981 the popular BBC consumer affairs programme *That's Life* ran a survey of women's reactions to the maternity services in the United Kingdom: a massive exercise of which the results were published with a commentary in 1982 (Boyd and Sellers 1982). The folklore was finding a voice; women who lacked the verbal skills or factual ammunition to question the medical professionals were at last being heard.

The most disheartening aspect of the resulting debate was the unwarranted adversarial tone brought to it principally by the medical profession. Too often legitimate complaints about questionable medical practices were treated as whining self-pity and women's desire for a humane and gentle birth was seen as callous disregard for their babies' welfare. It was therefore vital to test the central assumption behind this attitude: that the use of high technology rather than human skills always made birth safer. Were women really willing to trade their babies' health for a pleasant experience? Did their feelings about good and bad births have any validity? The answers to these questions assumed a personal importance for me as I began to plan for the birth of my own baby.

Received wisdom for the last couple of decades has been that a specialist unit in hospital is the safest place to give birth and it has been assumed that this is due to the increasing amount of technological intervention that has taken place in such units—the 'active management of labour' (I include electronic monitoring as intervention, since immobilizing a labouring woman in a supine position has a considerable effect on her labour). Individual procedures were questioned from time to time, especially after it began to emerge that electronic monitoring seemed to give rise to an increase in caesarean sections (Gordon 1982), that induction on grounds of dating alone enhanced rather than decreased the risk of morbidity and mortality (Dunn 1976), that episiotomy often generated more physical damage and unhappiness than natural tearing (Kitzinger 1981) and so on; but the general principle retained its authority. It seemed to be proved by the Registrar General's surveys of maternal and infant mortality, and was accepted uncritically by successive government inquiries into the maternity services (Cranbrook 1959; DHSS 1980; Peel 1970).

In the late 1970s however a professional statistician, Majorie Tew, began to look at these official statistics more closely. She found that the government reports which had used them to recommend 100 per cent hospital births had treated them so crudely and unscientifically that they had drawn many incorrect conclusions; for instance, she pointed out, the increasing hospitalization of birth had included ever more normal births in the hospital sample while leaving an increasing proportion of precipitate and premature births in the decreasing home-birth sample (Tew 1981). Her own more rigorous analysis of the figures made some telling points: that working-class babies still fared much worse than middle-class ones—hospitalization had not diminished the difference between socioeconomic groups; that the need for emergency and resuscitation facilities after delivery was often iatrogenic; that increased hospitalization in areas with high perinatal mortality rates had not improved those rates (Tew 1980). One of her conclusions from the readjusted statistics was that general practitioner maternity units had a better safety record than consultant units (Tew 1981).

Meanwhile various general practitioners were doing some research on their own account. Black (1982) comparing two areas in Oxfordshire, one with a 45 per cent general practitioner maternity unit delivery rate and one with a 12 per cent rate, found no significant difference in mortality and concluded, 'The support for the idea that GP deliveries constitute a risk . . . is largely based on belief rather than published evidence'. Marsh (1977) described a 15-year audit of his own practice in which 60 per cent of births were under his own supervision—he achieved a perinatal mortality rate of 8.5 per thousand births, compared with an area average varying between 19 and 30 per thousand births in the same period. He suggested some reasons: general practitioner obstetricians looking after normal pregnancies freed hospital consultants to concentrate on more problematic ones; general practitioners were better placed to pick up and give special care to high-risk pregnancies; general practitioner obstetricians were experienced in normal deliveries—'The general practitioner working in a normal unit cannot and does not overreact with drips, machines and other interventions to minor abnormalities or minor delays in potentially normal cases; he [*sic*] merely observes more acutely whether the natural process will see the patient through.'

Taylor *et al.* (1980) examined the perinatal mortality rate of babies transferred from general practitioner to consultant care. This was known to be high and it had been assumed that these babies would have fared better if their mothers had been booked for consultant care from the start. Taylor's study compared two groups: one group of women booked for general practitioner care under a very specific booking policy, and another group in a different area whom the same booking policy would have allocated to general practitioner care, but who were under consultant care because there were no general practitioner maternity units in the area. Two perinatal mortality rates were compared: that of the babies in the first group whose mothers were transferred to consultant care, and that of the babies in the second group whose mothers would have been so transferred had they been under general practitioner care. No significant difference was found: '[The] findings indicate that low-risk women (and their infants) booked with general practitioners experienced no greater risk of morbidity and mortality than those booked into consultant units'.

Some advocates of general practitioner care have suggested that even if it does carry a slightly higher risk it is women's right to choose to take the risk, just as they might choose to take risks in other fields of adventure and achievement, such as mountain-climbing or hang-gliding (see, for example, Rayner 1981). This approach is well-meaning but its implications are questionable. When I was pregnant, miscarriage or stillbirth seemed unthinkable horrors, and I believe most women would go through almost anything to ensure the best outcome for their babies. General practitioner care can be justified on grounds of safety alone, leaving the quality of the experience aside (for the moment).

There is a body of opinion, rapidly gaining adherents in this country and the United States, that most obstetric care should be in the hands of skilled midwives, with hospital and consultant care responsible only for looking after abnormal pregnancies and labours, and providing emergency back-up in 'normal' cases. It has been stated with particular force in the United States, where active management of labour has become almost universal and midwives are not allowed, in most states, to practise without a doctor. This situation demands a high degree of personal commitment and professional skill (to avoid malpractice suits) from the midwives who do practise alone, and this dedication is expressed in books which combine inspirational descriptions of gentle, 'graceful' births with good basic midwifery primers (for example, Davis 1981; Gaskin 1980). Such a maternity system is not a pipedream; in Holland, which has an excellent perinatal mortality rate, two-thirds of births take place at home with midwives as the only medical attendants. One of the chief UK proponents of such a system is Christine Beels of the Association of Radical Midwives; unfortunately, in her enthusiasm for the rehabilitation of midwifery, she denigrates the role of the general practitioner (partly because she feels that general practitioner obstetrics is a dying art) (Beels 1980). Nevertheless, in their quest for the ideal in childbirth, general practitioner obstetricians and radical midwives have much in common.

Why has there been such a decline in the amount of general practitioner obstetrics? Bull (1981) considered some of the reasons: insistence by government and the medical profession on the greater safety of consultant unit births, a falling birth rate and consequent lack of opportunity for obstetric experience in general practice, poor remuneration, poor coverage of obstetrics in medical education. He saw some hopes for reversing the decline, especially in the development of the primary health care team based on a group practice, perhaps with one or two of the doctors in the team carrying most of the obstetric caseload.

From my point of view, the growing enlightenment on the quality of general practitioner maternity care was singularly good news because I happened to be already on the list of an enthusiastic general practitioner obstetrician. Despite this, I would in the normal course of things have been booked for a consultant delivery as an elderly primigravida; but my general practitioner persuaded the hospital to agree to his looking after my pregnancy and labour (a departure from the norm which caused raised eyebrows and puzzled enquiries each time I visited the hospital) provided that no problems arose. None did, so apart from checks by a hospital consultant at 14 and 28 weeks I received all my antenatal care from my general practitioner and his team.

The clinic was a few minutes' walk from my house and on the bus route to my job, so I did not miss much work-time for antenatal visits. For women without cars—and this group probably includes many of the higher-risk women who most need antenatal care—it is important that the clinic should be close at hand, particularly if (as in my area) public transport is expensive and not very good. Sitting on cold, smoke-filled buses or trailing through rain and snow is not much fun at any time, especially not during pregnancy.

There was a pleasant waiting-room at the clinic and waiting time tended to be short—just long enough to chat with the other mothers-to-be, admire the new babies, and play with the toddlers. I had heard stories of 2 and 3-hour waits at hospital clinics; quite apart from the loss of earnings or effect on the nerves of a pregnant woman perhaps with a small child in tow, this represents an unacceptable level of contempt for the value of women's time. Nobody minds a reasonable wait in order to maximize the efficient use of staff time, but it is unpardonable not to operate the simplest appointment system.

The health care team approach seemed to produce a well-coordinated, personal system in which one saw familiar faces at each visit and knew whom to ask for information: the receptionists arranged appointments and antenatal classes; the midwives (I usually saw the same one) checked blood pressure, weight-gain and uterine growth and did other obstetric routines, and ran relaxation classes; health visitors called before and after the birth to keep an eye on the mothers' and babies' general wellbeing and answer questions; and a family planning nurse offered contraceptive advice after the birth. The system was flexible and responsive to particular needs; for instance, the receptionists arranged home visits for women who missed antenatals (a group of higher-than-average risk—presumably because of stress, overwork, or similar factors).

There were also available, if needed, social workers and marriage counsellors to help with familial and social problems, to counsel women considering termination or facing the possibility of handicap, and so on.

Antenatal classes included relaxation and breathing exercises, appropriate keep-fit routines, parentcraft, and a chance to discuss any queries that came up over a cup of tea. In the last few weeks, the midwife arranged a visit to the maternity department of the local hospital, where we had a chance to see some of the things we had heard about—the special care baby unit, the delivery room, an Entonox cylinder, an electronic fetal monitor (out of order), lithotomy posts, resuscitation equipment, etc.

I found continuity of care to be a morale-booster in pregnancy. Too often hospital antenatals leave women depressed and annoyed, with their questions unanswered. My general practitioner on the other hand had an infectious enthusiasm for the whole business and never deflated my own elation and excitement. He was very open to requests and questions, and did not treat them as impertinent or threatening. Women, in general, feel more confident in and at ease with their own family doctor whom they already know and who has perhaps looked after them and their families for several years. If they know their general practitioner will actually be at the delivery they can feel more relaxed about what is inevitably a fairly daunting event.

In the last couple of months, after leaving work, I did some preparation on my own account—not elaborate exercise or dietary regimes, for which I am too lazy and disorganized, but a few basic minimum steps to reassure myself I had done my best to prepare for birth: some relaxation and pelvic floor exercises, perineal massage with coconut oil to avoid tearing, a mainly vegetarian wholefood diet (which is what I eat normally anyway) to avoid piles, varicose veins and other miseries, and raspberry leaf extract daily for the last few weeks for an easy and quick birth—an ancient herbal aid currently making something of a comeback (ARM *Newsletter* 1982). (In the event I did dilate rapidly and give birth to a 7 lb (3 kg) baby over an intact perineum, though how much the raspberry leaves and coconut oil had to do with it is anybody's guess.)

As the expected date of delivery, 19 December, came and went, I became aware of another advantage of being with my own general practitioner: for more than 2 weeks after the due date he put no pressure on me to be induced. Not being a hospital obstetrician used to seeing pathology everywhere, he remained relaxed about the delay and helped me not to worry. He saw me every week to assess the situation, and found no indicators (apart from date) that the baby should be induced. Because he did not believe that 'lateness' alone was a valid ground for it, he was as determined as I to avoid induction if at all possible—a policy which was vindicated by the baby, when she arrived, showing no signs of postmaturity.

Christmas and then New Year offered their distractions from the long wait. I counted kicks and did not fret, since the baby continued active. I tried giving it a few hints with hot baths, castor oil and sprints round the block, but without result apart from a few inconclusive contractions. At my antenatal visits 3 and 10 days after the due date my general practitioner remained unworried; at 17 days he admitted that he was finally beginning to lose his nerve! By that time I too was becoming anxious despite myself, and longing to hold the baby and see all was well with it. I had looked up the various methods of induction, and hoped to be offered a prostaglandin pessary to help my cervix to dilate if it was ready, without the strong artificial contractions brought on by oxytocin; and this was what he suggested. I went into hospital that same evening to have it the next day.

This had some disadvantages—I was kept awake almost all night by a buzzing fluorescent light in the corridor, and given an irritating and completely ineffectual enema as soon as I arrived, over 12 hours before labour was due to start; and I had looked forward to spending most of the first stage at home, which was now impossible. However, it was infinitely preferable to an oxytocin induction with all that it entailed.

The pessary was put in at 9.0 a.m. the next day, and all morning I had light irregular contractions, while midwives and a couple of student nurses came in and out to feel my bump and listen to the fetal heart. One of the students asked why some patients were in the general practitioner unit and some in the consultant unit, and when the midwife answered I commented how glad I was to have stayed out of the consultant unit. She asked suspiciously if someone had been setting me against the consultant unit and I hastily denied this, saying it was only that I wanted to give birth with as little machinery as possible. She gave me a short lecture on the benefits of modern technology and I ventured on no further discussion, feeling very vulnerable in the knowledge that she might be delivering my baby a few hours later.

At lunchtime my general practitioner and my husband both visited; still nothing definite was happening. After lunch, however, the contractions began to be more strong and regular—I hardly took this in until I realized I had been reading the same page of *A Passage to India* for over an hour. Unlike the morning, nobody came near me for several hours but I found I did not mind being alone; I was concentrating on the work of breathing through the contractions, timing them and finding good positions to cope with them. They were coming every 2 minutes and lasting about 50 seconds, so there was not much time to think about anything else. About 5.30 p.m. the midwife realized that I might have started labour, and suggested breaking my waters (to which I had decided not to object if it offered the chance of speeding up a very slow labour). She found me only 4 cm dilated, the same as several hours before, and so ruptured the membranes. This had a dramatic effect; the contractions at once became chaotic and painful. The labour notes I had made for my husband said 'If I start groaning and clutching the bedhead, this is probably transition; help me with the Entonox mask and tell me it won't last long.' However, Rob was not there (he had not been contacted) and the midwife, who was, disregarded the obvious signs and persisted in asserting that I was still in early labour. I was in no position to contradict her, and had to assume that labour was going to be too painful for me to deal with without drugs, so asked for pethidine. This she gave me, without examining me again and without offering Entonox instead. She was still withdrawing the needle when the unmistakable urge to push surfaced in my consciousness.

All this would be hard to forgive if it had spoilt my awareness and enjoyment of labour and affected the baby's wellbeing, but fortunately it did neither, probably because she was born barely half an hour later (her Apgar score at birth was 9/10).

I found the second stage of labour very exhilarating—strong, compelling contractions to which I instinctively responded not with any method I had learned but with what felt right at the time: pushes interspersed with quick panting. A semisitting position suited me at this stage; I do not know how the midwife would have reacted if I had insisted on a less orthodox one.

My general practitioner arrived soon after second stage had started, somewhat to my relief as my faith in the midwife had been rudely shaken. It was good to see a familiar face when I was so close to delivering, having seen no-one but the hospital staff for several hours. It seemed a very short time later that he told me to look down, and I saw an oval of dark wet hair waiting to emerge. One more push, and Leila Madeleine slithered out into the world; she was put on to my stomach and I grasped her clumsily with both hands. I looked at her and she looked at me.

At this point poor Rob arrived, laden with sandwiches, Scrabble, ice-cubes, and other equipment for a long labour, just in time to see the placenta delivered. It was not yet 7 o'clock, scarcely half an hour since he had been told that labour had started. I grieved for his missing the birth, but there's always next time . . . the baby was feeding greedily, apparently unperturbed either by the pethidine or by her rapid journey. She turned out to be a friendly, bright, and relaxed infant, which I attribute at least in part to her good birth.

I had a tiny internal tear, which my general practitioner sutured straight away. I hardly noticed this; I was holding the baby and feeling inordinately pleased that much of what I had anticipated had turned out to be true. I found labour to be precisely that: hard work, exacting but not painful except for a brief period. As a keen but not very fit fell-walker I thought it very similar to climbing a 3000 foot (912 metre) peak—the long trudge up the lower slopes, the pain barrier two-thirds of the way up, the hard but triumphant scramble up the last few hundred feet, then the incomparable view from the top.

To enjoy labour it is essential to have as medical back-up—even if only to give reassurance that all is going normally—someone already known and trusted. A stranger, however competent, is a distracting and perhaps stressful presence. The hospital staffing may mean one or even two changes of staff while labour is in progress; and hospital staff too often are, or appear, uncaring and scornful. The general practitioner system is almost the only way of having with you someone who not only knows you but has looked after you in pregnancy. Providing intranatal care demands great commitment from general practitioners, since it means they must stay within a short distance of the general practitioner maternity unit day and night, but it offers some rewards in the shape of helping to deliver the babies they have already cared for in the womb, and sharing the parents' joy.

After photographs had been taken, congratulations exchanged and Leila dressed, Rob and I went back to the ward. He left at about 9 o'clock—it seemed strange that he had to say goodbye to his new daughter so soon—and I kept Leila with me till I was almost asleep. She was brought back to be fed at 2 a.m., then to stay with me at 6 a.m. Every time I saw her she seemed like a miracle.

A major perk of being a general practitioner patient is that even primigravidae can usually leave hospital after 48 hours, since the general practitioner and community midwife check up on them at home (I stayed an extra day because Leila choked up some mucus on her second day). Hospital offered the usual minor irritants: awful unhealthy food, a smoke-filled dayroom to eat it in ('After all they say about not smoking in pregnancy!' one of my room-mates remarked sardonically) and the string of unwritten rules which varied according to which staff were on and were impossible to avoid breaking. None of this made even a dent in my happiness, but I was glad to leave the artificial, strained atmosphere of hospital on the fourth day, and envious glances followed me from the less lucky mothers who had come in before me and still had several days to stay.

My general practitioner had been to see us twice in hospital and visited when we came home, to have a look at Leila and reassure me about her. Thereafter one of the community midwives visited every day for a week to do postpartum checks on me, keep an eye on Leila's slight jaundice and answer queries about bathing, breastfeeding, etc. We saw several different midwives and gathered a selection of useful hints. Ten days after the birth the health visitor called with information about the child health clinic, vaccination, etc. and the offer of help with any problems. It all added up to an unobtrusive, kind, and reliable background of support during a very exciting time.

'After an active birth, the mother feels that she has given birth rather than having had her baby extracted from her', says the Active Birth Manifesto (Balaskas 1982), and I can see the force of that. There is no substitute for a prepared, active birth—which may not necessarily be a totally 'natural' one. A friend described to me as 'enjoyable' her first labour which lasted 27 hours and ended in a high forceps delivery. Because she had known how to relax and cope with contractions, and had been fully consulted about the eventual delivery, it had been a happy experience for her. No-one minds essential intervention, and any regrets that labour has not gone according to plan are swallowed up in relief at the baby's safety. Unfortunately doctors have often taken advantage of this to impose unnecessary intervention by blackmailing women with stories of their babies being in danger when they are not.

The vehemence of the consumer movement in childbirth derives partly from the sadness of many women who have had a first labour turned into a nightmare of anxiety and pain by the medical procedure surrounding it. They often seek and achieve more self-determination and fulfilment in a second labour, but it is tragic that they should have been robbed of what might have been a straightforward first birth: 'Every time I look at my second child I swear I think of what I've missed out on with my first' (*Spare Rib* 1980). There is a quality of enchantment about a first pregnancy and labour which should be left intact if at all possible; it is part of the rite of passage which turns a couple (or single woman) into a family, and obstetricians should think hard and long before violating it.

Medics will argue, to counter this view, that many women are so scared of labour that they want to hand the whole thing over to the doctor, lie back and have their labour done for them. This is true, but whose fault is it? Doctors have introduced many of the elements of fear, stress, and pain, and must take some of the responsibility for breaking the vicious circle in which birth has such a reputation that women simply do not want to experience it.

This will involve both reducing intervention to a minimum and buoying up women's confidence in their ability to give birth. Too often a cheerful and optimistic attitude in a pregnant woman is greeted with suspicion by hospital staff, who interpret it as 'unrealistic expectations' which will give rise to false hopes and terrible disappointment. They see it as their duty to demolish such optimism and substitute gloom, like the midwife interviewed for the *Guardian* in 1982 who gratuitously sneered at 'emotional women, elderly primiparae who have read all the books . . .' (Junor 1982). Women are not fools or mental defectives; we can take responsibility for our own emotions, and we sensed before research on catecholamines proved it that the right attitude for childbirth is a happy and relaxed one.

The outcome of birth should be measured for months and years, not just the immediate postnatal situation. Postnatal depresssion has been explained in terms ranging from the clinical (hormones) to the sociological (environment), but it is impossible to rule out the birth experience as a contributory factor. A woman's first few weeks with her baby are bathed in the memory of the experience they have shared—like the first weeks after falling in love. She goes back over it, jealously claiming and reclaiming every moment. Unnecessary intervention will leave her with nagging regret and perhaps a blank spot in her feelings for her child: 'The most pernicious memory that a mother may be left with is that she simply was not there' (Oakley 1981). This can even be associated with bonding failure, which makes life sad and hard for mother and baby for months or years (Lynch and Roberts 1977).

Moreover, too many women in our culture already have a low sense of self-worth and a poor body image, because of social pressures to conform to a narrow and artificial range of physical types—slim, sexy, young—which give rise to widespread depression and dietary disorders such as anorexia and bulimia nervosa, overeating and obesity. Women need to experience their bodies as strong and competent. If birth is just a surgical procedure in which they are passive objects, this alienated self-image is worsened.

The alternatives that women have been seeking for childbirth—home births, the Pithiviers method, and so on—have two common features: they shun unnecessary interference, and they cherish the personal, emotional side of birth (both of which factors are now admitted to have medical advantages). In general practitioner care, both features have been preserved.

To return to the clinical measure of satisfactory outcome; the perinatal mortality rate. This has been so reduced in recent years that it now consists mainly of two elements: congenital defects and economic disadvantage (Taylor *et al.* 1980). Working-class babies run a much higher risk than middle-class ones, and this factor is fairly intractable to medical intervention. NHS medicine, as the Black Report pointed out, has reflected, not eroded, social inequalities. In so far as it can ameliorate this higher risk, it can probably only do so through general practitioners' primary health care teams.

One of my first thoughts after Leila's birth was 'Every woman has a right to a birth like that one'. Too ambitious a hope at present, perhaps; and no doubt other women have had less satisfying experiences of general practitioner obstetric care. Where a general practitioner is uninterested, or does not bother to develop his or her expertise in obstetrics, the results may be as disheartening as the hospital 'conveyor-belt'. Nevertheless, I have tried to show that the standard of general practioner obstetrics can be very high indeed, rightly outshining specialist obstetrics as the appropriate system for low-risk women. I hope more and more general practitioners will begin to consider obstetrics, for their patients' sake, as a vital part of their work.

REFERENCES

ARM *Newsletter* (1982). Raspberry leaf tea. *Assoc. Radical Midwives Newsletter*, **Spring**, 6.

Balaskas, J. and A. (1982). *Active birth manifesto.* Active Birth Movement, London.

Beels, C. (1980). *The childbirth book.* Granada Publishing, London.

Black, N. (1982). Better than expected. *Health Soc. Services J.*, **4796**, 592–4.

Boyd, C. and Sellers, L. (1982). *The British way of birth.* Pan, London.

Bull, M. J. V. (1981). The general practitioner accoucheur in the 1980s. *J. Roy. Coll. Gen. Pract.*, **31**, 357–67.

Cranbrook, the Earl of (1959). *Report of the Maternity Services Committee.* HMSO, London.

Davis, E. (1981). *A guide to midwifery; heart and hands.* John Muir, Santa Fe.

DHSS (1980). *Reply to the second report from the Social Services Committee on Perinatal and Neonatal Mortality.* Cmnd 8084. HMSO, London.

Dunn, P. M. (1976). Obstetric delivery today; for better or worse? *Lancet* **10** April.

Gaskin, I. M. (1980). *Spiritual midwifery.* Book Publishing Company, Summertown.

Gordon, Y. (1982). Choices in childbirth. *Paper given at the International Conference on Active Birth,* Wembly, London, 30 October.

Junior, P. (1982). In praise of special deliveries. *Guardian* 16 June, 8.

Kitzinger, S. (1981) *Some women's experiences of episiotomy.* National Childbirth Trust, London.

Lynch, M. A. and Roberts, J. (1977). Predicting child abuse: Signs of bonding failure in the maternity hospital. *Br. Med. J.* **1,** 624–6.

Marsh, G. N. (1977). Obstetric audit in general practice. *Br. Med. J.,* **2,** 1004–6.

Oakley, A. (1982). *From here to maternity,* p. 112. Penguin, Harmondsworth.

Peel, J. (1970). *Domiciliary midwifery and maternity bed needs.* Report on the subcommittee; DHSS and Welsh Office, HMSO, London.

Rayner, C. (1981). Defensive obstetrics: how we have let our patients down. *World Med.* 24 January, 25, 27.

Spare Rib (1980). Birth: home or hospital? *Spare Rib* September, 24.

Taylor, G. W., Edgar, W., Taylor, B. A. and Neal, D., (1980). How safe is general practitioner obstetrics? *Lancet* 13 December, 1287–9.

Tew, M. (1981). Facts, not assertions of belief. *Health Soc. Services J.* **4709,** 1194–7.

Tew, M. (1981). Effects of scientific obstetrics on perinatal mortality. *Health Soc. Services J.* **4734,** 444–6.

Section B
Antenatal care

2 Overall trends in obstetrics

G. M. Stirrat

INTRODUCTION

Childbirth in the United Kingdom has never been safer than it is today. The maternal mortality rate is, thankfully, less than 0.1 per 1000 births, the gross perinatal mortality rate for England and Wales for 1983 was just over ten per 1000 total births (OPCS 1983). Although these figures are encouraging, there is no room for complacency: firstly because the perinatal death rates in the areas where it is highest are still three times those of the areas where it is lowest. Secondly because life or death statistics do not accurately reflect the provision of good health care.

No matter the criteria used to judge the benefits and hazards of modern obstetrics, there is no doubt that the situation has improved dramatically for both mother and baby over the last 20 years. A brief retrospective look at those two decades would, therefore, help us to set 'overall trends' in their proper context.

The first of the two decades was the time of the highest postwar birthrate of 18 to 19/1000 home population compared to about 12 today. In 1960 the maternal and perinatal mortality rates were 0.31 and 33 out of 1000 total births respectively. By 1970 the former had fallen to 0.14 and the latter to 23 out of 1000 total births.

For those of us working in large maternity hospitals these were the days of hectic flying squad calls to women delivering at home because there was no alternative; of malnourished primigravidae 'grinding' their way through several days of occipito-posterior labour; of catastrophic placental abruptions with uncontrollable coagulation defects; of young women dying in renal failure thanks to the evil ministrations of the criminal abortionist. For those in general practice the memories will be similar. A family doctor who recently retired after 28 years in practice near York has spoken of some of his obstetric experiences. He tells of women dying suddenly and unexpectedly at home in irreversible cardiac failure; and of managing diabetic pregnancies 'before Clinistix made life easy when urines were not tested for sugar at every antenatal visit'. In one set of twins born at home both cords prolapsed in the second stage. Kielland's forceps had to be used with 'no better anaesthetic than gas and air'. Two infants born at 32 and 33 weeks failed to survive when today we might expect them to do so.

Of course, these anecdotes are neither fully representative of a dedicated practice nor of childbirth as a whole at that time. They do, however, serve to highlight problem areas and perhaps show that at that time we seemed very much to be controlled by events rather than controlling them. What has brought about these changes? The first and foremost influence has, undoubtedly, been a dramatic drop in the birthrate, and the second better social conditions. I do not think the importance of the former can be over-emphasized. This can be illustrated by taking the city of Glasgow as an example where social conditions improved for most families at a time when the traditional sources of wealth were at the beginning of a rapid decline. Along the Clyde the docks were still full of ships being loaded and unloaded. The sounds of hammering, riveting and welding rose from every shipyard where yet another cargo ship or tanker was gradually taking shape. Today, the wharves are empty, the shipyards are silent, the towering cranes long since gone. What was it, then, that allowed social conditions to improve despite all this? Nothing more nor less than the lessening of the burden of childbearing on the womenfolk, backed up by the benefits of the national health service and the welfare state.

In relation to the practice of midwifery, the reduction in the birthrate brought much-needed room to move and time to think. The old technology was dying, the new beginning to bear fruit.

New, powerful pharmacological agents became available. Although the decline in birthrate began before the introduction of the combined oral contraceptive pill, it was the general acceptance of the latter which accelerated things. The routine use of ergometrine allowed better control of postpartum blood loss. The production of synthetic oxytocin allowed the obstetrician to proceed to induce labour with a reasonable expectation of success. More and more new antibiotics were introduced.

Anaesthetic agents became less noxious and our anaesthetic colleagues more skilled in their use, particularly in obstetrics. Caesarean section became very much safer for the mother, to the baby's benefit.

Epidural anaesthesia was introduced into obstetrics and the horrors of the prolonged labour became manageable almost overnight. The new electronics began to make continuous observation of the fetal heart possible. The use of the wartime Asdic submarine detection equipment, transferred to industrial use in the shipyards and observed there by Professor Ian Donald, led to his consideration of the potential value of ultrasound in obstetrics and gynaecological diagnosis. The rest is history.

Other flashes of genius or the application of marvellously simple techniques also helped to transform things. The introduction of anti-D immunoglobulin by Sir Cyril Clarke for the prevention of rhesus disease comes into the first category, and the partogram by Hugh Philpott and others for the graphic display of progress in labour is an example of the second.

Other changes relied on a better understanding of physiological mechanisms, particularly perhaps in developmental physiology. We, therefore, began to be aware of our perinatal responsibilities and opportunities, and neonatal paediatrics was born.

Nor were our chemical pathology colleagues far behind. New techniques such as radioimmunoassay were increasingly improving our ability to diagnose and monitor disease processes.

The benefits from a thousand and one advances were considerable but it was not without cost! As, for example, the penalties of intervention became less, the indications for them became less clear. In consequence by the mid-1970s the incidence of induction of labour exceeded 50 per cent in some units and reached 75 per cent among some individual consultants.

In addition, too great a specificity and sensitivity were ascribed to the newly developed diagnostic methods: and although their introduction was undoubtedly of clinical benefit, their uncritical and universal application as *the* answer to the problem in question led, in some cases, to the ascribing of pathology where none existed and, in others, to the failure to detect it when it did.

The same relatively uncritical acceptance pertained to our use of increasingly powerful drugs. 'I don't think it will do harm, therefore it must do good' was, and is, the argument. This was despite the example of late, severe complications in the offspring of women treated with diethylstilbestrol in the 1950s for a whole variety of pregnancy problems.

In addition, the increasing application of 'machinery', biochemistry and pharmacology to the management of the pregnant women was lessening the role of the midwife and making her subservient to the obstetricians. At the same time and perhaps for the same reason the involvement of general practitioners in the total care of the pregnant woman fell inexorably. In 1963 in England and Wales 45 per cent of women were delivered in the care of their general practitioners and another 30 per cent had some antenatal and/or postnatal care from theirs. In 1980 the respective figures were 15 and 80 per cent. The potential reasons for that have been discussed by Bull (1981) and Stirrat (1983) and are considered elsewhere in this book. However, we are not yet up to date for, despite the inertia within the system and the economic stringencies which we face, there is a new spirit abroad among those involved in the maternity services. The aim is to define and provide appropriate levels of care to the woman who needs it most, using personnel with whom she is able to develop a personal relationship and who have the skills most appropriate to her needs. The ideal may not be achievable but that should not prevent us from pressing towards it using guidelines which are already established. The general practitioner and his midwife are vital to this scheme and they must be encouraged to play as full a part as possible in the care of the pregnant woman antenatally, intrapartum and postnatally.

FUTURE TRENDS

In looking into the future, overall trends in obstetrics can be considered as follows:
  (i) Trends in attitudes
  (ii) Trends in care
  (iii) Trends in technology
  (iv) Trends in outcome

Trends in attitudes

It is easy to talk of such changes but more difficult to demonstrate that they are widespread. In addition to what can be perceived from the 'grass roots' the recent report on training for obstetrics and gynaecology produced by a joint working party of the Royal College of Obstetricians and Gynaecologists and the Royal College of General Practitioners (1981) provides evidence of changes for the better. In it the Colleges 'are agreed on the need to provide realistic and satisfactory education for general practitioners so that they can play a *full part* (my italics) in a service that will deliver a high standard of humane care to women and their babies'. They then set out an admirable and comprehensive list of training objectives for basic medical education, shared antenatal and postnatal care, intranatal care and gynaecology (including genitourinary conditions and family planning). The recent vigorous assertion of 'the role of the midwife' by the Central Midwives Board (1983) is also to be welcomed. Who can disagree with their view that 'it makes good sense and is in the interests of effective use of scarce resources that all concerned cooperate to ensure that midwives' skills are being utilized to the full for the benefit of mothers and babies wherever maternity care is given— in the home, in general practitioner surgeries, in health centres and in general practitioner and specialist maternity hospitals'.

There is also a new sense of realism among those working in maternity hospitals. They would readily agree with the Maternity Services Advisory Committee (1982) that 'a major problem is the sheer volume of work which hospitals now attract', and that standard patterns of care need to be examined. One danger of such an exercise in an era of severe financial pressures on health authorities is that options will be chosen because they are cheaper and not because they are beneficial to mothers, babies or the caring staff involved.

It is also important that general practitioner-based care is not idealized and romanticized to the extent that the expectations of women are raised beyond realizable levels. If, for example, appointments for hospital visits were merely decanted on to the community-based services without fundamental reappraisal of the aims and effectiveness of different patterns of care, the problem of the hospital would merely be displaced into the community. Gutteridge (personal communication 1981) has pointed out that 'in the context of specific fears and anxieties of pregnancy and childbirth a "good relationship" (with a general practitioner) does not necessarily boil down to very much'. It is our responsibility to ensure that the pregnant woman obtains first-class care *and* enjoys a good relationship with those looking after her.

Trends in care

Personnel

Reading the Report of the RCOG Working Party on antenatal and intra-partum Care (Royal College of Obstetrics and Gynaecologists 1982) one is aware of a consistent theme running through it—namely that of teamwork. As it states 'the essence of care is cooperation'. The importance of an effective maternity services liaison committee is emphasized 'to organize and monitor maternity care', and clear recommendations are made which, if followed, would undoubtedly produce true integration of perinatal care among obstetrician, paediatrician, general practitioner, midwife and health visitor. This report is essential reading for all involved in providing this care.

Co-operation leads to communication and most of the errors of omission and commission which occur in perinatal care arise as a result of failure in communication. This applies especially to many of the problems which arise between the carers and the cared for. We must involve the mother and father at all stages and be adaptable enough to respond to their reasonable wishes as well as clinical circumstances.

Patterns of care

As Johnstone (1980) has pointed out, 'at the beginning of this century any special care deliberately devoted to the aspect of preserving the health of the expectant mother, of treating any unhealthy conditions during pregnancy, and of foreseeing and, if possible, forestalling dangers likely to arise in her labour . . . was virtually unknown'. In her fascinating discussion of the origins and development of antenatal care Ann Oakley (1982) demonstrates that 'the ideological stimulus of the antenatal care movement in Britain in its formative years was the prevention of maternal mortality but in the past two decades the stimulus has become the prevention, not only of mortality but also of morbidity in babies'. Over the same period the doctor and midwife have been able to move away from merely responding to antenatal or intrapartum crises as they occurred to patterns of care designed to prevent and pre-empt problems. It has been suggested, and is likely to be true, that even more attention to the health of a woman before she undertakes a pregnancy would help to reduce perinatal morbidity, and perhaps mortality, even further (RCOG 1982). This *preconceptual counselling* is discussed in Chapter 4. Although individual consultants in some hospitals have started prepregnancy clinics, such preparation is undoubtedly best achieved in the community by nurses, midwives, health visitors and general practitioners.

As far as *antenatal care* itself is concerned, Enkin and Chalmers (1982) remind us that its basic pattern has remained unchanged and largely unchallenged for well over half a century. They note that 'superimposed on this basic structure, a variety of investigations, procedures, prescriptions and proscriptions have been introduced, developed or phased out as ideas, knowledge and fashion have changed. In the course of the evolution of antenatal care there has been a growing tendency to apply to all women measures which are of unquestionable benefit to only a minority.' An awareness of this underlies the discussions in the whole of this section of the book and in particular Chapter 6 on antenatal programmes by Marian Hall. She and her colleagues in Aberdeen (Chng, Hall and MacGillivray 1980; Hall, Chng and MacGillivray 1980) have already questioned the value of the first antenatal visit and routine antenatal care as presently carried out.

The first priority is, of course, to define the aims of antenatal care. The Maternity Services Advisory Committee (1982) define it as being 'to ensure as far as possible the health and wellbeing of the woman and the unborn child'. For Chamberlain (1978) 'antenatal care should be designed to maintain and improve the health of the mother and the fetus so that they are brought to labour in a good state of health'. Looking at it from a different perspective, the aim of antenatal care is to assess risk of harm to mother and baby, and apply the appropriate level of surveillance to minimize or eradicate its effects. Although there is good evidence that antenatal care is of great benefit in women at high risk of developing problems as a result of, for example, age, past, or family history, or pre-existing illness, Enkin and Chalmers (1982) point out that the majority of women are not at above-average risk of an adverse outcome. In women who are already at low risk there is little room for improvement. Indeed intervention can do more harm than good. The emphasis must therefore be on appropriate care in the appropriate place.

One of the most exciting developments in antenatal care in recent years centre around the comprehensive schemes of community antenatal care which have sprung up in several centres throughout the country. The scheme which has received the greatest attention is that in the Sighthill District of Edinburgh. There, close liaison between consultant and general practitioner teams has produced a system of care that is not only subjectively pleasing to all but seems to have been associated with a real decrease in, for example, preterm delivery, low birthweight and intrapartum problems. The main characteristics of the scheme are:

(i) Each pregnant woman is formally assessed by noting features of the pregnancy against a checklist of risk factors and appraising their significance.

(ii) A replanned programme of management automatically follows the eliciting of particular factors and assessment is updated.

(iii) Through the operation of points i and ii, there is a focus of attention on possible, probable or proven problems of the pregnancy, which promotes a high standard of care.

(iv) Having a structured scheme and agreed protocols for the investigation and management of pregnant women provides the framework of understanding and cooperation between general practitioner and specialist.

There is little doubt that this pattern of care, in which personal attention backed up by appropriate technology is given in the community to those women who need it most should be our blueprint for the future. For women at highest risk hospital-based clinics will still have a major role.

We have already noted that the involvement of general practitioners in intrapartum care fell from 45 per cent of deliveries in 1963 to 15 per cent in 1980. It is, however, important to note that deliveries by general practitioners in integrated maternity units rose from 6 to 9 per cent of all confinements between 1970 and 1975 (Bull 1981). The way in which the general practitioner and consultant teams can work together to produce optimal care for the pregnant woman is illustrated by the results from Oxford reported by Klein (1983 a, b). Nulliparous women booked for shared-care came into hospital at a less advanced state of cervical dilatation than those booked for the general practitioner unit and spent longer (11 compared with 8 hours) in hospital before delivery; the comparable durations in multiparae were 6 and 4 hours. Both the first and second stages of labour were longer in the general practitioner unit-booked women but they received less pethidine and fewer had epidural analgesia; they received less electronic fetal monitoring, augmentation and forceps delivery, and fetal distress was diagnosed less often. The 1-minute Apgar score was less than 6 in 17.5 per cent of infants of nulliparae booked for the shared-care system compared with 1.6 per cent of those booked for the general practitioner unit. The intubation rate of infants of nulliparae was 11 per cent in the shared-care system compared with no intubations in the general practitioner unit. When problems arose in those booked for general practitioner unit confinement the prompt and effective response of the consultant unit team contributed to the excellent outcomes. Thus, an integrated approach by the community and hospital-based teams produced optimal care for mother and baby.

The RCOG Working Party on Antenatal and Intrapartum Care (1982) 'remains convinced that all confinements should take place in hospital'. They quote an incidence of 10 per cent for abnormalities arising unexpectedly in justification for this, but it is not clear how they arrive at this figure or what abnormalities are encompassed. They also note that the Peel report (1970) provided a major impetus for confinement being in hospital. What it does not say is that the Peel report wished to see 100 per cent hospital delivery achieved by *integration of general practitioner and consultant beds.* What actually happened was that women were transferred for delivery under consultant supervision but the pattern of hospital care hardly changed at all. The current patchy trend for more deliveries to occur in integrated general practitioner units is merely a belated implementation of Peel's recommendations. The limiting feature is the confidence of the general practitioner and his midwife. They have been told so often that mothers and babies are not safe in their hands during labour that they have long since come to accept it. However, most studies on place of delivery and perinatal outcome have failed to show the clear association between general practitioner deliveries and adverse outcome that has been implicitly accepted by the profession and successive governments (Black 1982; Taylor 1980). This theme is expanded in Chapter 14. The view expressed by the RCOG Working Party is primarily an emotional one bolstered by a selective view of the statistics. It is a perfectly understandable position to adopt. The obstetrician feels (or has been made to feel) that the ultimate responsibility for the welfare of the mother and child rest with him or her. Therefore he or she must keep matters within their sphere of influence, especially at such a crucial moment as labour. Although one can argue that these views are not wholly valid, they have undoubtedly been reinforced by recent trends in litigation. In addition, they now seem to be enshrined within government policy and, with so many other battles to be fought in the Health Service strong support for economically non-viable isolated general practitioner maternity units is not going to be forthcoming.

Trends in technology

We have already noted that the primary aim of antenatal, as for all other, care is to assess risk. The days when simple clinical measures or mere intuition could be relied upon for an adequate assessment are long since gone. That is not to say that clinical judgement is no longer important, but rather that techniques are now available to us which extend our ability to perceive deviations from normality and thus better assess risk to mother and baby. The problems of specificity and sensitivity of diagnostic tests have already been alluded to. By specificity is meant how many in whom the test is positive have the condition being looked for (in other words, what is the false-positive rate)? By sensitivity is meant in how many with the condition being looked for is the test negative (in other words, what is the false-negative rate)? These two concepts and their impact on antenatal care have recently been examined by Grant and Mohide (1982).

The first realization which is gradually dawning is that most of the biochemical and physical assessments used to monitor fetal welfare are not diagnostic of disease but indicative of an increased risk of a particular condition being present (such as intrauterine growth retardation). The distinction is an important one for, when applied clinically, it can guide us to the appropriate level of care for each pregnant woman. This is illustrated in Fig. 2.1 in which three levels of screening are illustrated. For most women 'first phase screening' is all that is necessary throughout pregnancy. The ultimate intervention, that is to achieve delivery, is only indicated when the balance of risk suggests that the baby would be better off in the cot than the uterus. Fig. 2.1 also illustrates that it is necessary to obtain information from several sources using a variety of techniques, each of which tries to assess a different aspect of fetomaternal wellbeing.

Advances in technology have been rapid over the last decade. They will continue to be so over the next. This will occur in two ways. Firstly, previously large, complex and expensive instruments will become smaller (and therefore portable), easier to use, and cheaper. They will therefore become more generally available for us in, for example, health centres and

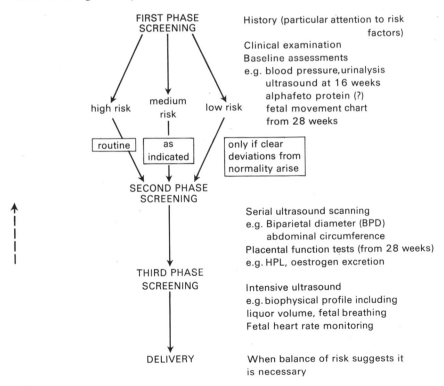

Fig. 2.1. Risk assessment and levels of antenatal surveillance.

community clinics. This applies particularly to real-time ultrasound scanning and fetal heart rate recording. Training in the interpretation of the information they provide is, therefore, urgently needed. There are few things more dangerous than a machine badly used or wrongly applied. The second development will be in entirely new techniques which will allow us to assess the intrauterine milieu more directly but non-invasively. The phenomenon of nuclear magnetic resonance (NMR) is the most likely early candidate for this role, but formidable difficulties remain to be overcome before it becomes practicable.

Trends in outcome

We have already seen how mortality rates for both mothers and babies have dropped dramatically over the past 20 years. Indeed it is now almost taken for granted that a woman will not only survive pregnancy and childbirth but will do so intact. We have almost reached the point at which it is also taken for granted that the baby too will survive intact. The decision not only to have children but when and how many is now a matter of choice rather than chance. When, therefore, one orders a baby one expects it to be perfect.

Achievements in this area have been considerable, but expectations have outstripped them. As a consequence, when catastrophe strikes there is a general feeling that something could and should have been done to prevent it. If we are to make any significant further reductions, it is important that we try to look at this highly emotionally charged area through dispassionate eyes. There are several lessons still to be learned:

(i)   'Avoidable factors' still contribute to over 40 per cent of all maternal deaths.

(ii)   The greatest single contribution to the reduction in perinatal mortality in the last 5 years has been survival among very low birth weight babies (less than 1000 g). This is illustrated in Figs. 2.2 and 2.3.

(iii) The two commonest single causes of perinatal death are preterm delivery and lethal congenital malformations. The incidence of the former has not changed significantly since the 1940s and is unlikely to do so until we find out more about its causes. The new techniques in molecular genetics might gradually help us to unravel the reasons for at least some of the commoner congenital anomalies.

What is sure, however, is that these problems will not be solved merely by doing more and more of what we have been doing for years. New initiatives and research insights are going to be necessary.

(iv)   We are still 'hung-up' on mortality when in reality we should be concentrating to a far greater extent on morbidity and handicap. That, of course, is more easily said than done. Death is an endpoint which can be measured and from which firm data can be obtained. Handicap is much

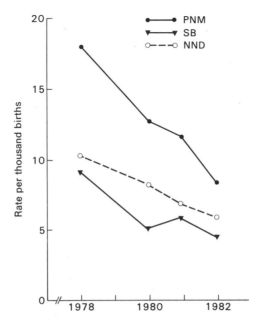

Fig. 2.2 Perinatal mortality in Bristol Maternity Hospital 1978–82. The improvement in perinatal mortality between 1980 and 1982 was due to increased survival of very low birth-weight infants.

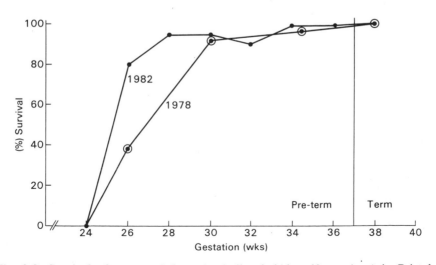

Fig. 2.3. Survival of preterm infants (excluding lethal malformations) in Bristol Maternity Hospital: 1982 compared with 1978.

more diffuse and has many antecedents other than what has happened during pregnancy.

One overriding consideration for which it is impossible to legislate in such an overview is the extent to which economic stringency will affect matters. The cake is finite; the demands for a share of it almost infinite. As our population ages, more health service resources will need to be spent on the elderly. However, neglecting the maternity service strikes at the very root of the nation's health. Severe competition for funds means that is what is happening in some areas. Standards of care are all too often being sustained only by the dedication and goodwill of the over-committed staff. There is a real danger that we will find ourselves returning to the 'shooting from the hip' approach from which we have gradually managed to extricate ourselves over the past two decades.

It is, of course, the responsibility of each and every one of us to make sure that we care for our patients in the most effective and economic manner available to us. What follows in the remainder of the book is an attempt to see how that can best be done by all of us in relation to the pregnant woman. At the heart of this is the general practitioner and his midwife. That is how it must remain.

REFERENCES

Black, N. (1982). Do GP deliveries constitute a perinatal mortality risk? *Br. Med. J.* **284**, 488–90.

Bull, M. J. V. (1981). The GP accoucher in the 1980s. *J. Roy. Coll. Gen. Pract.* **31**, 357–7.

Central Midwives Board (1983) *The role of the midwife.* C.M.B., London.

Chamberlain, G. (1978). A re-examination of antenatal care. *J. Roy. Soc. Med.* **71**, 662–8.

Chng, P. K., Hall, M. H. and MacGillivray, I. (1980). An audit of antenatal care. The value of the antenatal visit. *Br. Med. J.* **281**, 1184–6.

Enkin, M. and Chalmers, I. (eds.) (1982). *Effectiveness and satisfaction in antenatal care.* Spastics International Medical Publishers, London.

Grant, A. and Mohide, P. (1982). Screening and diagnostic tests in antenatal care. In *Effectiveness and satisfaction in antenatal care* (eds. M. Enkin and I. Chalmers). Spastics International Medical Publishers, London, pp. 22–59.

Hall, M. H., Chng, P. K. and MacGillivray, I. (1980). Is routine antenatal care worthwhile? *Lancet* **2**, 78–80.

Johnstone, R. W. (1980). Fifty years of midwifery. *Br. Med. J.* **1**, 12–16.

Klein, M., Lloyd, I., Redman, C., Bull, M. and Turnbull, A. C. (1983a). A comparison of low-risk pregnant women booked for delivery in two systems of care: shared care (consultant) and integrated general practice unit. I: Obstetrical procedures and neonatal outcome. *Br. J. Obst. Gynaecol.* **90**, 118–122.

Klein, M., Lloyd, I., Redman, C., Bull, M. and Turnbull, A. C. (1983b). A comparison of low-risk pregnant women booked for delivery in two systems of care: shared care (consultant) and integrated general practice unit. II: Labour and delivery management and neonatal outcome. *Br. J. Obst. Gynaecol.* **90**, 123–8.

Maternity Services Advisory Committee (1982). *Maternity care in action*. I: Antenatal Care, HMSO London.

Oakley, A. (1982). The origins and dvevelopment of antenatal care. In *Effectiveness and satisfaction in antenatal care* (eds. M. Enkin and I. Chalmers). Spastics International Medical Publishers, London.

Office of Population Censuses and Surveys (1983). Government Statistical Service, Ref. VS83/3-8.

Peel, J. (1970). *Domiciliary midwifery and maternity bed needs*. Report of the Sub-committee; DHSS and Welsh Office, HMSO London.

Royal College of Obstetricians and Gynaecologists (1982). *Report of RCOG Working Party on antenatal and intrapartum care*.

Stirrat, G. M. (1983). The general practitioner's role in obstetrics. *Update* January.

Taylor, G. W., Edgar, W., Taylor, B. A. and Neal, D. G. (1980). How safe is GP obstetrics? *Lancet* **2**, 1287–9.

3 Women's expectations of pregnancy

Catherine Boyd

INTRODUCTION

'Too sacred an office to be held unwillingly'
Marie Stopes (1925)

Marie Stopes' vision of motherhood and her lifelong efforts to make pregnancy a choice rather than an unavoidable act of God or affliction demonstrates women's changing expectations of pregnancy over the past century. The control which women have acquired over their fertility has enabled a questioning of previous values to take place. The assumption that life must be accepted as it is, has been replaced by a greater desire to plan and to direct events. With an increasing capacity to decide *when* to get pregnant, women have not however rejected motherhood; but rather pregnancy and motherhood are seen as one life event of immense significance but not one that will exclude all other activities.

Women's expectations of pregnancy can be viewed from various perspectives. Firstly a historical perspective will shed some light on current attitudes and behaviour. How much have attitudes changed? Is it possible to pinpoint reasons for these changes? Secondly a review of some demographic data on contemporary family and social life will show how far changing attitudes are reflected in actual behaviour. Thirdly a look at current ideologies, and feminism in particular, will focus attention on present problems and possible future trends. Safety and satisfaction in pregnancy and childbirth are more and more seen to be in conflict with one another. How does the general practitioner fit into this changing situation? Is the general practitioner (like the midwife) particularly well suited to meet the changing expectations of women for care and support during pregnancy?

A discussion of women's expectations of pregnancy needs to take into account three problems. First, it is difficult, if not impossible, to separate pregnancy from childbirth expectations. A woman's feelings about being pregnant are so intimately bound up with her feelings about giving birth and becoming a mother that it is unrealistic to isolate one part of this continuous process from another. However, an attempt will be made to concentrate on the earlier parts of the process by asking what women's needs are during pregnancy and whether or not they are met. This will be an underlying theme of the paper.

Second, it is important to recognize that women who become pregnant are not a homogeneous group. Of the three-quarters of a million or so women a year who are conscious of being pregnant 40 per cent have conceived unintentionally, one in five have their pregnancies terminated or miscarry, around 45 per cent are pregnant for the first time, and 12 per cent are unmarried, separated, or divorced. A woman's attitude to her pregnancy will be profoundly influenced by the background to the pregnancy. The expectations of a woman anticipating a second pregnancy will be coloured by the experience of her first. A woman discovering an unplanned pregnancy may not have given much thought at all to what pregnancy entails. How are women's feelings about pregnancy affected by having had a previous miscarriage or termination of pregnancy? In a recent survey of 6000 new mothers 19 per cent said they had had a miscarriage previously and 6 per cent a termination (Boyd and Sellers 1982).

Third, it is necessary to clarify what is meant by expectations. The dictionary defines 'expectation' as 'the action or state of waiting' or 'the action of mentally looking for something to take place; anticipation', but in expectations of pregnancy more is meant than simply the act of waiting for something to happen. The hopes and fears that women have about pregnancy are also a part of expectations of pregnancy as is an anticipation of the kind of care and support she will have.

In addition some expectations will be repressed while others will be very consciously felt. The romantic picture of radiant pregnancy and motherhood may serve a useful purpose in encouraging women through the grimmer aspects of pregnancy. But it needs to be stressed that even in women with very positive feelings about becoming and being pregnant there may be a multitude of unexpressed fears and doubts present as well.

Pregnancy and childbirth, like no other experience in the lives of women, is prepared for, fantasized about, and thought about, even from earliest childhood when cushions will be stuffed under jerseys and pregnancy acted out. An understanding of the hopes and fears that women bring with them to pregnancy will help those whose task it is to provide help, care, and support to women during this crucial period in their lives and to do it in the most appropriate way. Further, an awareness of this background may help professionals anticipate those women who may subsequently succumb to emotional or psychological difficulties after the birth.

Pregnancy is an event of the greatest significance both for the women herself and for the wider family unit. Just as an awareness of any previous medical problems is regarded as a prerequisite to good antenatal care so should 'care givers' and health professionals be conscious of the hopes and fears, the needs and expectations that women bring to their pregnancies.

THE HISTORICAL PERSPECTIVE

Women's expectations of pregnancy have developed and changed in response to fundamental shifts, in the last two or three centuries, in the nation's social and economic life. Although, even today, women still talk in a fatalistic way of having 'fallen' for a pregnancy, most women now regard pregnancy as something to be planned and prepared for, often several years after marriage, rather than an automatic and immediate consequence of marriage. What are the social and economic factors which explain the changing roles of husband and wife as productive and domestic workers and the loosening of the bond between wifehood and motherhood.

Preindustrial, industrial and postindustrial Britain

In preindustrial Britain the position of women was in marked contrast to their situation following industrialization. 'Productive' work was carried on in, and around, the home by both men and women. The arrival of children did not radically affect the lives of either mother or father. Children were cared for in a closeknit community with little distinction being made between domestic and productive work.

The industrial revolution profoundly changed the family lives of men and women and, consequently, the arrival of children had a much greater impact on the lives of women than it did on men. In the years 1750–1840 the home was increasingly displaced by the factory as the main place of productive work. The needs of new processes and technology required ever larger units of production.

Up to a point, women joined in with this change but with the Victorian age came a decline in the employment of women outside the home and a rising belief in the idea of women's 'natural domesticity'. In 1851 one in four married women were employed. By 1914 this had fallen to one in ten. The connection between the new idea of women's 'natural domesticity' and the changing organization of economic life has been described by one historian this way: 'the doctrine that a woman's place is in her home is peculiarly the product of a period in which men had been lately displaced from the home as his work place' (Oakley 1974). Pressure was exerted at this time (nineteenth century) to restrict women's employment in the factory with the argument that factory work would impair reproductive performance. Thus the nineteenth century saw the emergence of the concept of a private family-centred life as a primary social value. The child began increasingly to occupy a more central role. For these changes to take place it was necessary, as Ann Oakley has cogently argued, for the 'privatization and domestication' of women to occur. In fact as she points out the most important and enduring consequence of the industrial revolution has been the emergence of the modern role of housewife as 'the dominant mature feminine role'. The needs of the industrial revolution and the new morality of Victorian England resulted in women functioning more and more in the private world of domestic life leaving the world of 'productive' work to their husbands. Women in Victorian England were expected to bear and raise large families and to restrict their activities to those things which strengthened and enhance the family as the basic unit of society. Dr Jack Dominian in his study of marriage in Britain described the change thus:

one of the most important factors in marriage in the last two centuries has been the industrial revolution which, for the first time in the history of man, separated spouses from each other during the day in large numbers and also stopped men from being gainfully employed at the site of the home (Dominian 1980).

Current discussions about reproductive hazards at work echo this argument although many of these hazards can affect men's reproductive capacity as well as womens. For thousands of years men and women worked side by side in predominantly argicultural settings, but technology removed men to the site of the industry and women to other industry if she worked, or kept her at home if she did not.

The twentieth century saw further changes in the division of the sexes into productive and domestic workers. Ann Oakley (1974) describes the effect of the two world wars as a time when 'women's domesticity had, for the time being, ceased to be a masculine convenience'. The requirements of the war effort brought millions of women back into the labour force. There was a 25 per cent increase in the employment of women in the First World War.

Despite efforts to re-establish pre-First World War patterns (men had a right to reinstatement, women did not) women increasingly attempted to join the labour force, while, for the majority, the role of housewife was still the primary role. By the end of the years between the wars the number of women in paid employment had doubled. Two million additional women were now in paid employment. The Second World War gave a further boost to this trend; in 1939 27 per cent of the work-force was female. By 1945 this had risen to 39 per cent.

The 1960s and 1970s had seen a fourth phase emerge. The earlier expansion in women's employment just noted was mainly amongst young women who still tended to stop work, if not at marriage then with the birth of the first child and were then unlikely to return to work at all. In contrast, in the last 20 years there has been a great expansion in the employment of married women and older women who are either caring for children simultaneously or who have completed the job of child rearing. Of the current labour force 40 per cent are female, and three-quarters are also housewives and mothers. Recent high levels of unemployment have caused a questioning of the trend towards women combining wifehood and motherhood with paid work. Some argue that when paid work is scarce it should be kept for men who are accepted as being responsible for the family income. Others argue that a wife's wage is frequently crucial to the family budget. In addition it is pointed out in defence of mothers working that the two-parent/two-children family model is becoming less and less common. One in five children today will see their parents divorce before they reach the age of 18. Many mothers at work now are consequently providing the main income for the family unit.

Looking ahead to a fifth phase it seems likely that the segregation between the roles of men and women will further diminish, that flexible working patterns will become more common and that fathers will take a more active part in the rearing of children and the running of the home. Just as pregnancy and childbirth have had a decreasing effect on the lives of women in terms of stopping paid work so perhaps it is having an increasing effect on the lives of men. Statutory paternity leave is now under discussion by the EEC and some trades unions have already negotiated such arrangement in this country. The pattern can be set in the weeks after the birth whereby the care of the baby is no longer regarded as the exclusive preserve of the mother. Thus pregnancy is less and less regarded by women as the beginning of a lifelong commitment to the domestic role. The arrival of the first baby will change her life, but is unlikely to remove her from the world of paid work. She may stop work or reduce her hours for the years of childcare, but she no longer assumes either that marriage means immediate pregnancy or that pregnancy means an exclusively domestic life.

For all these changing expectations on the part of women to become a reality one thing has been essential. If women were to become active determinants of their own futures the capacity to control when pregrancy occurred was vital.

COMPULSORY PREGNANCY OR FERTILITY CONTROL?
BREAKING THE LINK BETWEEN BECOMING A WIFE AND BECOMING A MOTHER

Although women with children have been coming back to work since the 1920s it has only been in the last 20 years that the real expansion has occurred. It was the advent of the contraceptive pill, the first safe and effective method of birth control, at the beginning of the 1960s which partly accounted for this change.

The observation that the expansion in employment of mothers had taken place since the early 1960s was made in a Department of Employment research paper (Hakim 1979). Dr Hakim reports that the 1961 census recorded for the first time the trend of women returning to work after having children. This trend was confirmed by the 1971 census when for the first time economic activity was higher for women over 35 than under 24—a complete reversal of the 1901 picture. Dr Hakim writes 'This change has been termed the "2 phase" working life or the bi-modal pattern of female employment and is due almost entirely to the re-entry of women into the labour market after their children have reached school age'. Dr Hakim concludes 'over a period of 20–30 years the profile of the typical working women has completely changed. Before the second world war she was typically single and young. By 1971 she was typically married and of mature age.'

The impact of the contraceptive pill was not simply to speed up a trend towards more mothers returning to work. At the same time a change occurred whereby women, particularly from the more educated groups, delayed the birth of their first child following marriage. As Karen Dunnell (1979) has observed, the proportion of women working after marriage increased from 17 per cent in the prepill cohort (1956–60 marriages) to 86 per cent in the 1970–75 cohort: 'Much of this change would seem to be due to a lengthening of the interval between marriage and first birth that was observed for women marrying after 1960, and the correspondingly larger proportion of women married in those years and later who were still childless'.

The connection between the availability of effective contraception (and abortion which increased greatly after the 1967 Abortion Act) and the participation of women in the labour market seems clear when a review is made of international comparisons. This shows that countries with the most liberal contraception and abortion policies are those with the highest proportion of women in the labour force. OECD figures for 1977 show the top four countries for female economic activity to be:

Sweden	70 per cent	
Denmark	67 per cent	per cent of women in
Finland	65 per cent	paid employment
Norway		
United Kingdom	57 per cent	

These can be compared with:

Greece	27 per cent	
Luxembourg	31 per cent	per cent of women in
Ireland	33 per cent	paid employment
Spain	33 per cent	

As Madeleine Simms, writer and sociologist, has remarked 'the availability of contraception and abortion is a sensitive indicator of the position of women in any society'. The fact that family planning provision has been a part of the NHS since 1975 has made contraception in general and the pill in particular even more widely available and has given control of fertility to millions of women who previously depended on only the most unreliable methods.

Women may want to choose how many children they have and when they have them—indeed falling fertility rates were in evidence long before the pill—but it was only when safe, effective, and convenient birth control became easily available to all women that it was possible for 'ideal' family patterns to become a widespread reality.

Controlling fertility is not just important because it enables women to plan their lives, establish their careers, choose the optimum moment to stop work (albeit temporarily) and to achieve financial security before losing the wife's wage, but also because it changes women's attitudes to their pregnancy.

Widely available birth control means that each pregnancy is more likely to have been prepared for and looked forward to. Each pregnancy is therefore a more significant event and the subsequent birth of a healthy and normal baby even more important than it was in the past. Many obstetricians will bear witness to the fact that couples, who are now more likely to have only two children, have higher expectations that all should be normal. Ann Oakley (1981) has described these expectations of normality like this: 'women expect every pregnancy to produce a healthy baby. Embarking on a first pregnancy seems like a safe course, the horizon of the first healthy cry easy to navigate and the entire journey to desired family size seems well charted and free of the hazards that beset past generations of mothers.'

In the days of 'compulsory pregnancy', as Marie Stopes described, it a mother's tears when a baby died were sometimes tears of relief as well as grief . . . if she had not already engineered an abortion. The change that has been brought about by the widespread availability and use of birth control can be demonstrated by a reminder of how things used to be. Marie Stopes (1925) wrote in *The First 5000* of poor women who, 'driven to despair and to madness by the incessant horrors of pregnancy they dread, will by hook or by crook, from the street corner or the gutter, find out how to strangle the life which should never have began'. Four years later in *Mother England* Marie Stopes (1929) published this modest request from two sisters-in-law with between them 22 children (two dead) and one on the way 'we would like it if you would kindly oblige us with a little knowledge on birth control, as we are practically old women before we are middle aged'. For women such as these, pregnancy brought no joy and no hope—just the dread of another birth to endure and another mouth to feed. The desperate wish to control family size was there but the knowledge and appropriate methods were not. From 1916 to 1945 birth control use amongst the poorer classes hardly changed. In 1945 only 15 years before the pill, fewer than one-half of the poorer classes used any form of birth control (mostly the condom and withdrawal). The better-off classes were much more likely to have access to birth control and to use the safer methods such as the diaphragm. The advent of the pill provided efficient birth control for poorer women for the first time and enabled a much wider sector of society to realize their unmet aspirations for fertility control. These aspirations were in sharp contrast to Marie Stopes' description of her opponents' vision of pregnancy as 'one of the accidents or hazards of life to be endured, like the weather or some natural disaster'.

By 1976 28 per cent of all married women were currently using the pill and another 25 per cent were either using the coil or had been sterilized (Dunnell 1979). Of the younger married women (age 20–24) an astonishing 67 per cent were currently using the pill, showing how important a part the pill has played in breaking down the automatic bond between marriage and motherhood.

The particular impact of reliable birth control on the lives of poorer women is borne out by the greater reduction in family size observed among poorer women than among the better off. During the decade 1965–75 pill use doubled 'while the average family size of women in social class one dropped by only 8% . . . that of social class 4 women fell by 20% and social class 5 women by 25%' (from 2.9 to 2.2) (Dunnell 1976). Legalized and more easily available abortion has also played a part.

Women given the choice want to decide with their partners how many children they wish to have and when to have them. The impact of the pill (and other forms of reliable contraception) on the lives of married women is reflected in its corresponding impact on single women. Here the desire not to conceive is greater than among married women. The pill has enabled these women to match their hopes of delaying pregnancy until they are older and married (usually) with their need to explore relationships and gain self-knowledge. In 1976 73 per cent of single sexually active women were using the pill (one-quarter of all single women) (Dunnell 1979). As many as 87 per cent of single women in the premarriage years of 20–24 in 1976 were on the pill. So it seems that by and large women, given the choice, regard pregnancy as a state not to be lightly entered into. Their expectations of pregnancy entail a recognition of the repercussions and responsibilities involved combined with a desire to enjoy some of the other experiences of life from which motherhood will inevitably cut them off. A picture emerges then of reliable contraception being increasingly used in the last 20 years firstly to delay pregnancy after marriage and secondly by sexually active single women to prevent pregnancy. In later years, married women will then turn again to reliable forms of birth control to limit family size and return to work.

UNPLANNED PREGNANCY

So pregnancy now takes its place in the lives of women in contrast to its previously dominating role. Sexual activity is no longer automatically associated with the possibility of conception, but as something which can be a pleasure in its own right. That pregnancy now occurs more in response to a positive decision to start a family than it did is to the benefit not just of women but to their families and the wider community as a whole. As the bond between marriage and motherhood has become looser, so too has the bond between sexual activity and pregnancy. But how true is it that pregnancy is more likely to be a positive choice than in the past? Are there fewer unplanned pregnancies than there were? Evidence suggests that wider use of contraception is reducing unwanted conceptions (Francome 1983). Young people are more knowledgeable than they were and birth control is more freely available.

Dr Francome points out that 'the number of live births for teenagers age 15–19 has declined from 51 per 1000 in 1971 to only 31 per 1000 in 1980. This is a remarkable trend and a larger percentage decline than in other' groups.' He goes on to show that only one-third of this decline can be accounted for by abortion, and that improvements in the efficiency of birth control use must be the most plausible explanation for the remainder of the decline.

In contrast to the decline in unwanted conceptions, has been perhaps surprisingly a parallel increase in births to unmarried women, which have doubled in the period 1961–81 and are now about 12 per cent. Out-of-wedlock conceptions are now much less likely to lead to a 'shotgun' wedding, especially among younger mothers. The rise in the divorce rate has lead to more 'single' women in the older age groups who may still have a child; more single older women are choosing to get pregnant whether or not they have a partner to support them and more couples are entering parenthood without marriage. The children of this last group, while technically illegitimate, do not suffer from the financial disadvantages of having only one parent. The distinction between legitimate and illegitimate is becoming less and less useful as a pointer to disadvantage since the important factor is whether or not a mother is supported, not whether she is married or unmarried.

So the increasing illegitimacy rate does not mean that more unwanted children are being born. Rather that society has become more tolerant, and that unmarried couples now opt to have a baby in these circumstances. In addition, unplanned, out-of-wedlock conceptions that do occur are more likely to end in abortion than they were. The decreasing need for couples to resort to the shotgun marriage to legitimize their child is seen in Fig. 3.1. Looking at the outcome of pregnancy to women under 20 from 1970 to 1980 an increase in abortion and out-of-wedlock births has been matched by a sharp decline in births within 8 months of marriage. A teenager with an unplanned pregnancy is now more likely to continue her pregnancy out of choice rather than compulsion and she is less likely to marry the father of the child than 10 years ago.

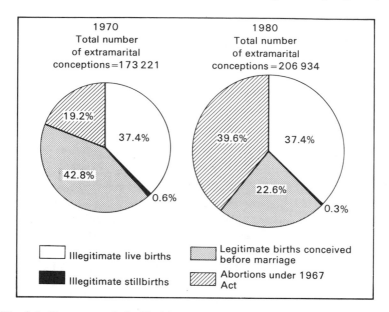

Fig. 3.1. Recent trends in illegitimate births and extramarital conceptions.

The impact of the 1967 Abortion Act on unmarried women (of all ages) has meant that women who have conceived out of wedlock, are increasingly able to regard the continuation of their pregnancy as a positive step. Between 1970 and 1980 the percentage of extramarital conceptions which resulted in termination doubled from 19.2 to 39.6 per cent while the number of such conceptions resulting in a shotgun marriage nearly halved, from 42.8 to 22.6 per cent (Fig. 3.1) (Werner 1982).

So the 1970s has seen a definite shift for the pregnant single women from the likelihood of her marrying the father towards the likelihood of her terminating the pregnancy, and from the stigma of illegitimacy to the present day where more than one in ten babies are born out of wedlock. In fact in some districts illegitimacy rates are as high as 25 per cent—a reflection often of the social and cultural values of particular ethnic groups which do not necessarily observe the two-parent family model to the same extent as the traditional British pattern dictates, preferring an extended family approach to the rearing of children.

Single women now have choices that were previously not available to them. Having a baby out of wedlock is more likely to be a positive decision and in any case many unmarried women having babies are increasingly supported by their partners. The distinction between married and unmarried, as far as pregnancy is concerned, becomes less and less important—although as will be seen most people still regard childbearing as the most important reason for getting married.

FEWER CHILDREN, OLDER MOTHERS

What effect does effective and available birth control (and freer abortion policies) have on the numbers of children people choose to have? It seems that women still want to have children as strongly as ever. Although there has been an increase in voluntary childlessness so too has there been an increase in the efforts devoted to help infertile couples conceive and bear children. The expectation that fertility can be controlled leads to the converse expectation that infertility too can be controlled.

People may still want to reproduce as keenly as ever, but given control of fertility they opt for smaller families. It has been pointed out that the most striking change that can be observed in recent family formation trends is that childbearing is 'occurring at a relatively slow pace' (Werner 1982). In fact the average family size for the generation of women born around 1950 may well fall short of replacement level.

Three trends have been observed to explain falling family size. First women are having their first child at an older age. Over the past decade the average age of mothers giving birth to their first child has increased from 23.8 (1968–70) to 25.0 in 1978, since when it has shown little change. This is still well below the figure of 26.4 recorded in 1938. Second, women in the older age groups (35–39) are having fewer children. The age-specific fertility rate for women in this age group fell from 47.3 in 1938 to 22 in 1981. The decline at these ages since the prewar period reflects the decrease in births of higher-order children and the long-term tendency towards an earlier age at childbirth. Third, there has been a shortening of the period during which women are actively engaged in childcare. Women born in 1935 had an average of 2.22 children by the time they were 35. Women born 10 years later had an average of 2.08 children by that age (OPCS 1982).

So women are opting (with their partners) for smaller families, started at a slightly older age, and completed earlier than in the past. Contraception and abortion have enabled childbearing increasingly to be planned in the context of family, financial and work considerations. Women are not turning away from childbearing. The drive to become pregnant is as strong as ever, with as many women as ever in our history having at least one child. The belief that pregnancy and childbirth will bring rewards greater than any sacrifice that has to be made is deepseated—but that price need no longer involve the separating of a mother from the rest of the world. Becoming a mother will change a woman's life forever, but pregnancy need no longer mean becoming a housewife forever. She is more likely to regard childbearing as something that will temporarily remove her from the outside world but that she can and will return to this world where she will combine motherhood with her own interests and aspirations.

THE PRESENT DAY

'A baby makes a family. A home is not a home without children. The drive to parenthood is felt but not understood' (Oakley 1982).

Little research has been done into why women want to become pregnant. What are women's hopes and fears about pregnancy? Most women would find it difficult to describe their feelings about a future pregnancy—especially a first-time pregnancy. Pregnancy is seen in terms of having a baby, not in terms of what it feels like to create that baby. Women, when pregnant, may say that they expect to feel sick, or tired, probably basing their ideas on their own mother's descriptions of pregnancy. But their main emotions and thoughts are geared to the prospect of becoming a mother and all the changes that this will entail for their lives.

Women anticipating a second pregnancy will base their feelings very much on their experience of a previous pregnancy. If pregnancy has been easy and without medical or other problems they are likely to enter a subsequent pregnancy with a more carefree attitude.

The decision to get pregnant is concerned primarily with the decision to have a child. Although some women will say that they felt a strong need to prove that they could get pregnant the predominant feeling for most women planning a pregnancy is that they want a baby and pregnancy is a means to that end. As women have tended more and more to enter pregnancy as a positive move, the expectations of the kind of care and support she will receive when pregnant has been changing. Women now expect and hope not just that pregnancy will result in a healthy baby, but also that the experience of pregnancy (and childbirth) will be emotionally and psychologically satisfying.

Women who have consciously chosen to become pregnant, aware of the implications for themselves and their lives do not wish their pregnancies to be turned into a medical event. Rather they look forward to an equal partnership with health professionals who will give care and support. Some women are disappointed in this. Ann Oakley (1981) has observed 'for the first time in her life since she was a child a woman having a baby is considered not to know what is in her best interests'.

WHY GET PREGNANT

The realistic expectations that couples increasingly have of pregnancy and parenthood was revealed in a study conducted by the Marriage Research Centre in 1976 of 68 recently married couples under the age of 30 (Mansfield 1982). Of these couples 80 per cent expected to wait at least a year before starting a family. The main reason given for postponing conception was economic. The wife's salary was a vital part of the family budget. The second most important reason was they wanted time for personal preparation. These couples wanted to build the foundations of their marriage both emotionally and psychologically before embarking on the challenges and disruptions of parenthood. They did not want to avoid parenthood, rather they stressed that having children was one of the most important reasons for getting married. But they were aware of the negative aspects of starting a family, and as the author of the report commented this is 'consistent with the prevailing ideology in society which highlights the needs of children and requires self sacrifice from mothers and fathers'. Creating a firm base on which to build a family was stressed. The realistic, almost negative image of parenthood expressed by some couples was in contrast to the days when wifehood and motherhood were intrinsically bound together and further the quality of the relationship between husband and wife were not regarded as such a high priority. One couple in the study were delaying the start of a family

to give us a really good chance of getting to know each other. I think it is wrong to say that children help a marriage. I think on the whole because you have got this extra burden you tend to be less available to help one another. So it is very important that you have a strong foundation yourselves before you start bringing children into the world.

The feeling that having children is not the only reason for getting married —after all the marriage will probably continue long after the childbearing years are completed—comes across clearly in this survey of young couples. This awareness is combined with an attitude to parenthood which reflects a commitment to and an understanding of the responsibilities of bringing up children in the modern world.

The concern expressed by these couples that parenthood does not necessarily enhance a marriage is also expressed in Jack Dominian's study of marriage since 1945 (Dominian 1980). He observes that many couples in difficulty date the deterioration in their marriage from the arrival of the first child. The wife loses the companionship of outside work, money is often scarce, and tiredness takes its toll. Will the greater tendency for couples to delay the first birth and to prepare for the disruptions ease the adjustment to parenthood? Or, alternatively, will couples who place increasing value on the quality of their marriage find having children even more disruptive?

The evidence, such as it is seems not to support the latter view. Rather it seems that pregnancy and childbirth strengthen and reinforce an already strong partnership while having the opposite effect on a vulnerable couple.

UNMET NEEDS, PRESENT PROBLEMS AND FUTURE CHALLENGES

What special needs do pregnant women have? Primarily, of course, a pregnant woman looks for reassurance that her baby will be well and normal. But she also needs the emotional and psychological support to guide her through the sometimes difficult transition to motherhood. As Ann Oakley (1981) points out in her study of 66 women who were pregnant for the first time: 'The problem is that motherhood is not a passive role. Brought up to regard herself as dependent on other people, a mother discovers that her children are dependent on her.' The shortcomings of present antenatal care were revealed in a study of 6000 mothers to be in 1981: 22 per cent of women in the survey found their visits to the antenatal clinic made them feel either 'unimportant' or 'anxious'; 49 per cent of women said they could only ask their hospital doctor questions 'to some extent' or 'hardly at all'; 37 per cent of women said their hospital doctor was 'sometimes helpful and sympathetic', and 19 per cent 'not very helpful or sympathetic'. When women were asked the same questions about midwives and general practitioners a rather different picture emerged. Half the number who had found their hospital doctor 'not very helpful or sympathetic' felt like this about their midwife (hospital or community) or about their general practitioner. 69 per cent of women found their general practitioner helpful and sympathetic, and 73 per cent felt like this about their community midwife. When asked 'who was the best source of information in your pregnancy? 'nearly a third of women mentioned their general practitioner, twice the number who mentioned either the hospital doctor or midwife (Boyd and Sellers 1982).

The general practitioner is able, it seems, to regard a woman's pregnancy in the context of her whole life, her other commitments and her wider needs. The hospital doctor in contrast, with his concentration on physical indices of success and the pressures of busy clinics with the centralization of antenatal care in to hospitals, does not usually have either the time or the inclination to consider a pregnant woman's wider needs. Indeed he does not really regard such matters as his job. One woman who wrote to BBC TV *That's Life* programme said 'it would be lovely to think that during my next pregnancy I would be treated as a person instead of another "case"; that everyone would be aware of feelings and have the time to listen, with interest, to how one feels.' Another respondent wrote

At the hospital clinic the four to five minutes actually spent not waiting was spent on BP, weight checks, and a quick prod round the abdomen. Conversation was kept to a minimum. At the GP clinic he gave me ample time to discuss anything worrying me and answered my questions fully. My GP gave me lots of support and comfort. The five visits I had to my hospital antenatal clinic I deemed necessary evils.

The general practitioner is providing for women's wider needs in pregnancy in a way that the hospital doctor is not, or cannot. To the extent that recent falls in perinatal mortality stem from better medical care of pregnant women the trend towards hospital care must be welcomed. But is it necessary for the general practitioner to be sacrificed in the process? For pregnant women the involvement of their general practitioner in caring for them, particularly in pregnancy, but also where possible at delivery is clearly satisfying. The continuity of being cared for by a doctor who is not simply interested in your abdomen and who will eventually care for the baby and child is vital to this satisfaction and all attempts to maintain or expand the role of the general practitioner in obstetric care should be encouraged.

The takeover of obstetric care by hospital doctors from midwives and general practitioners has come about as part of the medicalization of pregnancy and childbirth plus the general trend, away from community towards hospital care. The view that having a baby is a medical event has been gathering pace, even to the extent that as many as one in nine babies are now delivered by Caesarean section in this country (Maternity Alliance 1983). The women's movement of the last two decades with its emphasis on women controlling their own lives and their own bodies has criticized this trend in obstetrics. Ann Oakley (1982) has described the two approaches this way 'the superiority (of doctors over midwives) was that of scientific knowledge as opposed to the benefits of experience, the advantages of intervention in the process of pregnancy, labour and delivery as opposed to allowing events to take their natural course; it was also shaped by a belief that men know more about women than women do.' She continues 'for mothers, conversely, child bearing is more likely to be seen as a natural biological process; an event that is an integral part of their whole lives and development; an experience to be evaluated in its contribution to happiness in a more general way than mere survival.' With an underlying assumption that pregnancy and childbirth are pathological processes, something for which women must be treated, an attitude to care develops which neglects crucial needs, even creates anxiety and stress and, most importantly, can deprive women of the feeling that it was they who created and gave birth to their baby.

The challenge that is presented by this conflict is between physical health and safety and the fundamental needs of women to be given appropriate support through pregnancy and childbirth, so they can grow into their new role of mother.

This conflict between the passive, ill, hospital patient and the healthy self-determining adult must be faced, if women's changing expectations of pregnancy are to be met. General practitioners are ideally placed to help resolve this conflict. With the general practitioner's emphasis on health rather than illness, preventive rather than curative medicine, and with their much wider perspective of the lives and needs of pregnant women it is general practitioners who should provide increasing care (with midwives) leaving their hospital colleagues to concentrate on specific medical problems and high-risk cases. Close integration is required between hospital and primary health care team for this system to work well, but with such a service women could begin to look forward to a kind of health care in pregnancy which today looks like becoming increasingly uncommon.

In conclusion women today are more likely than in the past to have planned their pregnancy, and to have lived independent lives before becoming mothers. Maternity care needs to reflect these changes. However, current trends towards the downgrading of the midwife's role and the decreasing role of the general practitioner in maternity care makes it more difficult for these changing expectations of care to be met. Women have grown up and are increasingly unwilling to be passive recipients of care. They want, rather, to be in partnership with health professionals so that they can grow into the new responsibilities of motherhood.

REFERENCES

Boyd, C. and Sellers, L. (1982). *The British way of birth.* Pan, London.

Dominian, J. (1980). *Marriage in Britain 1945–80.* Study Commission on Family, London.

Dunnell, K. (1979). *Family formation. 1976* HMSO, London.

Francome, C. (1983). Unwanted pregnancies amongst teenagers. *J. Biosoc. Sci.,* **15**, 139–43.

Hakim, C. (1979). Occupation segregation. *Department of Employment Research Paper.*

Mansfield, P. (1982). Getting ready for parenthood. *Children and marriage, Special Issue of Int. J. Sociol. Soc. Policy,* **2**, (3).

Maternity Alliance (1983). '*One birth in nine—a study of Caesarean section rates.* Maternity Alliance, London.

Oakley, Ann (1974). *Housewife.* Pelican, London.

Oakley, Ann (1981). *From here to maternity.* Pelican, London.

Oakley, Ann (1982). *Subject Women.* Fontana, London.

OPCS (1982). Population Trends 30. Editorial: a review of 1981.

Stopes, Marie (1925). *The first 5000: Being the first report of mothers clinic for constructive birth control.* John Bale and Co, London.

Stopes, M. (1929). *Mother England: A contemporary history* (letters to Dr Stopes). (ed. M. C. Stopes). John Bale and Co, London.

Werner, B. (1982). Recent trend in illegitimate births and extramarital conceptions. *Population Trends,* **30**, 9. OPCS, London.

4 Pre-conception counselling

G. N. Marsh

THE GENERAL PRINCIPLES OF PRE-CONCEPTION COUNSELLING

Critics have dismissed pre-conception counselling as a 'middle class gimmick'. But the sporadic antenatal care given in the early years of the twentieth century was largely to middle-class women who began to realize that care during pregnancy would have an effect on its outcome. Gradually its advantages were appreciated and today the entire population looks upon antenatal care as a normal prerequisite to a satisfactory delivery and a healthy baby, and women not attending for antenatal care are even criticized by their lay peers. By the same token pre-conception counselling is currently being discussed at the 'middle-class level'. The principles on which it is based appear to be well founded and the idea appeals to common sense (*British Medical Journal* 1981; Chamberlain 1980, 1981). It is very possible that in another decade pre-conception counselling will be part of the conventional wisdom of British society (Maternity Alliance 1983). This chapter is written with that possibility very much in mind.

The fundamental thoughts underlying pre-conception counselling are, that healthy people are more likely to conceive a healthy fetus than unhealthy people, and that once conceived there are many early hazards to the fetus that can be prevented or avoided. A high proportion of congenital abnormalities begin almost as soon as conception has taken place, or in the very early differentiating cell mass stage. Anything that can be reasonably done to prevent babies being born with congenital abnormalities would seem worthwhile. Common sense would suggest that if mother and father are both extremely fit and well the chances of abnormal cell division in the early weeks of the developing embryo are less likely to occur than if they are sick, debilitated, undernourished or malnourished, on drugs, or in other ways 'unhealthy'. It is the aim of preconception counselling to rectify, or at least minimize these shortcomings.

There are now many preventable hazards in pregnancy and during preconception counselling the patients can be advised about their deleterious effects and can take steps to minimize these (for example, stop smoking, have a rubella vaccine, etc.). Some intending parents are unprepared psychologically for pregnancy, childbirth, and childrearing and some discussion of this can be beneficial. The perinatal mortality and morbidity of 'wanted babies' is reasonably assumed to be lower than that of 'unwanted babies'. These deleterious statistics can continue into infancy and childhood.

Low social class pregnancies have a higher perinatal mortality rate than higher social class and although social class cannot be changed immediately many of the 'qualities' of a higher social class setting can be offered to low social class women (for example, advice regarding diet or dietary supplements).

GENERAL COMMUNITY AWARENESS OF PRE-CONCEPTION COUNSELLING

Schools

It would be helpful in the context of pre-conception counselling if secondary education included emphasis on the importance of general physical fitness. More attention still needs to be given to the avoidance of smoking—never starting being the best prevention of all—and the importance of moderation in regard to alcohol. Discussions on the use and abuse of drugs, both proprietary preparations and also those prescribed by doctors, would be of value in instilling a reasonable yet healthy scepticism concerning the concept of a 'pill for every ill'. The coupling of the study of nutrition in schools with 'self-survival courses' (new style 'domestic science') should be aimed at maintaining general physical fitness and particularly an ideal weight for height. If such education were successful many more men and women than is currently the case would be fit to embark on a pregnancy.

Women's magazines, radio, and television

There is no doubt that the media have a considerable influence on the health 'norms' of a society. They should (and do) include contributions by health visitors, other health educationalists, general practitioners and specialists about the ideas behind prepregnancy counselling and how to implement them. As a result some couples would see their doctors prior to conception and the doctors themselves would be prompted to respond appropriately.

Postnatal examinations

The postnatal examination is now a well-established routine and does offer an opportunity for prepregnancy counselling directed towards the next conception (Chapter 21). 'Knowing what one knows now' can be a good way of opening a discussion aimed at appraising the recent pregnancy and delivery and particularly assessing whether any factors that caused problems or anxieties could be avoided next time. The simplest practical example would be the giving of rubella vaccine to women who had been found to be seronegative during the pregnancy. From a behavioural point of view women who had attended for the first time late in their pregnancy could be counselled to come earlier next time. Many of the items on the 'checklist' described later in this chapter could be appropriately discussed at a postnatal examination.

Patients who went into premature labour could have possible reasons discussed and advice suggested regarding prevention, and patients who had developed pre-eclampsia could be advised about weight control, salt intake and interval between pregnancies.

Post-abortion examinations

In some ways more important are patients attending following a spontaneous abortion (particularly in a first pregnancy). As well as some attempt to ascertain the cause (frequently not known), they often need considerable reassurance with regard to the next pregnancy as well as a run through the prepregnancy checklist.

Patients who had late abortions could have cervical encirclage discussed as a possibility in their next pregnancy. Patients who had termination of pregnancy will need advice particularly about contraception until they are in a situation where pregnancy is desired—or alternatively about sterilization if no further pregnancies are contemplated.

The primary health care team

Primary health care teams need to discuss as a matter of general principle the concept of prepregnancy counselling in order to make it part of their conventional wisdom. As leaders in health opinion the health visitors, social workers, midwives and nurses can promulgate the idea and discuss it in their frequent contacts with the community. The Health Education Council now produce leaflets and other literature on prepregnancy counselling which should be available in general practitioners antenatal and family planning clinics (Maternity Alliance 1982). General practitioners could annotate their records in such a way that childless married women could be given a resumé of advice coincidental with their attendances for other problems.

District family planning clinics

Family planning clinics are an obvious setting for preconception counselling. In particular women who have never conceived should have a special note made in their records that such counselling is needed, or has been given.

Medical school teaching

Medical students themselves need to be taught preconception counselling so that whether they become specialists in the obstetric field, general practitioners, or even work in other specialties they can be well informed of its value and able to show or generate interest during consultations about other matters.

CHECKLIST OF TOPICS THAT CAN BE DISCUSSED DURING PRE-CONCEPTION COUNSELLING

Age

Some general advice should be given to women regarding the 'ideal age' for pregnancy and the problems associated with 'older' pregnancies. It is customary in my practice for me to recommend women to have their first baby before they are 30 when this is socially appropriate. Older women are less fertile, they have more pairs of twins and they have a higher likelihood of hypertension. There is an increased incidence of chromosomal abnormalities presumably due to the primordial oocytes which have been present since birth being older and therefore more vulnerable to abnormality. To preclude the need for amniocentesis and other hazardous interventions I recommend that families are completed by the time the mother is 36 whenever possible.

Number and frequency of children

There is some evidence that pregnancies conceived within six months of an abortion or termination of pregnancy are slightly more likely to miscarry, so if there are no other social reasons for speed, and psychologically the woman is prepared to be patient, an interval of six months at least might be advisable. The social norm in Britain seems to be for one child to be walking before the next one is born and an interval of two years between children seems to be acceptable. Conventional wisdom is that 'two under two' is 'hard work' and avoidance of this desirable. Size of family is very much a matter of personal choice, but to replace the world's population at its present level it has been 'guesstimated' that western women should have approximately 1¼ children?

Body weight and diet

Overall, white women living in Britain have a thoroughly satisfactory and nutritious diet. Even 'junk food' contains reasonable amounts of iron and vitamins. Nevertheless, for an ideal state people should be advised to eat fresh fruit and vegetables daily and take an adequate amount of protein, carbohydrate and roughage. All women should be made aware of the normal weight for their height and charts usually based on life insurance statistics are available. Overweight women can be well advised to lose weight since stringent dieting during pregnancy is inadvisable regardless of the starting weight (Campbell 1982). Apart from the social disadvantage of being extremely heavy in pregnancy, obese women have a poor obstetric performance (Gross, Sokol and King 1980; Maeder, Barno and Macklenburg 1975). Similarly very thin patients produce poor obstetric scores and should be advised to increase their dietary intake in order to gain weight. Their possibly inadequate diet should be fairly carefully analysed and any 'faddism' can receive appropriate comment (Vinall 1983). Haemoglobin, serum iron and total iron binding capacity (particularly the latter two) will often be found to be low in the underweight group and can be corrected prior to conception. Ethnic groups, too, need a careful analysis of their diet and may well need supplements (Veigas *et al.* 1982a; 1982b).

Exercise

There is no evidence that exercise before conception affects the course of the pregnancy or its outcome, but the physically fit should theoretically stand pregnancy and labour better and have a far greater feeling of well-being. Exercise taken by expectant fathers and mothers may well form a habit after delivery and encourage both parents to inculcate exercise habits in their children and participate in these with them.

Exercise is extremely relevant in the control of obesity and is a means of minimizing the hazards associated with it.

Smoking

Intending parents should cease smoking prior to conception, well worth-while for their own health, as well as that of their baby. Women who smoke during pregnancy are twice as likely to have spontaneous abortions and also produce lighter babies (*British Medical Journal* 1978; *Lancet* 1979). The prevalence of cot deaths and respiratory tract infection in infants is higher in households where either parent smokes compared with non-smoking households. It is therefore important that both partners cease. There seems to be some synergistic effect between smoking and alcohol and the effects on the fetus. (Wright *et al.* 1983). Cigarette smoking is more dangerous in social class 4 and 5 patients than 1 and 2; they tend to smoke more anyway and the smoking adds to the deleterious effects of their other social disadvantages. Smokers are less likely to breast-fed their babies (Lyon 1983).

Alcohol

Alcohol readily passes the placenta and the fetal blood–brain barriers, but it is excreted only slowly by the fetal detoxicating mechanisms. The mother's rate is much quicker. The fetus is therefore 'drunk' longer and the effects are far greater. Accordingly alcohol intake should be minimized, or stopped entirely prior to conception (*Lancet* 1983). Heavy drinkers (those drinking more than 100 g of alcohol, or ten drinks, per week) have more spontaneous abortions, more low weight babies, and particularly so if they smoke as well

(Harlop and Shiono 1980; Kline *et al.* 1980; Wright *et al.* 1983). They have more babies with congenital abnormalities (4 per cent in abstainers and approximately 20 per cent in those drinking over 70 g of alcohol) and occasionally produce a baby with 'fetal alcohol syndrome' (Halliday, McCreid and McClane 1982; Jones and Smith 1975; Jones *et al* 1973). Fetal distress is commoner in labour and they have more children with a low IQ. Some studies have shown that women having as few as two drinks per week have two to six times as many spontaneous abortions. The weight of evidence against drinking in pregnancy is so colossal that the sensible advice to women (supported by a parallel behaviour in their partners) would be to stop altogether or at worst limit it to a very occasional drink.

Work

There are some hazardous occupations which can affect the fetus in its very early development. Classic examples are women working with radiation in X-ray departments, or checking luggage and passengers at airports with radioactive scanners. Women exposed to anaesthetics or other volatile gases may also be at risk (Cohen, Belville, and Browne 1971; Pharoah, Alberman, and Doyle 1977). Some chemicals and in particular defoliating herbicides can cause fetal abnormality (Farquharson, Hall, and Fullerton 1983). There are not many women at risk in this way, but those who are should be advised to contact the appropriate personnel at work responsible for environmental hygiene. Many firms will already have taken appropriate preventive procedures (Baker 1981).

Excessive work causing a woman's general tiredness and debility will be an inappropriate environment around the time of conception, but there is no definitive evidence that this causes any fetal abnormality.

Social class

Women in the lower social classes are already disadvantaged by virtue of poorer finance, nutrition, housing, hygiene and stature. Accordingly these groups need much more attention, and other correctable hazards attended to far more rigorously than women of a higher social class. They should be told that they will receive a more intensive antenatal programme than their counterparts in social classes I and II. By the same token social class I and II women can attend less frequently, since they are far less vulnerable (see Chapter 31).

Worry and anxiety

In the main, patients at a preconception clinic should be encouraged to relax, sustain enjoyable hobbies and take adequate rest and exercise. Most women expecting their first baby can proceed hopefully with a high expectation of a normal outcome both with regard to the labour and to the baby that they produce. Where there have been problems in earlier pregnancies or labours, however, anxieties mount and the preconception clinic, often taking place at the postnatal examination (see above, p. 47), can allay many worries. Indeed proffering good, or even fortified, antenatal care with perhaps more frequent attendance or more frequent appropriate tests will reassure women.

Psychological suitability

Some women have many ill-founded doubts and fears about pregnancy and these can be answered at a prepregnancy consultation. If the patients are well known to the general practitioner they may express anxiety regarding their maternal (or paternal) instincts. This can be explored and answered by reasonable common sense. For the most part patients can be reassured that 'anxieties are normal'.

Family and personal history

Enquiries should be made regarding congenital abnormalities in parents or siblings and hereditary illness in the family. Genetic counselling may be necessary—most of this merely simple reassurance of ill-founded anxieties by the general practitioner. Occasionally a geneticist will need to be involved (Weatherall 1982).

Women who will need accurate ultrasound dating and amniocentesis for the determination of congenital abnormalities such as mongolism or spina bifida can be told of these routines and their implications prior to pregnancy. At least such women will know in advance of the various tests that they may need and their 'moral' implications. They can read the appropriate literature and magazines to help them in advance with difficult choices. There is some evidence, but not totally conclusive, that given a family history of spina bifida, women should receive vitamins and folic acid before conception and in early pregnancy in order to prevent it (Smithells, Sheppard and Schorah et al. 1980). Confirmatory trials are under-way, but the results will not be available for several years.

With a history of congenitally abnormal babies either in themselves or their parents and siblings attendance for a prepregnancy consultation can at least lessen guilt if recurrence should take place. At least 'everything was done'.

Ethnic groups

Ethnic groups living in Britain are particularly liable to dietry shortcomings and deficiencies and resultant blood disorders, especially a low haemoglobin (Basu 1982). In addition such patients have special problems, for instance sickle cell anaemia, thalassaemia etc., and such illnesses need consideration and advice prior to as well as during pregnancy.

Drugs

Women taking medication for serious illnesses (such as diabetes, epilepsy, etc.) need their medication assessing to see whether any of their drugs could have teratogenic or other harmful effects on the fetus (Ashton 1983). Changes could be made to alternative therapy. Inessential drugs (such as tetracycline for acne vulgaris, tranquillizers for anxiety states etc.) and proprietary medicine from the chemists should be stopped well before conception.

Rubella

No patient attempting conception should be in doubt as to whether she has rubella antibodies, since exposure to the virus is extremely dangerous to the fetus in the first trimester. Since 2–6 per cent of 15-year old females are seronegative and 20–30 per cent of 15-year old boys, there is some evidence that the massive vaccination campaign at schools aimed at girls at the age of 13 is having its effect (Clarke *et al.* 1983). However, there is still a significant group of patients who are not vaccinated usually because they were not at school, or because the vaccine was declined. Such defects can be rectified at the preconception clinic. If a rubella injection has been given reasonably recently—say in the last 5–10 years—then it can be reasonably presumed that antibodies will be present, but all other women would be advised to have a blood test. If vaccine is given contraception must be rigorous for 3 months following the injection since there is a theoretical possibility of the vaccine damaging the fetus. This has not yet been actually proved in practice. Rubella antibodies should be estimated at the beginning of each pregnancy to make sure that those present at the previous pregnancy have not waned by the time the present pregnancy occurs.

Cervical cytology

Prior to conception all women ideally should have two negative cervical smears, the last within 3 years. This would preclude the need for taking a smear during pregnancy. If the last smear showed symptomless trichomonas or monilia infections it should be repeated and if positive treated (see below under vaginal discharge, p. 54). Evidence of virus (herpetic) infection on the smear would indicate gynaecological referral since the hazards to the fetus of vaginal delivery in the presence of overt herpetic infection is considerable (Adler and Mindel 1983).

The pill and other contraceptives

Women should be instructed to have two normal 'non-pill' periods in order to regulate ovulation prior to conception. This will facilitate estimation of date of delivery. It will also avoid any possibility of a 'hormonal hangover' on the embryo. I personally recommend two normal periods following removal of an intrauterine device in order to let the uterus 'settle down' to a normal menstrual cycle and flow prior to conception.

Dating periods

All women should be advised to record their menstrual cycle accurately for the few months prior to conception. Estimated date of delivery is facilitated and anxiety regarding postmaturity with its attendant dangers of ill-timed induction can be lessened. With the advent of routine confirmation of dates by ultrasound, period dates are less important, but nevertheless positive correlation between expected date of delivery from an accurately recorded period and an ultrasound at around 16 weeks of pregnancy is extremely reassuring both to the mother and the obstetrician.

Antenatal care itself

At preconception attendance women can be told of the importance of attending early once they are pregnant and given some idea of the schedule of attendances appropriate for them (Pearson 1982). If unable to attend they should know that they must inform the clinic of the reason.

Maternal disease

'Tiredness'

Although hardly a disease tiredness is a common symptom. Those complaining of tiredness disproportionate to their lifestyle may commonly be suffering from the results of either inadequate diet, menorrhagia, or the vicissitudes of low social class life—any or all of these. A low haemoglobin and low serum iron are commonly associated. Iron therapy, and vitamin C to improve absorption, should be instituted. To begin a pregnancy with a haemoglobin and iron deficit would seem to be unnecessarily arduous and possibly hazardous.

Vaginal discharge

Patients complaining of significant vaginal discharge should have a cervical smear and a vaginal swab taken, the latter being inoculated directly into culture medium. Since monilia and trichomonas vaginalis are difficult conditions to eradicate in pregnancy, and the former can carry risks to the baby at delivery, effective treatment prior to conception is advisable. 'Cure' should be based not only on an absence of symptoms, but also on a smear and swab check. Extremely rarely a gonococcus will be found and necessitate treatment.

Urinary tract infections

Symptomatic urinary tract infections should be treated prior to pregnancy and a post-treatment sterile urine culture obtained. Approximately 6 per cent of women have a positive bacteriuria in early pregnancy and appropriate preconception therapy could probably decrease this number. Urinary infections are more difficult to eradicate during pregnancy and carry an associated risk of pylonephritis and pre-eclampsia. The therapeutic armamentarium is limited since some of the drugs are possibly teratogenic or folic acid antagonists (co-trimoxazole, for example).

Hypertension

Known hypertensives, or those detected during the preconception consultation (diastolic blood pressure persistently over 90 mmHg on three separate occasions would be a reasonable definition), should be advised of the dual risks of older age and excessive parity. On the whole, women with hypertension should be advised to have their babies early and to have a small number of children particularly if the hypertension worsens during a pregnancy. Some antihypertensive drugs are more appropriate in pregnancy than others and therapy should be changed accordingly.

Diabetes

There is no such thing as a mild diabetic in pregnancy since the complication rates appear to be independent of the severity of the disease, particularly as measured by the amount of insulin needed. Meticulous control in the pre-conception period is vital since these women have a greater number of spontaneous abortions as well as more babies with congenital abnormalities. They can also produce large immature, often preterm, babies. Referral of diabetics prior to conception to a diabetic specialist for rigorous assessment of their diet, insulin dosage, and blood sugar levels should be mandatory. Some women who may become diabetic in later life manifest a 'prediabetic' syndrome in pregnancy with all the inherent dangers of overt diabetes. A strong family history of type II (non-insulin-dependent), diabetes would indicate a glucose tolerance test prior to the pregnancy. The heredity of type I (insulin-dependent) diabetes has not been fully defined (Creutzfeldt, Kobberling and Neel 1976). Those with abnormal results should be referred to a diabetic specialist for advice.

Diabetics must always be booked for specialist delivery units since the prevalence of abnormalities either in labour, or with the baby postpartum, are common.

Asthma

Oral steroid-dependent asthmatics will require careful control during pregnancy; their asthma may improve, worsen, or more commonly not change. Prior to pregnancy an attempt should be made to wean them onto inhaled bronchodilators, including inhaled steroids. If this is successful it could change their booking arrangements from specialist to general practitioner unit. Asthmatics dependent on oral steroids will require specialist booking in case of sudden respiratory or cardiovascular problems during, or immediately after, labour.

Heart disease

In women with heart disease the maternal mortality rate increases considerably after the age of 25 and also after having two children. At a pre-conception consultation early pregnancies and small families can be advised for this relatively rare group of women.

WR and Kahn tests

It is rare that these tests are ever positive in pregnancy, but if there is any suspicion of an appropriate history then they should be done prior to conception. Women with positive results need referral to a venereologist.

REFERENCES

Adler, M. W. and Mindel, A. (1983). Genital herpes: hype or hope? *Br. Med. J.* **286**, 1767–8.

Ashton, H. (1983). Teratogenic drugs. In *Adverse drug reaction bulletin*. Adverse Drug Reaction Research Unit, Shotley Bridge General Hospital, Consett, Co. Durham.

Baker, C. C. (1981). Correspondence on preconception clinics. *Br. Med. J.* **283**, 1055.

Basu, H. K. (1982). Cultural differences between immigrant Asians and native Britons. In *Obstetric problems in the Asian community in Britain*. RCOG, London, pp. 19–24.

British Medical Journal (1978). Leading article **1**, 259–60.

British Medical Journal (1981). Leading article: preconception Clinics **283**, 685.

Campbell, D. M. (1982). Dietary restriction in obesity and its effect on neonatal outcome. In *Nutrition in pregnancy*. Proceedings of the 10th Study Group of the RCOG. (eds. D. M. Campbell and M.D.G. Gillmer) *September*.

Chamberlain, G. (1980). The prepregnancy clinic. *Br. Med. J.* **281**, 29.

Chamberlain, G. (1981). The use of a prepregnancy clinic. *Mat. Child Health* **August**, 314.

Clarke, M., Schild, G. C., Miller, C., Seagroatt, V., Pollock, T. M., Finlay, S. E. and Barbara, J. A. J. (1983). Surveys of rubella antibodies in young adults and children. *Lancet* **March**, 667–9.

Cohen, E. M., Belville, J. W. and Browne, B. W. (1971). Anesthesia, pregnancy and miscarriage: a study of operating room nurses and anesthetists. *Anesthesiology* **35**; 343–47.

Creutzfeldt, W., Kobberling, I. and Neel, I. V. (eds.) (1976). *The genetics of diabetes mellitus.* Springer Verlag, Heidleberg, New York.

Farquharson, R. G., Hall, M. H. and Fullerton, W. T., (1983). Poor obstetric outcome in three quality control laboratory workers. *Lancet* **1**, 983–4.

Gross, T., Sokol, R. J. and King, K. C. (1980). Obesity in pregnancy: risks and outcome. *Obstet. Gynecol.* **56**, 446–50.

Halliday, H. L., McCreid, M. and McClane, G. (1982). Results of heavy drinking in pregnancy. *Br. J. Obstet. Gynaecol.* **89**, 829.

Harlap, S. and Shiono, P. H. (1980). Alcohol, smoking and incidence of spontaneous abortions in the first and second trimester. *Lancet* **2**, 173–6.

Jones, K. L., Smith, D. W., Streissguth, A. P. and Marianthopoulos N.C. (1973). Patterns of malformation in offspring of chronic alcoholic women. *Lancet* **1**, 1267–71.

Jones, K. L. and Smith, D. W., (1975). The fetal alcohol syndrome. *Teratology* **12**, 1–10.

Kline, J., Shrout, P., Stein, Z., Susser, M. and Warburton, D. (1980). Drinking during pregnancy and spontaneous abortion. *Lancet* **2**, 176–80.

Lancet (1979). Leading article, **1**, 536.

Lancet (1983). Leading article, **1**.

Lyon, A. J. (1983). Effects of smoking on breast feeding. *Arch. Dis. Child.* **58**, 378–80.

Maeder, E. C., Barno, A. and Macklenburg, F. (1975). Obesity. a maternal high risk factor. *Obstet. Gynecol.* **45**, 669–71.

Maternity Alliance (1982). 'Getting fit for pregnancy' (leaflet). Maternity Alliance, London.

Maternity Alliance and National Council for Voluntary Orgaizations' Health and Handicaps Group. (1983). Prepregnancy Care: a joint statement. **February**.

Page, R. (1981). Correspondence on preconception clinics. *Br. Med. J.* **283**, 858.

Pearson, J. F. (1982). Is early antenatal attendance so important? *Br. Med. J.* **284**, 1064–5.

Pharoah, P. O. D., Alberman, E. and Doyle P. (1977). Outcome of pregnancy among women in anaesthetic practice. *Lancet* **1**, 34–6.

Smithells, R. W., Sheppard, S., Schorah, C. J. *et al.* (1980). Possible prevention of neural-tube defects by periconceptional vitamin supplementation. *Lancet* **1**, 339–40.

Veigas, O. A. C., Scott, P. H., Cole, T. J., Mansfield, H. N., Wharton, P. and Wharton, B. A. (1982a). Dietary protein energy supplementation of pregnant Asian mothers at Sorrento, Birmingham, I. *Br. Med. J.* **285**, 589–2.

Veigas, O. A. C., Scott, P. H., Cole, T. J., Eaton, P., Needham, P. G., and Wharton, B. A. (1982b). Dietary protein energy supplementation of pregnant Asian mothers at Sorrento, Birmingham, II *Br. Med. J.* **285**, 592–5.

Vinall, P. S. (1983). Diet and pregnancy: why 'eating for two' is not necessary. *MIMMS Mag.* **15 August**.

Weatherall, D. J. (1982). *The new genetics and clinical practice*, Nuffield Provincial Hospitals Trust.

Wright, J. T., Barrison, I. G., Lewis, I. G., MacRae, K. D., Waterson, E. J., Toplis, P. J., Gordon, M. G., Morris, N. F. and Murray-Lyon, I. M. (1983). Alcohol consumption, pregnancy, and low birthweight. *Lancet* **March 26**, 663–5.

5 An updated view of the physiology of pregnancy

Malcolm Stewart

FERTILIZATION AND OVUM TRANSPORT

Fertilization takes place in the Fallopian tube, following which the ovum slowly travels along the tube entering the uterine cavity 3–4 days after fertilization as a morula which in its turn becomes a blastocyst. Although the time taken to traverse the Fallopian tube is thought to be critical for successful implantation, little is known of the factors controlling morula transport within the tube. It is likely that the cilia of the tubal epithelium are directly involved in transporting the fertilized egg; but the complementary roles if any, of the myosalpinx and tubal fluid remain to be defined. Speculation is that, in man, the fertilized ovum is retained at the ithmoampullary junction or other site (Klopper 1980): the so-called critical pause (and a prerequisite for successful ovum transport in some animal species) is borne out neither by selective resection of the rabbit oviduct nor indeed by experience of the human subject undergoing tubal surgery (Eddy, Antonim, and Paverstein 1977; Gomes 1977; Klopper 1980; McCormick and Torres 1976; Peterion, Musich, and Behrman 1977; Winston 1977). Likewise, speculation that ultimate control of tubal transport resides either within the ovary, or within the fertilized egg itself (Winston 1977), must remain for the time being, just that.

IMPLANTATION

By about 6 days following fertilization, the blastocyst has breached the surface epithelium of the endometrium. The outermost layer of the blastocyst has already proliferated to form the trophoblastic cell mass which will in turn form a trophoblastic shell surrounding the conception. Gonadotrophin secretion from the early trophoblast begins and sustains the corpus luteum in the ovary, thus interrupting the menstrual cycle; the ensuing higher levels of progesterone connecting the endometrial stroma to a sheet of glycogen-rich cell, a tissue now called the decidua.

Implantation takes place therefore, about 1 week after ovulation or, in menstrual terms, by about day 21 of a 28-day cycle and the endometrial glands will be showing clear evidence of secretory activity. The degree of secretory activity appears critical, earlier and later secretory change being hostile to successful implantation. There is 'an extraordinary gap in one's knowledge of endometrial morphology that is scarcely acknowledged' (Robertson 1981) and until this gap is filled a fuller knowledge of the pre-requisite for successful implantation will elude us.

EMBRYOGENESIS

Even before implantation the blastocyst has shown a striking degree of organization with separation of the inner cell mass from the trophoblast. By the time of implantation the inner cell mass, destined to form the embryo proper will have differentiated into two layers, primitive endoderm and ectoderm, to form a bilaminar disc. The formation of a midline heap of ectodermal cells near the posterior end of the disc, the primitive streak, is followed by the proliferation of cells within the streak which migrate downwards to form a new layer between the ectoderm and endoderm. Thus the bilaminar disc becomes a trilaminar embryo in which (1) ectoderm will differentiate to form the nervous system and the skin; (2) mesoderm will become the cardiovascular and urogenital systems, bone, muscle and con-nective tissue, and (3) endoderm will become the lungs and gastrointestinal tract. A full account of subsequent embryonic and fetal development can be found in any standard textbook of human development and has no place in this review. It should be noted that organogenesis is largely complete 12 weeks after the last menstrual period, and sexual differentiation by 16 weeks.

DEVELOPMENT OF THE UTEROPLACENTAL CIRCULATION

Soon after implantation a trophoblastic shell forms around the embryo. Two kinds of trophoblast can be distinguished: villous trophoblast which will differentiate to form the placenta, and non-villous trophoblast which will penetrate the decidua and the decidual terminations of the spinal arteries, converting the latter into distensible funnel-shaped vessels (utero-placental arteries) which supply the intervillous space.

The transformation of the spinal arteries into large low-resistance utero-placental vessels appears to have two distinct phases (Brosens, Robertson and Dixon 1967). In the first, trophoblast and fibrinoid progressively replace the musculoelastic components of the decidual segments of the spinal arteries with consequent enlargement of their lumen. This has taken place by the gestational age of 10 weeks. During this time villous trophoblast has formed first trabecular columns and then, by continued growth, villous stems from which the fine villi will develop. By the 3rd week of gestational age the villous stems have become vacularized; by the 4th week the fetal heart has started to beat and a rudimentary circulation between fetus and placenta established. At this stage trophoblast is sprouting circumferentially from the trophoblastic shell. From 4 weeks' gestational age onwards however, those sprouts facing the uterine cavity gradually atrophy while those villous stems penetrating the decidua proliferate and, in close apposition to the developing uteroplacental arteries, give rise to the villi of the placenta proper.

Thus by 10 weeks' gestation a space has formed into which the early villi of the placenta dip (the intervillous space) and which is filled by maternal blood supplied from the developing uteroplacental arteries. Fetal blood is therefore brought into intimate apposition with maternal blood, the two circulations being separated merely by endothelium and trophoblast.

By 16 weeks' gestational age a new wave of trophoblast advances up the uteroplacental arteries to initiate the second phase of their transformation; so that by 20 weeks' gestation vessel wall change and dilatation extends into the myometrial segments of these vessels. By the same time the placenta has to achieve its definitive form and indeed full thickness. Hitherto growth will largely be in circumference.

This then constitutes the full maternal vascular adaption to pregnancy in the placental bed and the establishment of a haemochorial placentation in which the fetal trophoblast is directly bathed in maternal blood. The intervillous space represents the site of gaseous and nutritive exchange for the fetus and will gradually increase in size from zero to about 250 ml by term. Likewise perfusion of the intervillous space will rise from zero to about 500 ml/minute by term. This is facilitated in the first instance by the adaptive change described. Later in pregnancy there is hypertrophy and hyperplasia of the entire uterine tree with the uteroplacental arteries now depleted of their muscular and elastic components, undergoing further passive distension probably in response to the intra-arterial pressure.

Impaired development of the uteroplacental vasculature with dilatation of the uteroplacental arteries confined to the decidual segments only, has been described both in preeclampsia (Robertson, Brosens and Dixon 1967) and some cases of 'idiopathic' growth retardation (Robertson, Brosens and Dixon 1981; Sheppard and Bonnar 1976, 1981). The significance of these changes in relation to fetal growth will be reviewed more critically later in this chapter.

PLACENTAL DEVELOPMENT AND PLACENTAL FUNCTION

The functional units of the placenta are the terminal villi. In early pregnancy these are few and have a simple structure with an outer layer comprising two quite distinct forms of trophoblast: outermost syncytiotrophoblast and innermost cytotrophoblast. As the placenta rapidly increases in size the villi multiply and mature in appearance. From 10 to 20 weeks' gestation just a placentation is being definitively established, and the villi become smaller but much more numerous. The syncytiotrophoblast thins, the cytotrophoblast becomes irregular and even absent in some villi and the fetal capillaries within the villi increase in diameter. These villous changes, together with the great rise in number, increase the exchange capability of the villous surface of the placenta, and at a time when the fetal growth rate starts to outstrip the placental growth rate. In the mature placenta the villi are even smaller in diameter and the trophoblast even thinner and more attenuated, with the development of membranous and non-membranous areas. These highly specialized areas almost certainly represent sites of transfer and of synthesis (Fox 1978, 1979).

A number of factors affect the rate of exchange from maternal blood to fetal blood for any given nutrient. Some, already described, include perfusion of the intervillous space, the total villous area available for exchange and the thickness of the trophoblastic barrier between the two circulations. Others include concentration gradients and the nature of the substance and its transport system. In general terms transport of highly diffusible substances such as blood gases which have a high coefficient of utilization (Meschin 1978) is determined by maternal plasma concentration and maternal plasma flow, while those which have a lower coefficient of utilization and are therefore exchanged more slowly are more dependent upon the membrane characteristics of the placenta.

Nutrient exchange

Oxygen

Oxygen passes to the fetus by a process of simple diffusion down a concentration gradient. Fetal uptake of oxygen is enhanced in the first instance by a higher haemoglobin concentration and haemotocrit, and in the second, by the higher affinity of fetal haemoglobin for oxygen.

Carbon dioxide and carbon monoxide

Carbon dioxide similarly follows a concentration gradient from fetus to mother. Respiratory readjustments within the mother lower her P_{CO_2} which further enhances its elimination. Carbon monoxide readily diffuses across the placenta and with chronic exposure, as in smoking, elevated fetal carbon haemoglobin levels have been found (Longo 1970). Because of the high affinity of fetal blood for carbon monoxide, fetal levels have been reported to be nearly twice those of maternal levels.

Glucose

Glucose is the principal nutritional substrate for the fetus. The mode of transfer is not one of simple diffusion, but rather of faciliated diffusion permitting much more rapid transfer than other hexoses. The system is stereospecific, hexose-specific and also allows for retrograde flow of glucose from the fetus back to the mother. The subject has been reviewed recently by Shelley (1979).

Amino acids

Every amino acid is found in higher concentration for fetal plasma than maternal plasma, and higher concentration for trophoblast chain than for fetal plasma. Transfer is therefore by active transport. The higher trophoblast levels, especially for the acidic and neutral straight chain amino acids suggests that they may at least in part be synthesized by the trophoblast. The only proteins transferred from mother to fetus are almost exclusively IgG. All other fetal proteins are synthesized from transferred maternal amino acids. Very little is known about the specifics of amino acid transfer in man. Extrapolation from the animal model is unwise. This subject too has been recently reviewed (Young 1979).

Fetal lipids

Fetal lipids largely derive from two sources, the first and largest being maternal free fatty acid transfer, the second and lesser being synthesis from acetate and carbohydrate. As for amino acids, most information has been derived from animal models. The balance of evidence favours free transfer of fatty acids across the human placenta. Role-limiting factors are uncertain but elevated maternal levels have a permissive effect. Together with carbohydrate and amino acid transfer, this subject has also been recently reviewed (Hull and Elphick 1979).

Water

Water distributes itself freely through all the tissues of the body. Water transport between mother and fetus occurs therefore as a result of live processes; the first and overwhelmingly the greater is by bidirectional diffusional exchange, the second is by net transfer which at most represents 23 g/day in late pregnancy, 'diffusional exchange exceeding net transfer by a factor of several thousand throughout most of pregnancy' (Hytten 1979).

Sodium exchange

The exchange of sodium is similar to that of water. Net exchange is in favour of the fetus but again there is an enormous bidirectional flux (Flexner *et al.* 1948). In animals at least there is a sodium–potassium (Na–K) pump in the syncytiotrophoblast which may protect fetal potassium levels. Chloride is found in similar concentrations on both sides of the placenta. Its transfer probably follows that of sodium.

Vitamins

Rather less is known about the transfer of vitamins. *Water-soluble* appear to be actively transported by complex mechanisms involving intermediate biochemical forms, and may be stored in the placenta. Even less has been written about *fat-souble* vitamins. Vitamin A is probably transferred as carotene which is then converted to vitamin A. Much work is greatly needed in this field.

Iron

Iron reaches the fetus by active transport across the placenta. Fletcher and Suter (1969) have speculated that there might be competition between receptor sites on the maternal developing red cells, and the placenta in favour of the fetus. However cord ferritin levels of babies born to iron-deficient mothers are depressed (Rios *et al.* 1975) suggesting that their neonates have iron depletion.

The syncyntiotrophoblast

Ultrastructural examination of the syncytiotrophoblast has demonstrated pinocytic vesicles, multivesicular bodies and dome-shaped protrusions all of which appear to have specific transport roles. It also has demonstrated within the syncytiotrophoblast a variety of organelles seen in association with both protein and steroid synthesis. There seems no doubt therefore that the syncytiotrophoblast also represents the major site of hormone production both polypeptic and steroid within the placenta (Fox 1978). These hormones are largely responsible for many of the further adaptive changes in maternal physiology that are now considered.

TOTAL BODY WATER AND CLINICAL OEDEMA

Total body water increases continuously through pregnancy. This increase is difficult to measure but is predominantly within the extracellular compartment, leading to increases both in circulating volume and interstitial fluid.

Although limit oedema represents the most tangible expression of increased interstitial fluid, the amount of water retained in this compartment is far more than can be accounted for by limit oedema alone. There is, rather, a generalized increase of water retained in association with the mucopolysaccharide of the ground substance of the connective tissue throughout the maternal body. This retention of water, probably an oestrogen-mediated phenomenon, causes softening and stretching of connective tissues in such disparate sites as the pelvis, cornea, vagina, gingiva, cervix and nipple, and accounts at least in part for antenatal complaints such as pelvic joint pain, problems with contact lenses and gingivitis.

Clinical oedema is reported in approximately 40 per cent of all uncomplicated pregnancies. There is a higher incidence in pregnancies complicated by hypertension, and this incidence reaches 90 per cent when the hypertension is associated with proteinuria (Thomson, Hytten and Billewicz 1967). It is not surprising, therefore, that when considering a total population there is a clear association between oedema and hypertension. But what is the significance of oedema when found in 40 per cent of a normotensive population? In a retrospective study of 24 079 singleton pregnancies from Aberdeen, Thomson, Hytten and Billewicz (1967) were able to show an increased incidence of clinical oedema with increased maternal weight for height. There was no effect of blood pressure upon the incidence of oedema until the final diastolic pressure was 90 mmHg or more. After controlling for height, weight, parity and blood pressure, women with clinical oedema were found to have larger neonates, fewer growth-retarded neonates and a lower perinatal mortality when compared to women with no detectable oedema. Although none of these differences achieved statistical significance, they lend convincing support to the idea that oedema in the normotensive pregnancy is a physiological rather than a pathological event.

PLASMA VOLUME

Plasma volume rises continuously from early pregnancy to term, from a non-pregnant value of 2500 ml to a peak value of 3750 ml in primigravidae and 4000 ml in multigravidae. It is unclear how soon after conception this rise starts but speculative reports put it as early as 4 or even 3 weeks. A maximal rate of increase is achieved by 12–16 weeks gestation and a peak value obtained by 32–36 weeks after which it is maintained until term. An early report that peak values were attended by a subsequent drop of 200 ml by term has not been confirmed and was probably due to measurements being undertaken in the supine position.

Not only does plasma volume expand to a greater degree in multigravid than primigravid women, it also expands to a greater degree in multiple pregnancy (Fullerton *et al.* 1965; Rovinsky and Jaffin 1965), and adversely to a larger degree in women with poorly growing fetuses (Duffus, MacGillivray and Dennis 1971; Gibson 1973). In short, there is an intimate association between degree of plasma volume expansion and size at birth. This even extends to the quasiexperimental situation where in women exposed to chronic diuretic therapy, both plasma volume and birth size is reduced (Campbell and McGillivray 1975).

The exact cause of plasma volume expansion is unknown. Certainly it is at least assisted by the increased blood levels of angiotensin II and aldosterone. Whether they are provoked directly by oestrogen-induced plasma remain substrate (Dusterdieck and McElwee 1971) or reflexly evoked by a drop in peripheral resistance or both is not clear. The development of the uteroplacental vasculature, and the effects of progesterone upon the smooth muscle in the vascular tree, lower peripheral resistance. This is seen at its lowest mid-pregnancy with a marked fall in diastolic blood pressure (Bader *et al.* 1955; Pyorala 1966; Rovinsky and Jaffin 1966; Schwarcz, Aramendia and Taguine 1964). High levels of oestrogen and progesterone do not appear to be necessary to provoke circulatory change. Increases in the plasma volume of non-pregnant women have been reported after only short courses of oestrogen therapy (Witten and Bradbury 1951). Elevated blood levels of angiotensin II have been found in women taking the combined oral contraceptive pill (Walters and Lim 1970) and such women have also been reported to have an increased plasma volume and cardiac output. It is tempting to speculate that by its endocrine output, the fetoplacental unit is controlling the increase and maintenance of plasma volume that so closely mirrors its own size.

RED CELL MASS AND HAEMOGLOBIN CONCENTRATION

Red cells mass, like plasma volume, rises progressively through pregnancy from 1400 ml in the prepregnant woman to 1750 ml in later pregnancy. The mean increment is thought to be less (250 ml) in those women not taking iron supplements than in those on iron supplements (400 ml). Progressively larger increments in red cell mass have been reported in twin, triplet and quadruplet pregnancy (Fullerton *et al.* 1965; Rovinsky and Jaffin 1965).

Corpuscular size and haemoglobin concentration remain more or less constant throughout pregnancy in an iron-sufficient population. As the incremental change in plasma volume outstrips the incremental change in red cell mass, the net result is that red cell count and haemoglobin concentration fall in pregnancy.

The World Health Organization (1972) accepts 12.0 g/dl as the lowest normal haemoglobin concentration for the healthy non-pregnant adult and 11.0 g/dl for the pregnant adult. This latter value is just a little higher than one would calculate allowing for a prepregnancy haemoglobin concentration of 12.0 g/dl and normal plasma volume and red cell mass expansion. Haemoglobin concentration reaches its nadir at about 34 weeks' gestation and it may be that a lower acceptable limit of 10.4 g/dl is more appropriate. Some of these patients will however be making an iron or folate deficiency at this level and cord ferritin levels are lower in infants born to iron-deficient mothers (Gibson 1973). This may have important implications for the neonate. The greater part of fetal iron stores are acquired in the last trimester when maternal depletion is likely to be greatest, and a little under half the body iron in a 2-year-old is still of maternal origin (Castaldi 1979).

IRON AND IRON PROPHYLAXIS

The arithmetic of iron requirement in pregnancy is not simple. Iron is required for transfer to the fetus, placenta and cord, for expansion of the red cell mass, and to meet normal daily adult losses. Further iron will be required to cover blood loss at delivery and for lactation. The total pregnancy requirement excluding lactation has been calculated to be in the order of 890 mg. Pregnancy amenorrhoea saves approximately 120 mg iron. The balance, 770 mg, represents the net cost of pregnancy in terms of iron. This cost is not incurred at a steady rate throughout pregnancy, but is least in the first trimester, and most in the last, when as much as 6–7 mg iron/day are required (Letsky 1980). Such a requirement has to be met from the maternal diet.

An average western diet yields 10–15 mg iron/day of which at best 10 per cent is absorbed. Absorption of iron is still poorly understood but it is enhanced when iron stores are depleted and reduced when iron supplements are given. Absorption is increased when there is new red cell formation, and decreased when combined with phytates. There is evidence of enhanced absorption in the second half of pregnancy when iron requirements are greatest and maternal stores most likely to be depleted (Apte and Nenger 1970; Svanberg 1975). Even with absorption rates as high as 40 per cent many women in late pregnancy will be unable to match the daily iron requirement for their diet; the balance, therefore, will have to be met from their iron stores which if already depleted will become more so.

Is iron supplementation in pregnancy really necessary? There is persuasive evidence that dietary iron is commonly insufficient to meet the pregnancy demand, and that low haemoglobin concentrations are in some cases associated with unequivocal iron deficiency (Fenton, Cavill and Fisher 1977).

This latter is a difficult diagnosis to establish; serum iron and iron binding capacity estimations are unreliable. Marrow aspiration presents incontrovertible evidence of iron deficiency when present, but is not welcomed by the patient. Estimations of plasma ferritin, a glycoprotein (normal range: 15–300 ns/litre) which is stable and unlike serum iron does not fluctuate with recent intake, seem to accurately reflect iron stores (Jacobs *et al.* 1972), at least in the non-pregnant woman.

Both low haemoglobin concentrations and maternal iron deficiency matter: the former not because oxygen carriage to the fetus is affected (anaemia has to be profound for this to happen) but because the risk to the mother from haemorrhage is increased; and the latter because as already seen, neonatal iron stores may be endangered. That iron supplementation may reduce iron depletion as measured by ferritin levels has been clearly shown (Fenton, Cavill and Fisher 1977). This establishes a rationale for prophylaxis. There is, however, no evidence that treating a whole population rather than selecting those patients displaying evidence of iron deficiency for therapy optimizes results. This latter must represent the preferred strategy.

FOLATE AND FOLATE PROPHYLAXIS

Megaloblastic anaemia in pregnancy is nearly always due to folate deficiency. A true estimate of the incidence cannot be made. A far greater number of women have megaloblastic change in their marrow than in a peripheral blood film, and there is no simple test which will reveal true folate deficiency. This can only be diagnosed on examination of marrow aspirate. It is probable that the incidence of folate deficiency in any given population will reflect its nutritional status.

Folate requirements in pregnancy are approximately 800 mg/day for a singleton pregnancy and more in multiple pregnancy. The average western diet contains between 500 and 700 mg/day of folate but a large proportion of this can be lost in cooking. The pregnancy requirement is unlikely to be met from dietary folate alone, particularly in multiple pregnancy when Chanarin (1969) has reported an incidence of megaloblastic anaemia as high as 1:11.

Even more important is the possible association of folate deficiency with pregnancy complication and outcome. There is no convincing evidence that folate deficiency increases the risk of spontaneous abortion and abruptio placenta. There is, however, some evidence that folate when given with other vitamins is associated with a reduced incidence of neural tube defects, such as spina bifida (Leck 1983; Smitheus, Sheppard and Schorah 1976; Smitheus *et al.* 1977). Unfortunately the nature of this evidence precludes any firm conclusion as to whether folate, other vitamins or indeed some other uncontrolled confounding factor was responsible. There is a real need, both scientifically and ethically, to resolve the vexed question of whether periconceptual folate deficiency is a preventible cause of congenital abnormality. In the meantime a case can be established for folate prophylaxis at least in those with multiple pregnancy, or who are nutritionally at risk.

COAGULATION FACTORS

Coagulation problems are uncommon in normal pregnancy but disseminated intravascular coagulation (DIC) and fibrinolysis can complicate the abnormal pregnancy. The major changes to coagulation factors observed during pregnancy involve the prothrombin complex, especially factors VII and X, as factors VIII and fibrinogen. Fibrin degradation products (FDP) are also found in slightly increased amounts (Castaldi 1979).

Labour is attended by a decrease in fibrinogen and factor VIII levels with markedly elevated levels of fibrin degradation products (Kleiner *et al.* 1970). This is also seen with placental abruption, intrauterine death and amniotic fluid embolism.

CARDIAC OUTPUT

Cardiac output rises in pregnancy from a prepregnant value of 4.5 l/minute to 6.0 l/minute. This rise occurs early in pregnancy, is largely achieved by the end of the first trimester and remains elevated until term. Previous investigators who had shown an apparent drop in cardiac output from mid-trimester values to term have failed to allow for the effect of the gravid uterus upon the vena cava when the woman assumes the recumbent position.

Cardiac output further rises in the first stage of labour by as much as a further 2 l/minute although effective analgesia will reduce this, and peak values as high as 10 l/minute may accompany the voluntary expulsive efforts of the second stage. The effect of the third stage of labour upon cardiac output is the product of, on the one hand, loss of circulating volume from the placental bed at the time of placental separation, and on the other an increment in right-sided return subsequent to oxytocin administration.

Cardiac output is the product of stroke volume and heart rate. Clearly both can and do increase in pregnancy. Although authors differ as to the relative importance of these two components (de Swiet 1980; Walters 1979), the balance of evidence favours a greater proportionate increase in heart rate.

The pattern of change in cardiac output has important implications for the obstetrician. The rise in output takes place earlier and to a greater extent than is often realized. Previously well patients who present with acute dyspnoea and decompensation for the first time in the second trimester, should always have included in their differential diagnosis an undiagnosed mitral stenosis or other cardiac lesion. Women with a reduced cardiac reserve benefit from epidural analgesia in labour and from an effective forceps delivery. The third stage of labour presents its own peculiar hazards. The risk of overloading the right side of the circulation in patients with a tight mitral stenosis through vigorous use of oxytocics, in particular egrometrine, is well known; although recent work suggests that venous occlusion by the myometrium rather than emptying into the circulation is the consequence of uterine contraction (Schwarz 1964). Against this risk has to be balanced the concomitant risk of excessive haemorrhage, which in patients with left-to-right shunts and pulmonary hypertension, can result in reversal of the shunt with grave consequences.

ARTERIAL BLOOD PRESSURE

Arterial blood pressure in pregnancy is most accurately measured in the brachial artery by the indirect sphygmomanometric method. When compared to simultaneous readings obtained by direct arterial cannulation, sphygmomanometry underestimates the systolic and overestimates the diastolic pressures, the former by about 4 mmHg and the latter by a little more. Brachial artery sphygmomanometry is a subjective technique susceptible to an almost encyclopaedic list of confounding factors and bias which include: different phases of the Korotkoff sounds (IV and V) taken as the diastolic point; application of the cuff; size of cuff; arm girth; speed of deflation of the cuff; posture of the subject; known previous readings and technical digit preferences. Blood pressure values vary also with emotional state, degree of physical activity and ethnic group.

It is perhaps surprising then that there is general accord as to the pattern of blood pressure through pregnancy. Systolic pressure changes little in pregnancy whereas diastolic pressure drops appreciably by up to 15 mmHg reaching a nadir from 12 to 16 weeks' gestation and thereafter rising to about prepregnancy values by term (MacGillivray, Rote and Rowe 1969). Less clear is the effect of changed posture with contradictory findings from different investigators (MacGillivray, Rote and Rowe; Schwarz 1964). However, there seems to be unequivocal evidence that in the last trimester of pregnancy, some women upon assuming the recumbent position, suffer occlusion of the vena cava, reduced cardiac output and consequent hypotension. The hypotension, severe enough to cause syncope, also impairs perfusion of the intervillous space and will cause marked fetal anoxia. The reported incidence of the supine hypotension syndrome varies from 4–11 per cent (Holmes 1960; Howard, Goodson and Mengert 1953). The probable spacing factors are the degree of vena caval occlusion, the ability to establish a collateral circulation via the azygous and vertebral veins, and the power to maintain blood pressure in the face of falling cardiac output by reflex vasoconstriction. While protracted abdominal examination may be sufficient to provoke the syndrome in late pregnancy, epidural analgesia with its attendant automatic blockade significantly increases the incidence of intrapartum hypotension.

It is difficult to define a level at which either systolic or diastolic pressure should be regarded as abnormal. Both systolic and diastolic pressures rise with increasing age and parity. Pregnancy-acquired hypertension is much commoner than pre-existing hypertension. Although the majority of obstetricians would regard a pressure of 140 mmHg systolic and 90 mmHg diastolic as the upper limits of normality, a rise in diastolic pressure to 90 mmHg or more is found in about 20 per cent of all primigravidae (MacGillivray 1979). Data from Aberdeen suggests that late pregnancy hypertension in the absence of proteinuria is neither associated with reduced birth weight nor indeed with increased perinatal loss. This is in contradistinction to hypertension with proteinuria where birth weight was significantly reduced and a threefold increase in perinatal mortality observed (MacGillivray 1979). Page and Christiansen (1976) presenting data on mean arterial pressure (diastolic pressure and pulse pressure × 3) on the other hand have shown a progressive rise in perinatal mortality with increasing mid-pregnancy pressure. The implications are: first, that a rigid definition of normal and abnormal levels is inappropriate; second, that mid-trimester hypertension and hypertension with proteinuria have a significant detrimental effect on pregnancy outcome; but third, that mild late pregnancy hypertension in the absence of proteinuria may be associated with optimal outcome.

VENOUS BLOOD PRESSURE

Studies of central venous pressure in pregnancy yields conflicting results. The balance of evidence suggests, however, that there are no significant changes in venous pressure. Those changes that have been observed are more likely to be due to posture rather than to the pregnancy.

On the other hand, there is unequivocal evidence of a rise in lower limit venous pressure, which appears to be progressive throughout pregnancy (McLennan 1943). A number of factors help account for this and include occlusion of the vena cava by the gravid uterus, venous return (much augmented) from the gravid uterus, and increased venous distensibility. This probably explains the increased tendency to, and exacerbation in pregnancy of, lower limit varices, vulval varices and haemorrhoids.

PERIPHERAL RESISTANCE

Total peripheral resistance is the product of mean arterial blood pressure divided by cardiac output. It is principally affected by small vessel size and by blood viscosity. This latter alters little in pregnancy, but there is a general decrease in peripheral vascular tone, largely as a result of progesterone. We would expect therefore to see a decrease in peripheral resistance in pregnancy. This has been reported by many investigators (Bader *et al.* 1955; Pyorala 1966; Rovinsky and Jaffin 1966; Schwarcz, Aramendia and Taquine 1964). This decrease is maximal in mid-pregnancy.

REGIONAL BLOOD FLOW

Regional blood flow increases throughout pregnancy. In particular, there is increased perfusion of the skin, kidney, lung and uterus.

Skin flow increases 2 to 5-fold in pregnancy, particularly in the hands and feet (Ginsburg and Duncan 1967). Also increased is flow through the nasal mucosa which becomes hyperaemic and congested. This is the likely explanation for the characteristic nasal 'stuffiness' of pregnant women and their propensity for epistaxes. Such generalized cutaneous hyperaemia undoubtedly helps dissipate extra heat generated by the fetus.

Renal blood flow rises in the first trimester of pregnancy to about 1200 ml/minute by the early second trimester, and exceeds non-pregnant values by nearly 50 per cent (Walters 1979). There is uncertainty as to the timing of this change in the first trimester and dispute as to whether second trimester levels are maintained or drop to term. It seems more probable that the timing of this change and its pattern reflect in general that of cardiac output, and that drops in renal flow towards term are a posture-related artefact (Davison 1980).

Pulmonary blood flow mirrors cardiac output. The increase in pulmonary flow seen in pregnancy is achieved without an increase in right ventricular and pulmonary artery pressure (Bader *et al.* 1955). This must mean that peripheral resistance is lowered probably by dilatation of the pulmonary vasculature

Both uterine blood flow and flow through the intervillous space increase during pregnancy. A number of techniques have been employed to make these measurements. All of them involve assumptions often of some dubiousness, most are invasive and some have been made under the most unphysiological of circumstances. Methods employed include placement of an electromagnetic flowmeter on the uterine artery, nitrous oxide and 4-amino-antipyrine variations on the Fick principle, and a variety of isotope accumulation and washout techniques variously requiring inhalation, intravenous or transabdominal injection of the marker. There is consequently an enormous discrepancy between published results. Two features do however seem clear. First, there is a precise and almost constant relationship between uterine and uteroplacental flow and total conceptual size irrespective of gestational age (Assali, Ravramo and Peltonen 1960); second, there is a progressive increase in flow with increasing gestation, an increase which mirrors that of plasma volume rather than cardiac output. Little is known of the factors which regulate uteroplacental flow. It seems probable that autoregulation is not possible once the full vascular adaption to pregnancy has taken place. The uteroplacental vessels appear to be in a state of passive vasodilatation, and although Zuspan *et al.* (1981) have demonstrated catecholamine fluorescent nerve endings in the uteroplacental arteries, their competence is under considerable doubt. More probable is that uteroplacental flow in the human as in other animals is primarily pressure-dependent. This would fit with the previously described clinical observations.

THE EFFECT OF WORK AND REST UPON PREGNANCY OUTCOME

This is largely unknown. Morris has shown decreased uteroplacental clearance of a labelled isotope in women undergoing vigorous exercise, and it seems reasonable to assume that strenuous exercise might result in diversion of blood from the uteroplacental circulation. Regular exercise in pregnancy, however, has not been shown to affect outcome in normal western populations, and rest, although widely assumed to be beneficial, when combined with hospital admission has yet to be shown to improve outcome. Low birth weight in the developing countries is probably due to synergistic effects of the haemodynamics of vigorous exertion, suboptimal nutrition and an increased caloric requirement from the work.

PULMONARY FUNCTION

In pregnancy there is a continuous rise in tidal volume from a prepregnant value of about 500–700 ml in late pregnancy. Respiratory rate remains relatively unaffected so that the minute volume increases from 7.25 l/minute to 10.5 l/minute. This is achieved by increased movement of the diaphragm and flaring of the ribs.

   This increased alveolar ventilation affects both Po_2 and Pco_2. The effect on Po_2 is trival under normal circumstances (de Swiet 1980). The effect of Pco_2 however, with a drop of 4–8 mmHg from prepregnant values is greater and will facilitate the elimination of CO_2 from the fetus by establishing a steeper concentration gradient across the placenta (de Swiet 1980). Increased breathing may be stimulated by progesterone, to a lesser extent by oestrogen, and to a greater extent by the two in concert (Doring, Loescheke and Ochwadt 1950). The mechanism by which this obtains is unclear, but is presumed to involve the respiratory centres.

CARDIAC AND RESPIRATORY FUNCTIONAL RESERVE

Both cardiac output and minute volume increase by about a third in pregnancy. But, whereas maximum cardiac output can increase threefold in exercise, minute volume can increase by a factor of 10. This suggests that pregnancy change represents a far greater proportion of the functional reserve for cardiac output than for minute volume, and that patients with cardiac disease are more likely to decompensate in pregnancy than patients with respiratory disease.

RENAL FUNCTION

Renal anatomy and physiology is markedly altered in pregnancy. The principal changes concern the renal pelvis, ureters and bladder, increased flow and glomerular filtration, and changes in electrolyte, protein and other nutrient excretion.

There is a progressive dilatation of the calyces, pelvis and ureters throughout pregnancy. This has traditionally been attributed to a progestational effect upon smooth muscle, and is said to be associated with stasis of urine in the collecting systems. This is oversimplistic. Ureteric smooth muscle hypertrophies and ureteric tone is increased rather than decreased in pregnancy (Rubi and Sala 1968). The dilatation of the ureters evident in pregnancy is probably a consequence rather of partial obstruction of the ureters by the uterus at the pelvic brim. The insertion of the ureters into the bladder become displaced as pregnancy progresses leading to an increased incidence of vesicoureteric reflux (Mattingly and Borkowf 1978). These changes persist after delivery for as long as 3 months. Radiological investigation of the urinary tract should therefore be avoided for 3 months post-delivery, if possible, rather than the 6 weeks commonly advocated (Davidson 1980).

Renal blood increases throughout pregnancy as already described. Unlike renal blood flow, there seems to be a consensus as to the pattern of glomerular filtration rates in pregnancy which progressively increases with advancing gestation. It is likely that the rise in glomerular filtration rate exceeds the rise in renal blood flow at least by term, thus increasing the filtration traction. One result of these changes is a progressive drop in levels of plasma urea and creatinine which is of course further compounded by the dilatational effect of plasma volume expansion and possibly by reduced deamination. Thus normal non-pregnant values may represent abnormal pregnant values.

During a normal pregnancy there is cumulative retention of salt and water. Between 460 and 900 mEq/l of sodium are retained and distributed between fetus, placenta and the maternal extracellular compartment. This retention occurs despite increased glomerular filtration and can ensue only from a major increase in tubular reabsorption. The factors controlling sodium excretion in pregnancy are many and complex and have been summarized by Lindheimer and Katz (1974). Water excretion is principally determined by plasma osmolality which falls in pregnancy by 10 mOsm/kg when compared to prepregnant values. It is likely that there is a major readjustment of the balance between osmolality and antidiuretic hormone (ADP) as urine volume is reduced rather than increased in pregnancy (Davidson 1980). Attempts to manipulate sodium and water retention, even in the presence of peripheral oedema by diuretic therapy have little place. Diuretic decrease, plasma volume expansion and uteroplacental transfer and are all associated with a reduced birth weight (Campbell and MacGillivray 1975; Gant and Madden 1975, 1976).

GLYCOSURIA IN PREGNANCY

Glycosuria in pregnancy is found in anything up to 60 per cent of all women, depending upon the frequency of urine testing (Soler and Mains 1971). The principal reason for glycosuria is the increased presentation of glucose to the tubule as a result of an increased glomerular filtration rate (GFR). Other factors will include elevated levels of plasma glucose after an oral load and decreased tubular reabsorption. The traditional concept of a maximal tubular reabsorptive capacity for glucose which was exceeded by increased glomerular delivery has been discredited. Tubular reabsorption of glucose appears to have no finite ceiling. Current concepts of pregnancy glycosuria include frankly diminished tubular reabsorption in response to the sex steroids and the possibility of tubular damage (Davidson and Hytten 1974, 1975). The sporadic nature of glycosuria however suggests that it is the effect of increased delivery to the tubule that is predominantly responsible.

With such a high incidence, it is not surprising that glycosuria is a poor predictor of abnormal glucose tolerance in pregnancy. Employing an intravenous glucose tolerance test to define abnormal tolerance, and taking a large number of indicators for tolerance testing Sutherland, Stowers and Fisher (1979) have clearly shown the formidable difficulties in deriving a satisfactory screening strategy for diabetes in the antenatal clinic. Their recommended strategy is to arrange for a glucose tolerance test (GTT) on all women who present with one or more indicators on history, or who are found to have glycosuria in a second testing specimen. It must be observed that the greater the number of single indicators that are utilized for glucose tolerance testing, the greater the number of tests that are performed, and the least number of diabetics who will be missed. On the other hand, restricting testing to those with more than one at-risk factor will increase the pick-up rate per cent of tests performed, reduce the overall number of tests, but increase the number of diabetics missed. No strategy yet devised avoids this dilemma.

BACTERIURIA IN PREGNANCY

Of all women attending antenatal clinics, who book with sterile urine, 1 per cent will develop acute pyelonephritis in the course of their pregnancy (Peckham and Marshal 1983). Further, women with frank urinary tract infections have an increased incidence of preterm delivery (Sever 1980). Asymptomatic urinary infection ($>10^5$ cal/ml of bacteria) occurs in about 6 per cent of pregnant women and was first shown by Kass (1960) to predispose to pyelonephritis and prematurity. It is now clear that some 25 per cent of women with asymptomatic bacteriuria will develop pyelonephritis if left untreated, but only 3 per cent if treated (Williams 1980), and so vigorous treatment of asymptomatic bacteriuria in early pregnancy will prevent most (but not all) pyelonephritis in pregnancy. The effect of treatment of asymptomatic bacteriuria in preterm delivery is harder to evaluate because of a multiplicity of confounding factors.

ALIMENTARY FUNCTION

Pregnancy is marked by a variety of well-documented changes in alimentary function, though remarkably few physiological measurements exist in the literature. The principal effects to be noted are reduced acid secretion and a generalized decrease in gut motility. This latter has important implications.

There seems good evidence that gastric acid secretion is reduced in pregnancy, particularly in mid to late pregnancy (Hunt and Murray 1958; Murray, Erskine, and Fieldin 1957). Peptic ulcer is rare in the antenatal period but it is not clear whether this effect is mediated by reduced acid secretion or increased mucus secretion.

As in the cardiovascular and urinary system there is general relaxation of smooth muscle, leading to decreased gut motility and incompetence of the cardiac sphincter. Although contradictory accounts of gastric emptying are present in the literature, it seems likely that solid meals at least are retained in the stomach for longer. Gastric emptying is further delayed in labour, and even more so if the patient is given narcotic analgesia (Davison, Davison, and Hay 1970; Nimmo, Wilson and Prescott 1975).

It would seem that a delay in gastric emptying, incompetence of the sphincter at the cardia, and an increase in intra-abdominal pressure associated with uterine enlargement, all predispose to gastric acid reflux up the oesophagus, causing oesophagitis and heartburn. Certainly heartburn is reported most commonly in late pregnancy when these effects are maximal, and certainly it is experienced most often when patients lie down. Equally, heartburn will often respond to simple supportive measures such as sleeping with more pillows, obviating in many cases the need for antacid medication.

Potentially more serious, however, is the risk of gastric acid reflux and aspiration during obstetric anaesthesia. Although in Mendelsohn's original account of the syndrome which now bears his name no patient died, a mortality of as high as 25 per cent is reported. Therapeutic manoeuvres aimed at reducing the incidence of this worrying condition include altered posture for induction of anaesthesia and antacid therapy. Anaesthesia has been induced with the patient in both 'head up' and 'head down' positions. Not perhaps surprisingly, neither endeavour has been effective. Current emphasis is towards skilled intubation, using a curled endotracheal tube with a working sucker at hand. Antacid therapy, commonly employing magnesium trisilicate is avidly employed as prophylaxis in labour wards. Regimens differ, 'high-risk' patients in some wards, all patients in others, receiving antacids at 2–4 hourly intervals. It seems clear that the effect of antacid therapy upon pH is transient, elevated levels being reported for little more than 30 minutes after antacid injection. Thus many patients receive such therapy but do not need it. Others who do, do not receive it, and in all the probable duration of effect is for 30 minutes out of every 2–4 hours; hardly efficient prophylaxis! A preferred approach would be to abandon guessing games as to who will require general anaesthesia, and restrict therapy only to those patients in whom a decision to induce anaesthesia had been made, and to administer it immediately prior to anaesthesia. Thus antacid is given to the right patient at the right time. Sodium citrate is probably the drug of choice.

There is delayed transport through both the small and large intestine. The former might be expected to enhance nutrient absorption from the gut. But although increases have been reported in the absorption of iron (Apte and Nenger 1970) and calcium (Haeney and Skillman 1971), this appears to occur through mechanisms independent of transit time, and there is as yet no convincing evidence that nutrient absorption in pregnancy is specifically enhanced in this way. More convincing is the evidence for increased water absorption in the large colon (Parry, Shields, and Turnbull 1970) which would justify frequent complaints of constipation. Levy, Lemberg, and Sharf's (1971) commonly quoted study apparently refuting this is confounded in the first instance by its retrospective design.

WEIGHT GAIN IN PREGNANCY

Weight gain differs widely in pregnancy, but in the majority of studies has a mean of about 12.5 kg. Optimal outcome has been reported with a mean weight gain of 9 kg in the second 20 weeks (Hytten 1980). It is traditional to present weight gain as an analysis of its component parts but maternal stones almost certainly represent depôt fat.

Neither increased nor decreased weight gain in pregnancy is incompatible with normal outcome. Nevertheless there is consistent evidence that women with reduced weight gain tend to have lighter neonates.

NUTRITION IN PREGNANCY

Pregnancy is characterized by significant change both in maternal energy balance and in the levels of plasma nutrients.

In pregnancy a woman's energy balance becomes strongly anabolic and analysis of her weight gain displays both tissue growth and fat deposition. This latter, already some 3 kg by 30 weeks' gestation and deposited characteristically in the abdomen and thighs, accrues under the influence of progesterone and is mobilized under the influence of hPL. The principal function of this fat depôt appears to be energy storage, and mobilization in the last trimester reduces what would otherwise be disproportionately high pregnancy specific energy costs to about 400 kcal/day.

Apart from glucose little is known about the metabolism of individual nutrients and knowledge is largely restricted to plasma levels (Hytten 1983). One change is clear, the lipid-soluble fraction tends to rise and the water-soluble fraction tends to fall, but the reasons for these changes remain for the most part obscure. Mobilization of the fat depôt would be expected to yield higher levels of non-esterified fatty acids and glycerol, and expansion of the plasma volume will result in reduced plasma concentration of many substrates. Hytten speculates that these altered levels represent a resetting of homeostatic mechanisms that favours placental uptake, arguing that at lower plasma concentrations the placenta is relatively more efficient than maternal tissues, the ensuing balance therefore favouring the fetus.

If the foregoing seems beset with uncertainty, the same is certainly true when dietary intake is considered. There is no objective 'gold standard' against which maternal diet can be assessed and various figures from values observed in healthy populations have been produced; however, they do not tell us either the needs specific for one person or, more importantly, at what level of underachievement compromised outcome will occur. It is not surprising that for many nutrients the calculated requirements vary significantly from source to source.

There is a common illusion that in postwar Great Britain malnutrition is a thing of the past. Doyle *et al.* (1982) in a dietary survey carried out in pregnancy upon a low socio economic group of East End Londoners, demonstrated disturbing low energy intakes (only 6 per cent of the mothers' intake were within the recommended daily allowance in any one trimester); 50 per cent of the infants born to these mothers weighed 3000 g or less and there was a significantly decreased energy intake in those mothers delivering infants weighing 2500 g or less when compared to the rest of the cohort. If not evidence of malnutrition, this represents at least severe undernutrition which is probably still endemic in most urban centres. It is tempting to infer that the low birth weight evidenced by the group was principally due to dietary deficiency, but other confounding factors were not adequately controlled. The role of dietary deprivation in the genesis of low birth weight infants is not clear. Observation of disasters such as the Dutch hunger winter of 1944–45 (Stein *et al.* 1975) suggests that an effect on birth weight is maximal when deprivation occurs in the second half of pregnancy. It is noteworthy, however, that here the infants were not shorter, just lighter by 300 g and they caught their anticipated weights up within 6 weeks of delivery. Hytten (1983) speculates that this effect was due to a lack of 'the luxury of 300–400 g subcutaneous fat'. Supplementation experiments in general have been disappointing and Viegas *et al.* (1982) have shown differing results from supplementing either all mothers or those nutritionally at risk. Only in the latter group was any effect of supplement on diet noted and then only in that group receiving protein energy and vitamin supplements (vitamins alone have no effect). Again the increased crude birth weight was probably accounted for by increased fat as determined by skinfold thickness.

In general, evidence is lacking that vitamin supplementation is necessary or even desirable in pregnancy. There are exceptions to this statement. The role of folate and or other vitamins in preventing the development of neural tube defects remains to be established but may be relevant. Asian mothers are significantly at risk of developing vitamin D deficiency in pregnancy (Brooke *et al.* 1980), and supplementation with 400 units/day of vitamin D may be beneficial.

DETERMINANTS OF FETAL GROWTH

A number of changes in maternal physiology have been reviewed, and have unashamedly been presented as adaptation to facilitate fetal growth. A simple model encompassing some of these is presented below (Fig. 5.1):

Normal fetal growth requires an adequate amount of nutritional substrate to be presented to the intervillous space and thence to the placenta and fetus. Constraint can operate at any of the sites shown and there appears to be considerable interdependence. Perfusion of the intervillous space depends upon development of the full vascular adaptation to pregnancy in the vessels of the placental bed, and an adequate blood pressure. Defective development of these vessels has been described in women destined to show the clinical features of pre-eclampsia, and in women with so-called idiopathic growth retardation. In both clinical conditions intervillous perfusion is impaired, and birth size reduced. However in both conditions plasma volume expansion is also reduced. The relationship between incremental change in plasma volume and birth size has already been described and is

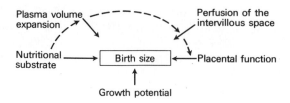

Fig. 5.1. Factors determining birth size.

intimate. It is tempting to speculate that it is plasma volume expansion through the second half of pregnancy that is responsible for the sustained rise in blood pressure from mid-pregnancy nadir to third-trimester peak, which constitutes the second prime determinant of intervillous flow. Experimental evidence suggests a relationship between nutritional status and plasma volume expansion (Rosso and Streeter 1979), starved rats fail to expand their plasma volume and the same may obtain in human pregnancy. Further interdependence is in respect of placental transfer. Whereas the placenta has an enormous functional reserve—up to one-third of its villi may be coated with fibrin in normal pregnancy (perivillous fibrin deposition) and thus remain functionally inert whilst the fetus shows no stigmata of growth retardation or fetal distress—reduced intervillous flow in the complicated pregnancy is associated with interaction of the placenta and markedly impaired function.

The growth potential of the fetus is largely determined by its genetic composition, although *in utero* it is the maternal rather than the paternal gene which is expressed in terms of birth size. Fetuses with major anomalies will evidence growth retardation in the middle trimester while the effect of vascular insufficiency is not usually seen until the third trimester.

Placental size varies from pregnancy to pregnancy and although compensatory hyperplasia may be noted in patients who smoke, live at high altitudes or are profoundly anaemic, by and large being a fetal organ it reflects rather than causes fetal size. Thus, to return to the model, although manipulation of nutritional substrate, plasma volume expansion, perfusion of intervillous space, and placental function can each individually affect birth size, in both the normal and abnormal pregnancy, change in one brings change in another. In human pregnancy where studies are largely observational, it is difficult to determine whether these relationships are of association or causation.

REFERENCES

Apte, S. V. and Nenger, L. (1970). Absorption of dietary iron in pregnancy. *Am. J. Clin. Nutr.* **23**, 73.

Assali, N. S., Ravramo, L. and Peltonen, T. (1960). Uterine and fetal blood flow and oxygen consumption in early human pregnancy. *Am. J. Obstet. Gynecol.* **79**, 86.

Bader, R. A., Bader, M. E., Rose, D. J. and Braunwald, E. (1955). Haemodynamics at rest and during exercise in normal pregnancy as studied by cardiac catheterisation. *J. Clin. Invest.* 34, 1524.

Bleker, O. P., Kloosterman, G. J., Mieras, D. J., Oosting, J. and Salle, H. J. A., (1975). Intervillous space during uterine contractions in human subjects. An ultrasonic study. *Am. J. Obstet. Gynecol.* **123**, 697.

Bonnar, J., Davidson, J. F., Pidgeon, C. F., McNicol, G. P. and Douglas, A. S. (1969). Fibrin degradation products in normal and abnormal pregnancy and parturition. *Br. Med. J.* **3**, 137.

Brooke, O. G., Brown, I. R. F., Bone, C. D. M., Carter, N. D., Cleeve, H. J. W., Maxwell, J. D., Robinson, V. P. and Windser, S. M. (1980). *Vitamin D Supplements in Pregnant Asian Women; Effects on Calcium Status and Fetal Growth.*

Brosens, I., Robertson, W. B. and Dixon, H. G. (1967). The physiological response of the vessels of the plancental bed to normal pregnancy. *J. Pathol. Bacteriol.* **93**, 569.

Campbell, D. M. and MacGillivray, I. (1975). The effect of a low calorie diet or a thiazide diuretic on the incidence of pre-eclampsia and on birth weight. *Br. J. Obstet. Gynaecol* **82**, 572.

Castaldi, P. A. (1979). *Haemopoiesis and haemostasis in human reproductive physiology.* (ed. R. P. Shearman) Blackwell Scientific Publications, Oxford, p. 410.

Chanaizin, I., (1969). *The megaloblastic anaemias.* Blackwell Scientific Publications, Oxford.

Davison, J. M. (1980). The urinary system. In *Clinical physiology in obstetrics.* (eds F. E. Hytten and G. V. P. Chamberlain) Blackwell Scientific Publications, Oxford, p. 289.

Davison, J. M. and Hytten, F. E. (1974). Renal handling of glucose in pregnancy. In *Proceedings of a Symposium on Carbohydrate Metabolism in Pregnancy and the Newborn* (eds H. W. Sutherland and J. M. Stowers) Churchill Livingstone, Edinburgh, p. 2.

Davison, J. M. and Hytten, F. E. (1975). The effect of pregnancy on the renal handling of glucose. *J. Obstet. Gynaecol. Br. Commonw.* **82**, 374.

Davison, J. S., Davison, M. C. and Hay, D. M. (1970). Gastric emptying time in late pregnancy and labour. *J. Obstet. Gynaecol br. Commonw.* **77**, 37.

Doring, G. K., Loescheke, H. H. and Ochwadt, B. (1950). Weitere untersuchungen uber die wirkung der sexualhormone auf die atmung. *Pflugers Archiv. Gesamte Physiol. Menschen Tiere* **252**, 216.

Doyle, W., Crawford, M. A., Laurance, B. M. and Drury, P. (1982). Dietary survey during pregnancy in a low social economic Group. *Hum. Nutr. Appl. Nutr.* **36A**, 95.

Duffus, G. M., MacGillivray, I. and Dennis, K. J. (1971). The relationship between baby weight and changes in maternal weight, total body water, plasma volume, electrolytes and proteins, and urinary oestriol excretion. *J. Obst. Gynaecol. Br. Commonw.* **78**, 97.

Dusterdieck, G. and McElwee, G. (1971). Estimation of angiotension II concentration in human plasma by radio immunoassay: some applications to physiological and clinical states. *Europ. J. Clin. Invest.* **2**, 32.

Eddy, C. A., Antonini, R. Jr and Paverstein, C. J. (1977). Fertility following mircrosurgical removal of the ampullary-isthmic junction in rabbits. *Fertil. Setil.* **28**, 1090.

Fenton, V., Cavill, I. and Fisher, J. (1977). Iron Stores in pregnancy. *Br. J. Haematol.* **37**, 145.

Fletcher, J. and Suter, P. E. N. (1969). The transport of iron by the human placenta. *Clin. Sci.* **36**, 209.

Flexner, L. B., Cowie, D. B., Hellman, L. M., Wilde, W. S. and Vorsburgh, G. J. (1948). The permeability of the human placenta to sodium in normal and abnormal pregnancies and the supply of sodium to the human fetus as determined with radioactive sodium. *Am. J. Obstet. Gynecol.* **55**, 496.

Fox, H. (1978). Placental structure in scientific basis of obstetrics and gynaecology. (ed. R. R. Macdonald) Churchill Livingstone, Edinburgh, p. 28.

Fox, H. (1979). The correlation between placenta structure and transfer function in placental transfer. (eds G. V. P. Chamberlain and A.W. Wilkinson) Pitman Medical, Tunbridge Wells, p. 15.

Fullerton, W. T., Hytten, F.E., Klopper, A. I. and McKay, E. (1965). A case of quadruplet pregnancy. *J. Obstet. Gynaecol. Br. Commonw.* **72**, 79.

Gant. N. F. Madden, J. D., Siiteri, P. K. and MacDonald, P. C. (1975). The metabolic clearance rate of dehydroiso and posterone sulfate. III: The effect of thiazide diuretics in normal and future pre-eclamptic pregnancies. *Am. J. Obstet, Gynecol.* **123**, 159.

Gant, N. E., Madden, J. D. Siiteri, P. K., MacDonald, P. C. (1976). The metabolic clearance rate of dehydroiso and posterone sulfate in acute effects of induced hypertension, hypotension and naturesis in normal and hypertensive pregnancies. *Am. J. Obstet. Gynecol.* **124**, 143.

Gibson, H. M. (1973). Plasma volume and glomerular filtration rate in pregnancy and their relation to differences in fetal growth. *J. Obstet. Gynaecol. Br. Commonw.* **80**, 1067.

Ginsburg, J. and Duncan, S. L. B., (1967). Peripheral blood flow in normal pregnancy. *Cardiac Res.* **1**, 132.

Gomes, V. (1977). Tubal reanastomoses by microsurgery. *Fertil. Steril.* **28**, 59.

Haeney, R. P. and Skillman, T. G. (1971). Calcium metabolism in normal human pregnancy. *J. Clin. Endocrinol.* **33**, 661.

Holmes, F. (1960). Incidence of the supine hypotensive syndrome in late pregnancy. A clinical study in 500 subjects. *J. Obstet. Gynaecol. Br. Emp.* **67**, 254.

Howard, B. K., Goodson, J. H. and Mengert, W. F. (1953). Supine hypotensive syndrome in late pregnancy. *Obstet Gynaecol.* **1**, 371.

Hull, D. and Elphick, M., (1979). Transfer of fatty acids in placental transfer. (eds G. V. P. Chamberlain and A.W. Wilkinson) Pitman Medical, Tunbridge Wells, p. 159.

Hunt, J. N. and Murray, F. A. (1958). Gastric function in pregnancy *J. Obstet. Gynaecol. Br. Emp.* **65**, 78.

Hytten, F. E. (1979). Water transfer. In *Placental transfer* (eds G. V. P. Chamberlain and A.W. Wilkinson) Pitman Medical, Tunbridge Wells, p. 90.

Hytten, F. E. (1980). Weight gain in pregnancy. In *Physiology of obstetrics.* (eds F. E. Hytten and G. V. P. Chamberlain) Blackwell Scientific Publications, Oxford, p. 193.

Hytten, F. E. (1983). Nutritional requirements in pregnancy. In *Nutrition in pregnancy.* RCOG, London, p. 1.

Jacobs, A., Miller, F., Worwood, M., Beamish, M. R. and Wardrop, C. A., (1972). Ferritin in the serum of normal subjects and patients with iron deficiency and iron overload. *Br. Med. J.* **4**, 206.

Kass, E. J. (1960). *Arch. Int. Med.* **105**, 194.

Kleiner, G. J., Mershey, C., Johnson, A. J. and Markus, W. M. (1970). Defibrination in normal and abnormal parturition. *Br. J. Haematol.* **19**, 159.

Klopper, A. (1980). *The ovary in clinical physiology in obstetrics.* (eds F. Hytten and G. V. P. Chamberlain) Blackwell Scientific Publications, Oxford, p. 432.

Leck, I. (1983). *In prevention of spina bifida and other neural tube defects.* (ed. J. Dobbing) Academic Press, London, p. 155.

Letsky, E. (1980). *The haematological system in clinical physiology in obstetrics.* (eds F. E. Hytten and G. V. P. Chamberlain) Blackwell Scientific Publications, Oxford, p. 43.

Levy, N., Lemberg, E. and Sharf, M. (1971). Bowel habit. In *Pregnancy digestion* **4**, 216.

Lindheimer, M. and Katz, A. I. (1974). Sodium and diuretics in pregnancy. *Obstet. Gynecol.* **44**, 434.

Longo, L. D. (1970). Carbon monoxide in the pregnant mother and fetus and its exchange across the placenta. *Ann. NY Acad. Sci.* **174**, 313.

MacGillivray, I., Rote, G. A. and Rowe, B. (1969). Blood pressure survey in pregnancy. *Clin. Sci.* **37**, 395.

MacGillivray, I. (1979). *The effects of hypertension in placental transfer.* (eds G. V. P. Chamberlain and A. Wilkinson) Pitman Medical, Tunbridge Wells, p. 195.

Mattingly, R. F. and Borkowf, H. I., (1978). Clinical implications of ureteral reflux. *Clin. Obstet. Gynecol.* **21**, 863.

McCormick, W. G. and Torres, J. (1976). A method of Pomeroy tubal ligation reanastomsis. *Obstet. Gynecol.* **47**, 623.

McLenn, C. E. (1943). Antecubital and femoral venous pressures in normal and toxaemic pregnancy. *Am. J. Obstet. Gynecol.* **45**, 568.

Meschin, G. (1978). Substrate availability and fetal growth. In *Abnormal fetal growth: biological bases and consequences.* (ed. F. Naftolin) Dahlem Konferenzen, p. 221.

Murray, F. A., Erskine, J. P. and Fieldin, J. (1957). Gastric secretion in pregnancy. *J. Obstet. Gynaecol Br. Emp.* **64**, 373.

Nimmo, W. S., Wilson, J. and Prescott, C. F. (1975). Narcotic analgesics and delayed gastric emptying during labour *Lancet* **1**, 890.

Page, E. W. and Christianson, R. (1976). The impact of mean arterial blood pressure in the middle trimester upon the outcome of pregnancy. *Am. J. Obstet. Gynecol.* **125**, 740.

Parry, E., Shields, R., Turnbull, A. C. (1970). The effect of pregnancy upon the colonic absorption of sodium, potassium and water. *J. Obstet. Gynaecol. Br. Commonw.* **77**, 616.

Peckham, C. S. and Marshal, W. C. (1983). Infections in pregnancy. In *Obstetrical epidemiology.* (eds S. L. Barron and A. M. Thomson) Academic Press, London, p. 210.

Peterion, E. P., Musich, J. R. and Behrman, S. J. (1977). Uterotubal implantation and obstetric outcome after previous sterilisation. *Am. J. Obstet. Gynecol.* **128**, 662.

Pyorala, T. (1966). Cardiovascular response to the upright position during pregnancy. *Acta Obstet. Gynecol. Scand.* **45** (Suppl 5), 1.

Rios, E. R., Lipschitz, D. A., Cook, J. D. and Smith, N. J. (1975). Relationship of maternal and infant iron stores as assessed by determination of plasma ferritin levels. *Pediatrics* **55**, 694.

Robertson, W. B. (1981). *The endometrium.* Butterworths, London, p. 75.

Robertson, W. B., Brosens, I. and Dixon, H. G. (1967). The pathological response of the vessels of the placental bed to hypertensive pregnancy. *J. Pathol. Bacteriol.* **93**, 581.

Robertson, W. B., Brosens, A. and Dixon, H. G. (1981). Maternal blood supply in fetal growth retardation. In *Fetal growth retardation.* (eds A. F. Van Assche and W. B. Robertson) Churchill Livingstone, Edinburgh, P. 127.

Rosso, P. and Streeter, M. R. (1979). Effect of food or protein restriction on plasma volume expansion in pregnant rats. *J. Nutr.* **109**, 1887.

Rovinský, J. J. and Jaffin, H. (1965). Cardiovascular hemodynamics in pregnancy in blood and plasma volumes in multiple pregnancy. *Am. J. Obstet. Gynecol.* **93**, 1.

Rovinský, J. J. and Jaffin, H. (1966). Cardiovascular hemodynamics in pregnancy

II. Cardiac output and left ventricular work in multiple pregnancy. *Am. J. Obstet. Gynecol.* **95**, 781.

Rubi, R. A. and Sala, N. L. (1968). Ureteral function in pregnant women III. Effect of different positions and fetal delivery upon ureteral tonus. *Am. J. Obstet. Gynecol.* **101**, 230.

Schwarcz, S. B., Aramendia, P. and Taquine, A. C. (1964). Haemodynamic alterations in normal pregnancy. *Medecina* **24**, 113.

Schwarz, R. (1964). Das verhalten des kreislaufs in der normalen schwangerschaft i. Der arterieue Blutdruck. *Archiv. Gynakol.* **199**, 549.

Sever, J. L. (1980). In *Infections of the urinary tract.* (eds E. Kass and W. Brumfitt) Chicago University Press, Chicago, p. 19.

Shelley, H. J. (1979). *Transfer of carbohydrate in placental transfer.* (eds G. V. P. Chamberlain and A.W. Wilkinson) Pitman Medical, Tunbridge Wells, p. 118.

Sheppard, B. L. and Bonnar, J. (1976). The ultrastructure of the arterial supply of the human placenta in pregnancy complicated by fetal growth retardation. *Br. J. Obstet. Gynaecol.* **83**, 948.

Sheppard, B. L. and Bonnar, J. (1980). Uteroplacental arteries and hypertensive pregnancy. In *Pregnancy hypertension* (eds J. Bonnar, I. MacGillivray and E. M. Symonds) MTP Press, Lancaster, p. 213.

Skinner, S. L., Lumbers, E. R. and Symmonds, E. M. (1969). Alterations by oral contraceptives of normal menstrual changes in plasma renin activity, concentration and substrate. *Clin. Sci.* **36**, 67.

Smeaton, T. C., Andersen, G. J. and Fulton, I. S. (1977). Study of aldosterone levels in plasma during pregnancy. *J. Clin. Endocrinol. Metab.* **44**, 1.

Smitheus, R. W., Ankers, C., Carver, M. E., Lennon, O., Schorah, C. J. and Sheppard, S. (1977). *Br. J. Nutr.* **38**, 497.

Smitheus, R. W., Sheppard, S. and Schorah, C. J. (1976). *Arch. Dis. Child.* **51**, 944.

Soler, N. G. and Malins, J. M. (1971). Prevalence of glycosuria in normal pregnancy. *Lancet* **1**, 619.

Stein, Z., Susser, M., Saenger, G. and Marolla, F. (1975). *Famine and human development. The Dutch Hunger Winter of 1944–45.* Oxford University Press, Oxford.

Sutherland, H. W., Stowers, J. M. and Fisher, P. M. (1979). *Detection of chemical gestational diabetes in carbohydrate metabolism in pregnancy and the new born 1978.* Springer, Verlag, p. 436.

Svanberg, B. (1975). Absorption of iron in pregnancy. *Acta Obstet. Gynecol. Scand.* (Suppl 48), 7.

de Swiet, M., (1980). *The cardiovascular system in clinical physiology in obstetrics.* (eds F. E. Hytten and G. V. P. Chamberlain) Blackwell Scientific Publications, Oxford, p. 3.

de Swiet, M. (1980). *The respiratory system in clinical physiology in obstetrics.* (eds F. E. Hytten and G. V. P. Chamberlain) Blackwell Scientific Publications, Oxford, p. 79.

Thomson, A. M., Hytten, F. E. and Billewicz, W. Z. (1967). The epidemiology of oedema during pregnancy. *J. Obstet. Gynaecol. Br. Commonw.* p. 74, 1.

Viegas, O. A. C., Scott, P. H., Cole, T. J, Eaton, P., Needham, P. S. and Wharton, B. A. (1982). Dietary protein supplementation of pregnant Asian mothers at Sorrento. Birmingham II: Selective during third trimester only. *Br. Med. J.* **285**, 592.

Viegas, O. A. C., Scott, P. H., Cole, T. J., Mansfield, H. N., Wharton, P. and Wharton, B. A. (1982). Dietary protein supplementation of pregnant Asian mothers at Sorrento. Birmingham I: Unselective during second and third trimesters. *Br. Med. J.* **285**, 589.

Walters, W.A.W. (1979). *Cardiovascular function in pregnancy in human reproductive physiology.* (ed. R. P. Shearman). Blackwell Scientific Publications, Oxford, p. 336.

Walters, W.A.W. and Lim, Y. L. (1970). Hemodynamic changes in women taking oral contraceptives. *J. Obstet. Gynaecol. Br. Commonw.* **77**, 1007.

Weir, R. J., Paintin, D. B., Robertson, J. I. S., Tree, M., Fraser, R. and Young, J. (1970). Renin, Angiotension, and aldosterone relationships in normal pregnancy. *Proc. Roy. Soc. Med.* **63**, 1101.

Williams, J. D. (1980). Infections of the urinary tract. In *Proceedings Third International Symposium on Pyelonephritis.* (eds E. H. Kass and B. Williams) University of Chicago Press, Chicago, p. 8.

Winston, R. M. L. (1977). Microsurgical tubo-cornual anastomoses for reversal of sterilisation. *Lancet* **1**, 284.

Witten, C. L. and Bradbury, J. T. (1951). Hemodilution as a result of estrogen therapy. Estrogenic effects in the human female. *Proc. Soc. Exp. Biol. Med.* **78**, 626.

World Health Organization (1972). *Nurtritional anaemias* Technical Report Series No 503.

Young, M. (1979). Transfer of amino acids. In *Placental transfer.* (eds G. V. P. Chamberlain and A.W. Wilkinson) Pitman Medical, Tunbridge Wells, p. 142.

Zuspan, F. P., O'Shaughnessy, R. W., Vinsel, J. and Zuspan, M. (1981). Adrenergic innervation of uterine vasculature in human term pregnancy. *Am. J. Obstet. Gynecol.*

6 The antenatal programme

Marion H. Hall

The aims of the antenatal programme may be delineated as follows:

(i) Education, including preparation for labour and parenthood.
(ii) Diagnosis and treatment of symptomatic problems.
(iii) Recognition and management of asymptomatic but potentially harmful conditions.

EDUCATION

Preparation for labour and parenthood is usually offered to classes or groups of parents by midwives, health visitors or others with a special interest such as the National Childbirth Trust. Some doctors do take an interest in this field. It is important in early pregnancy to make sure that women know what classes are locally available, to discuss what style of education is most suitable for them, and to identify other methods of informing those women who will not attend classes of any kind, who drop out from classes, who cannot attend because of work or family commitments, or who miss classes scheduled for late pregnancy because they have been confined to bed, or admitted to hospital, or even delivered, because of a pregnancy complication or preterm labour.

Alternative sources of information for these women could be written material (nationally or locally produced), self-help groups (which could be organized by the practice or by the hospital antenatal clinic), videotape (viewed at home or in groups) and/or discussion during ordinary antenatal consultations. Such discussion should take place at least to a limited extent in all consultations to check on comprehension of class discussions, and to allow opportunities for clarification of points not fully understood and to offer reassurance and extended information if required.

DIAGNOSIS AND TREATMENT OF SYMPTOMATIC PROBLEMS

This is, of course, provided for all patients in general practice whether pregnant or not, but there is some evidence (Macintyre 1981) that some pregnant women consult their family doctor more frequently during pregnancy than at other times, though the threshold for doing so is very variable. Another important point is that complaints referable to the pregnancy may not be the subject of a patient-initiated consultation since they are 'saved-up' for the next routine antenatal visit. This may be inappropriate when the complaint is one that would have justified emergency admission to hospital, such as antepartum haemorrhage or premature rupture of the membranes, and it is important that the information supplied to expectant parents in the various educational assessments mentioned above should include recognition of potentially serious pregnancy complications. This is not always the case at the moment (Hall and Chng 1982).

DIAGNOSIS AND TREATMENT OF ASYMPTOMATIC PROBLEMS

This is of course the main justification of antenatal care as a preventive measure, since it is envisaged that many antenatal and labour complications can be averted, predicted by the identification of high-risk groups, diagnosed early, or at worst referred for appropriate treatment once they have occurred. Unfortunately, however, not all aspects of antenatal care have been rigorously evaluated, and an uncritical acceptance by health professionals of all antenatal care as being good and worthwhile has undoubtedly wasted a great deal of everyone's time and contributed to the dissatisfaction expressed by pregnant women (Oakley 1979). It is of interest that Coope and Scott (1982) recently advocated almost exactly the same schedule as was proposed by the Ministry of Health in 1929 (Oakley 1982). Coope and Scott deserve congratulations upon the idea of giving pregnant women a detailed account of what antenatal care would consist of, but the schedule itself cannot be justified merely on the grounds that it has been done for the last 50 years. Critical appraisal is required.

WHO SHOULD GIVE ANTENATAL CARE?

Different health professionals have different styles of care and advantages to offer. The midwife is expert in the supervision of normal pregnancy, and, though not normally required in the United Kingdom to undertake total care, can take responsibility for most of the antenatal care of women who have shown no abnormality. Referral back to the general practitioner or specialist obstetrician when an abnormality is diagnosed is well within the province of the midwife, but the doctor may in the case of some women wish to specify in advance some circumstances in which referral back would be advisable. Many general practitioners could usefully consider how they could integrate community midwives into their antenatal care programme. Midwives should certainly not be used only as chaperones and urine testers.

The general practitioner often knows the woman and her family outside of pregnancy, has good rapport with her and may be best equipped to understand both the social background and any medical problems. General practitioners often offer much better continuity of care than hospital clinics (Thornhill Neighbourhood Project, 1982). However, the above advantages are no substitute for adequate training and expertise and only those general practioners who are on the obstetric list and have been properly trained, should give antenatal care (RCOG and RCGP 1981).

The specialist obstetrician has most experience of pregnancy complications and of the use of modern technology and should of course see all complicated cases, often for most if not all of their antenatal care. This should not of course preclude a continuing interest and involvement of the general practitioner (see Chapter 12).

Local arrangements vary as to whether all women (or all primigravidae) are seen by obstetricians or whether the general practitioner decides whom to refer, and when (Roseveare and Bull 1982; Taylor, Edgar, Taylor, and Neal 1980). This chapter discusses the information that will be of value in making referrals and in deciding upon the ideal regime for care in general practice.

RECORDING OF INFORMATION

It is most important that information should be sought and recorded in such a way that:

(i)   No essentials are missed out.

(ii)   All the information collected is available when clinically required, i.e., during the pregnancy, the confinement and the puerperium, to all concerned. (An immaculate general practitioner record is largely wasted if it does not accompany the pregnant women during her confinement.)

(iii) Information is recorded in a systematic way so that any new attendant (e.g. duty obstetric registrar or midwife who may be meeting the patient for the first time) may easily identify salient points.

The above objectives are best met by the use of a structured record following an agreed national pattern, to facilitate recording of essential information with a minimum of writing, but with some space for unusual problems. Where care is to be shared between the general practitioner and/or the midwife and/or the obstetrician, interprofessional communication may be achieved by the use of a shared-care card, by letter, or by the use of an integrated record, used by all the professionals and carried by the pregnant woman. The last method has been found satisfactory in many centres. (see Chapter 13). It causes least confusion and promotes communication with the pregnant woman, though there will occasionally be highly confidential information that must be withheld from such notes. Fears that

pregnant women would frequently lose their case records have proved unfounded (Zander 1982).

First visit

Previous obstetric history

When a woman has been pregnant before previous history may have a
predictive value, since certain patterns and pathologies have a tendency to
recur, or to cause subsequent problems.

Habitual abortion (usually defined as two or more consecutive) can be
usefully assessed only after subdivision into first-trimester abortion, which
is usually accounted for by fetal causes, and second trimester abortion,
which is more likely to be due to maternal causes such as incompetent cervix
or bicornuate uterus. Very little can be done to prevent first-trimester abortion apart from bedrest of which the value remains unproven. Support and
encouragement will, of course, be very necessary. With a history of preterm
labour, which may have a similar aetiology and tendency to recur (Bakketeig and Hoffman 1981) or second-trimester abortion, the woman should
be referred early to a specialist in case cervical cerclage is indicated.

It was thought that therapeutic abortion predisposed to problems in subsequent pregnancies but this belief was based on poorly controlled or uncontrolled studies, and there is no reason to suppose that a woman with one
previous abortion induced by methods current in Britain has any greater
risk of complications than a primigravidae (Savage and Paterson 1982).

Smallness for gestational age (SGA) which may be due to intrauterine
growth retardation (IUGR) is more likely to occur in the case of a woman
who has previously had a baby with the same condition (Chng, Hall, and
Macgillivray 1980). Since women with a high risk may be screened by, for
example, serial ultrasonic scanning, the woman should be referred early to
a specialist so that gestation can be confirmed, an appropriate plan for
antenatal supervision made, and booking for a specialist unit made (since
small-for-dates babies may well require intensive monitoring and care during and after labour). Similarly, largeness for dates may recur; in addition
to possible neonatal problems, difficulty during delivery, including shoulder
dystocia, may be anticipated, and specialist confinement is essential.

The significance of a previous history of caesarean section depends entirely
upon the indications for the procedure. If the indication was cephalopelvic
disproportion, elective repeat section will be necessary, whereas fetal distress as an indication is unlikely to recur and normal vaginal delivery can be
expected. There are many intermediate or less clearcut cases, and all women
with a previous caesarean section should be referred to a specialist for
review of the history and planning of confinement. Specialist confinement
is neccessary even if vaginal delivery is hoped for, because of the risk of scar
rupture.

A previous forceps delivery on the other hand does not always bode ill for the present pregnancy. Obviously if there was a difficult rotation, there may be a possibility of cephalopelvic disproportion, and labour needs specialist supervision, but if the previous forceps was a simple lift-out on account of maternal exhaustion or fetal distress, then spontaneous delivery should be expected next time.

From time to time, a woman's personal experience of labour may determine the next booking; she may have had inadequate pain relief and require specialist booking so as to have an epidural block, or on the other hand she may wish to deliver in a general practitioner unit to avoid 'unnecessary' interference. Provided there is no contraindication and bed occupancy permits, arrangements should be made to suit her.

Third stage complications (retained placenta and postpartum haemorrhage) are considerably more common in women who have had them before. Because these complications are so dangerous a previous history should be an indication for specialist hospital confinement.

The significance of a previous perinatal death depends entirely upon the cause and referral to the obstetrician is essential so that a suitable programme of care may be arranged to suit the circumstances.

The general practitioner will usually be completely familiar with details of the infancy of previous children. Certain congenital deformities such as those of the central nervous system or metabolic disorders, may tend to recur. Genetic counselling should have been done prior to this pregnancy but the conclusions may need to be reiterated. Sometimes antenatal diagnosis by amniocentesis will be possible and early referral to a specialist therefore necessary. Where a deformity is unlikely to recur or where previous perinatal death is due to a non-recurrent condition, or where there has been an infant death from non-obstetric causes, the practitioner will understand the apprehension of the patient, and offer as much reassurance as possible.

It is important to recognize that although many obstetric complications do tend to recur, in a woman with a previous history having a risk two to four times that of the woman without such a history, the 'at-risk' woman is more likely than not to escape the condition, and on a population basis most cases of the condition will occur in the group of women without the added risk (because there are so many more of them, albeit with a very low risk). This means that the woman with an extra risk should not be unduly alarmed, but the low-risk woman should not be led to suppose that normal confinement is guaranteed.

Medical history

Any serious condition that might jeopardize the pregnancy will clearly require early referral to an obstetric specialist. The latter can then enlist the help of an appropriate physician. Examples could be epilepsy (epileptic fits cause transient fetal anoxia), diabetes (insulin requirements may be increased) or thyrotoxicosis (the necessary drugs and/or radioiodine may have adverse fetal effects).

Confinement will be in a specialist unit and often (as in the case of diabetes) antenatal care will almost always be in specialist hands. The pregnant woman will often already be aware of this necessity as some diabetic clinics have a prepregnancy service (Steel *et al.* 1982). In any event the other reasons for it should be discussed. Previous medical history of surgery to the uterus (such as myomectomy, especially if the cavity was involved) may be relevant to the mode of delivery in the present pregnancy; referral to a specialist is necessary to discuss this, usually after scrutiny of the operation notes, etc.

A previous history of infertility is important, partly because of the fact that the woman may have little chance of further childbearing if there is a perinatal loss, and because such women may have physical problems impairing obstetric performance. Furthermore, ovulation may have been induced by clomiphene with an increased risk of multiple pregnancy.

Family history

Ideally the identification of familial disorders will precede the pregnancy, so that the individual or couple can have genetic counselling at leisure and make an informed decision as to whether to have children at all. However, it is not unusual for family discussion about familial disorders to be scanty or non-existent, sometimes due to ignorance and sometimes to misplaced guilt or shame. (The use of a questionnaire which the pregnant woman can take home to discuss with her family can sometimes identify familial problems of which the pregnant woman was unaware.) The family doctor is sometimes ideally placed to identify previously unrecognized familial problems. If the significance of a history is not clear the earliest possible referral to an appropriate specialist is indicated, since antenatal diagnostic procedures often have to be initiated by 16–18 weeks' gestation. With the exception of multiple pregnancy and pre-eclampsia, both of which show a familial pattern, little is known of the inheritance of other obstetric conditions.

Present pregnancy

Perhaps the most significant feature of the first visit is the confirmation of the pregnancy (often not really registered by the woman till medically confirmed), the clarification of the gestation and the expected date of delivery which will usually be possible by taking a detailed menstrual history with careful attention to recent oral contraceptive use. Where there is any doubt (and this includes all women whose last menstrual period is a pill-withdrawal bleed) an ultrasonic scan measurement of crown–rump length or biparietal diameter is indicated. This must be done in early pregnancy to be reliable, and to give a baseline for subsequent assessment of fetal growth and of the appropriate time for any intervention in early or late pregnancy.

Age is a significant factor. Very young girls rarely present in early pregnancy unless they are seeking termination. When they do book, attention must be given to the problems of continuing with school or further education. Social work help will usually be enlisted in connection with family adjustments, financial problems, and possible adoption.

Older women, being at greater risk of bearing a child with a chromosomal abnormality, will need counselling about possible amniocentesis. The age at which this is made available varies throughout Britain from about 35 to 40 years. It is important for the general practitioner to make sure that all women in the appropriate age group are referred early to establish the gestation prior to amniocentesis. Perinatal and maternal mortality are also increased in women over 35 years of age and uterine dysfunction more common, so these women will usually be referred for hospital confinement in any case. It is important to recognize, however, that they may have other health advantages and be very well-adjusted to a much-wanted pregnancy. It is not helpful to stigmatize them as 'elderly'.

Physical examination

Height is recorded since short stature (<1.52 m) may be associated with a contracted pelvis and some degree of cephalopelvic disproportion. Short primigravidae should be referred for specialist confinement.

Weight is recorded (with no shoes and minimal clothing) to identify very thin women, who are at risk of having smaller babies, very fat women, who are subject to diabetes and pre-eclampsia, and in whom the lie and presentation may be difficult to ascertain, and to give a baseline for later assessment of weight gain, which helps to predict baby size and the development of pre-eclampsia.

A general examination is, of course, also indicated although it is to be hoped that the days of discovering previously unsuspected rheumatic or congenital heart disease are past. Blood pressure must be recorded. Examination of the breasts is usual in women intending to breast-feed, to detect any remediable problem with the nipples such as retraction. However, it may be better to postpone this examination till the end of the second trimester since feeding intentions may not be definite till late pregnancy.

The size of the uterus is assessed by abdominal and vaginal examination, and correlated with menstrual data. Other pelvic masses can also be excluded, and a cervical smear taken (Draper 1982). Macgregor (1979) has pointed out the high pick-up rate of cervical intraepithelial neoplasia in antenatal patients. Some primigravidae may be nervous or embarrassed about a pelvic examination. If so, this need not be done unless there is a specific indication. If all women are referred to hospital it may most suitably be left to the obstetrician.

Investigations

It should be routine to test the haemoglobin, the blood group, the presence or absence of rhesus or other antibodies and hepatitis B surface antigen (HBsAg) (Table 6.1). It is now usual to test HBsAg positives for the presence of e-antigen which denotes a greater risk of infection for the baby and for birth attendants. It is usual also to test for VDRL positives (though the pick-up rate is very low in many areas) for rubella immunity (though ideally that should have been done before the pregnancy), and at 16–18 weeks for serum alphafetoprotein (αFP). A high alphafetoprotein level indicates an increased risk of central nervous system deformities, and thus the need for further tests, including ultrasonic scan and often amniocentesis. Alphafetoprotein screening is probably not cost-effective in areas of low incidence of central nervous system (CNS) deformity, and its routine use is still controversial (Brock 1982; Standing *et al.* 1981), since there are some false positives and false negatives. In any event screening should not be commenced without the full knowledge of the pregnant woman, since she may not wish to be tested if she has a conscientious objection to pregnancy termination. Mediterranean, Asian and African women should routinely have haemoglobin electrophoresis to detect any haemoglobinopathies.

Table 6.1 Investigations at the first visit

	Essential	If appropriate
Blood	Full blood count Blood group Antibodies VDRL Rubella HAI HBsAg	Hb electrophoresis Alphafetoprotein
Urine	Albumin Sugar	Bacteriuria
Other		Cervical smear Ultrasonic scan

Urine should routinely be tested for sugar and albumin. Testing for asymptomatic bacteriuria by urine culture and organism count is widely advocated to identify women who might benefit from prophylactic antibiotics. However, it has been argued (Chng and Hall 1982) that it would be more profitable to test only those women with a previous history of clinical urinary tract infection.

Some obstetric units (and some general practitioners) have a policy of offering a routine ultrasonic scan to all women in early pregnancy and this opportunity will be welcomed by most women who will enjoy visualizing the fetus. The gestation can usually be clarified by measurement of crown–rump length before 14 weeks' gestation (Adams and Robinson 1980). If the examination is postponed till 16–18 weeks' gestation, the biparietal diameter can be measured to assess the gestation and the diagnosis of multiple pregnancy and certain fetal malformations is more secure (Campbell and Little 1980).

Where routine scanning is not available care must be taken to refer early the minority of women who really require a scan, in other words those whose menstrual dates are uncertain, those where the uterine size is not compatible with dates, where the uterus does not seem to be growing or where fetal movements have not been felt by 20 weeks' gestation. From time to time a situation may arise of a woman who has difficulty in believing or adjusting to the fact that she is really pregnant, or who has irrational fears about the pregnancy. A real time scan, showing fetal features and movements, may be very reassuring. It is important, however, not to interpret scan results too literally; neither estimates of gestation nor exclusion of abnormality can be considered fool-proof.

General

Smoking and alcohol intake should be the subject of enquiry and discussion. Complete abstinence from both is usually advised but it must be recognized that this will not be possible for all women, and that in fact the risks of minimal exposure are probably very small. Also, exhortations for abstinence are less helpful than practical advice as to how this might be done.

There is little agreement as to what constitutes the ideal diet for pregnant women (RCOG Study Group 1983), but a balanced varied diet would seem sensible. There is virtually no place for weight reduction or serious restriction upon weight gain in pregnancy as this may result in a diminution of birth weight and does not prevent pre-eclampsia.

Most primigravidae and some multigravidae work during pregnancy and it is good practice to record their occupation in sufficient detail to identify any possible hazard (such as exposure of a laboratory technician to solvents, or a nurse in an orthopaedic ward to heavy lifting.) A move to safer work may be negotiable. Occupational risks are discussed by Chamberlain and Garcia (1983).

The general practitioner will know about any drugs he has prescribed but he should of course review any regular long-term prescriptions, such as anticonvulsants. Self-medication is also common; women should be advised to restrict this as much as possible in pregnancy, but need guidance as to what preparations it would be safe to take in the event of minor illnesses.

Many of the above matters may (and perhaps should) have been discussed before conception, but it is unrealistic to suppose that all pregnancies are planned (see Chapter 4). In any event, women may be more receptive to advice when they are actually pregnant.

Booking for confinement

It is common practice to book all primigravidae for confinement under specialist supervision on the grounds that they are an unknown quantity. However, the majority of primigravidae deliver spontaneously with a mid-wife in attendance. Suitable arrangements will depend upon the expertise and interest of local midwives and general practitioners and on the functional relationship between the general practitioner and the specialist unit. It may often be quite appropriate to book for a general practitioner unit the young fit tall primigravidae, provided that it is recognized by all concerned that transfer to specialist care on account of complications may be necessary during the pregnancy in as many as 30 per cent and during labour in as many as 14 per cent of the remainder (Chng *et al.* 1980; Dixon 1982).

Appropriate booking for multigravidae will usually be determined mainly by the previous obstetric history, and most multigravidae will be suitable for confinement in a general practitioner unit and indeed may be better managed there (Klein *et al.* 1983).

The wishes of the pregnant woman and her partner must be considered when the booking is made, and a full discussion and explanation can usually be concluded by a plan which is agreed as appropriate by all concerned. If however, the woman decides not to take the advice offered and insists on, for example, a home confinement, the position of a practitioner who is not suitably qualified or experienced or does not feel confident to undertake a home confinement is difficult. Referral to a colleague may be best but the woman (and her midwife) should not be left without medical back-up even if she has been uncooperative.

Where early discharge from hospital is usual, the practitioner will be expected to give puerperal medical care at home and should confirm with the midwife that home circumstances are suitable.

Schedule of antenatal care (return visits)

The schedule of care which is appropriate for a pregnant women may vary enormously according to her circumstances. It therefore seems most rational to agree upon a minimum schedule to which can be added an individual prescription according to the woman's needs. Every visit should have a purpose which should normally be explained to the pregnant woman. Specification of objectives allows later analysis of whether and how often these objectives are achieved, of the relative skills of different health professionals in achieving them, and is useful for training purposes.

Table 6.2 shows a suggested minimum schedule for normal multigravidae (other logical plans are clearly possible). The rationale for the booking visit has already been extensively discussed. The RCOG Working Party (1982) on antenatal and intrapartum care has recommended that it should be performed by a specialist obstetrician but this may not always be possible. The visit should certainly take place early, if possible by 12 weeks' gestation, both for clinical reasons and to allow high-risk women to be booked for hospitals with suitable facilities (Lewis 1982).

Table 6.2 *Minimum schedule of antenatal care for normal multigravidae*

Gestation in weeks	Main purposes of visit
12	Booking for care and confinement Clarification of gestation
22	Diagnosis of twins Baseline weight
30	Diagnosis of potential growth retardation and potential pre-eclampsia
36	Detection of malpresentation and potential pre-eclampsia
40	Assessment for delivery

If routine alphafetoprotein screening is practised this may be done between 16 and 18 weeks' gestation, but there is certainly no need for a medical practitioner to do the venepuncture.

Diagnosis of multiple pregnancy may of course, be suspected by fundal height assessment at any gestation time, but the earlier the diagnosis is confirmed the better so that some prophylaxis of complications may be attempted. Routine scanning and/or alphafetoprotein screening will diagnose most but not all twin pregnancies, but it is important always to consider the diagnosis. Poor weight gain (less than 0.3 kg/week in the second trimester of the pregnancy) is associated with an increased incidence of smallness for gestational age (SGA). However, there is no advantage in frequent weighing since the correlation with birth weight is more consistent the longer the interval between the measurements. High weight gain, on the other hand, often precedes and accompanies pre-eclampsia and may also be a sign of multiple pregnancy or polyhydramnios. At 30 weeks' gestation, weight gain may be taken together with booking weight, fundal height, smoking habit and previous obstetric history to identify women who need serial ultrasonic scan to identify smallness for gestational age at a gestation when intervention (bedrest or early induction) might be helpful. A full blood count is also necessary and an antibody check in rhesus-negative women.

At 36 weeks' gestation, high weight gainers can be selected for extra blood pressure measurements, a full blood count performed, and malpresentation can be diagnosed in time to change the booking and arrange scan for placental site or pelvimetry if appropriate. If external cephalic version is to be practised, the best time for this diagnostic visit might be 34 weeks' gestation.

More than half of the pregnant women will, of course, deliver spontaneously by 40 weeks' gestation, but those who are undelivered by 40–41 weeks should be seen to check whether there is any indication for induction. Blood pressure and urinalysis should of course be performed at each visit.

Routine visits

Routine visits in excess of this minimum schedule are very unproductive (Hall *et al.* 1980) if their objective is to detect asymptomatic abnormality, though other reasons may be adduced, such as social problems, educational aims, reassurance of anxious women. It is likely, however, that such objectives may be better achieved by seeing pregnant women less frequently but for a longer time on each visit.

It is impossible to specify all possible situations which might necessitate additions to the minimum schedule but some examples would be:

(i)　previously hypertensive multigravidae who should have extra (say weekly) blood pressure measurements, especially from 34 weeks' gestation;

(ii)　multigravidae with a previous intrauterine death who will need serial scans and cardiotocography from before the gestation at which death occurred last time;

(iii) women in whom pregnancy complications such as threatened abortion, antepartum haemorrhage, or pre-eclampsia, have already occurred, where a combination of rest, extra supervision and investigation may be indicated;

(iv) primigravidae, who are at greater risk of pre-eclampsia, should have a blood pressure check at 26, 34, 38, and 41 weeks, in addition to the minimum schedule already discussed. If they gain weight excessively and/or are older, weekly or even twice weekly measurement of blood pressure may be indicated from 34 weeks onwards.

The approach suggested here is not intended to be dogmatic, since most screening tests and procedures have not been adequately evaluated. Grant and Mohide (1982) have reviewed the subject and identified many of the pitfalls. However, practitioners should cease to justify numerous visits simply because they have always been recommended but try to construct a realistic schedule of antenatal care adjusted to the particular needs of the individual woman. It goes without saying that she should request an extra visit when she feels it to be necessary.

REFERENCES AND FURTHER READING

Adam, A. H. and Robinson, H. P. (1980). An evaluation of real time scanning in the first trimester of pregnancy. In *Real time ultrasound in obstetrics.* (eds. M. J. Bennett and S. Campbell) Blackwell Scientific Publications, Oxford, pp. 39–48.

Bakketeig, L. S. and Hoffman, H. J. (1981). Epidemiology of preterm birth; results from a long term study of births in Norway. In: *Preterm labour.* (eds. M. G. Elder and C. H. Hendricks) Butterworths, London.

Brock, D. J. H. (1982). Impact of maternal serum alpha-fetoprotein screening on antenatal diagnosis. *Br. Med. J.* **185**, 365–7.

Campbell, S. and Little, D. J. (1980). Clinical potential of real-time ultrasound. In *Real time ultrasound in obstetrics.* (eds. M. J. Bennett and S. Campbell) Blackwell Scientific Publications, Oxford. 27–38.

Chamberlain, G. and Garcia, J. (1983). Pregnant women at work. *Lancet* **1**, 228–30.

Chng, P. K. and Hall, M. H. (1982) Antenatal prediction of urinary tract infection in pregnancy. *Br. J. Obstet. Gynaec.* **89**, 8.

Chng, P. K., Hall, M. H., and Macgillivray, I. (1980). An audit of antenatal care; the value of the first antenatal visit. *Br. Med. J.* **281**, 1184.

Coope, Jean K. and Scott, Alison V. (1982). A programme for shared maternity and child care. *Br. Med. J.* **284**, 1936–7.

Dixon, E. A. (1982). Review of maternity patients suitable for home delivery. *Br. Med. J.* **284**, 1753–5.

Draper, G. J. (1982). Screening for cervical cancer: revised policy. The recommendations of the DHSS Committee on Gynaecological Cytology. *Health Trends* **14**, 37–40.

Grant, A. and Mohide, P. (1982). Screening and diagnostic tests in antenatal care. In *Effectiveness and satisfaction in antenatal care* (eds. M. Enkin and I. Chalmers). Spastics International Medical Publications, Heinemann, London.

Hall, M. H. and Chng, P. K. (1982). Antenatal care in practice. In *Effectiveness and satisfaction in antenatal care* (eds. M. Enkin and I. Chalmers). Spastics International Medical Publications, Heinemann, London.

Hall, M. H., Chng, P. K. and Macgillivray, I. (1980). Is routine antenatal care worthwhile? *Lancet* **ii**, 78.

Klein, M., Lloyd, I., Redman, C., Bull, M. and Turnbull, A. C. (1983). A comparison of low risk pregnant women booked for delivery in two systems of care shared care (consultant) and integrated general practice unit. II: Labour and delivery management and neonatal outcome. *Br. J. Obstet. Gynaecol.* **90**, 123–8.

Lewis, E. (1982). Attendance for antenatal care. *Br. Med. J.* **284**, 788.

MacGregor, J. E. (1979). Abnormal smears in pregnancy. *Br. Med. J.* **2**, 1002–3.

Macintyre, Sally (1981). Expectations and experiences of first pregnancy. *MRC Institute for Medical Sociology. Occasional Paper.*

Marsh, G. N. (1982). The 'specialty' of general practitioner obstetrics. *Lancet*, **1**, 669–72.

Oakley, Ann (1979). *Becoming a mother.* Martin Robertson, Oxford.

Oakley, Ann (1982). The origins and development of antenatal care. In *Effectiveness and satisfaction in antenatal care.* (eds. M. Enkin and I. Chalmers). Spastics International Medical Publications; Heinemann, London.

RCOG (1982). *Report of the RCOG Working Party on Antenatal and Intrapartum Care.* **September**. RCOG, London.

RCOG and RCGP (1981). Joint Working Party Report on Training for Obstetrics and Gynaecology for General Practitioners. RCOG and RCGP, London.

RCOG Study Group (1983). *Nutrition in pregnancy*. RCOG, London.

Roseveare, M. P. and Bull, M. J. V. (1982). General practitioner obstetrics; two styles of care. *Br. Med. J.* **284**, 958–60.

Standing, S. J., Brindle, M. J., Macdonald, A. P., and Lacey, R. W. (1981). Maternal alphafetoprotein screening; two years experience in a low risk district. *Br. Med. J.* **283**, 705–7.

Steel, Judith M., Johnstone, F. D., Smith, A. F., and Duncan, L. J. P. (1982). Five years experience of a 'pre-pregnancy' clinic for insulin dependent diabetics. *Br. Med. J.* **285**, 353–6.

Savage, W. and Paterson, I. (1982). Abortion. Methods and sequelae. *Br. J. Hosp. Med.* **October**, 364–84.

Taylor, G. W., Edgar, W., Taylor, B. A. and Neal, D. G. (1980). How safe is general practitioner obstetrics? *Lancet* **2**, 1287–9.

Thornhill Neighbourhood Project. (1982). *Antenatal care—who benefits?* A report by Thornhill Neighbourhood Project. Orkney House, 199 Caledonian Rd, London N1.

Zander, L. (1982). The challenge of antenatal care. A perspective from general practice. In *Effectiveness and satisfaction in antenatal care* (eds. M. Enkin and I. Chalmers) Spastics International Medical Publications; Heinemann, London, pp. 247–53.

7 The psychology of pregnancy and some common psychiatric states

B. M. N. Pitt

INTRODUCTION

Conception must for most women be an experience of some moment. Despite the widespread availability of both contraceptive advice and contraceptives it is not always planned or welcome. Pregnancy is psychologically and physiologically remarkable, though commonplace. Feelings about its implications for the future and such early effects as morning nausea, weight gain, backache, frequency, and fatigue are generally mixed. The awareness of two beings in one flesh, especially after quickening, is blissful for some women, but unnerving for others.

Yet there is no evidence that women who are pregnant are any more likely to see psychiatrists than those who are not (see Kendell *et al.* 1976), while they are rather less likely to be admitted to psychiatric hospitals. It is not that they are more equable. On the contrary, pregnancy is associated with an increase in anxiety, depression, and emotional lability (Kumar and Robson 1978a; Nilsson and Almgren 1970). But psychiatric states, if these are regarded as conditions to be referred to a psychiatrist, are relatively rare, and so is suicide (Sim 1963).

It may be that the state of pregnancy alters a woman's attitude towards disturbed feelings, so that she allows for them, and that others do so too, and are more supportive than at other times. Caplan (1964) has suggested that during pregnancy material usually repressed into the unconscious is more accessible, enabling the mother-to-be to see her present state in the light of more of her past than she can usually recall, which she is better able to acknowledge: thus she may gain strength and maturity.

Again, a pregnant woman is especially precious, not only for what she is but for what she contains, and any emotional vagaries or disturbances of behaviour may be attributed to her unusual condition and humoured, tolerated, and accepted, arousing sympathy and concern where at other times there might be exasperation and rejection. Then, pregnancy is finite, so its snags in the form of psychological disorder might be regarded as troublesome but transitory. Psychiatrists, even, might take the view 'Let's see how things are after the baby's born', being reluctant to prescribe any drugs which might be seen as damaging to the fetus or in the later stages to be too involved when a delivery is imminent! Nevertheless, it is strange that psychosis, generally regarded as genetically determined and sometimes precipitated by notable life-events, should actually be underrepresented during pregnancy; it is somewhat akin to Sherlock Holmes' observations about the dog which did not bark.

AMBIVALANCE

Barely 50 per cent of pregnancies, it appears, are planned. The Thomas Coram Research Unit (Gould 1983) reported that only half the expectant parents in their survey of 110 couples expecting a first child could say without qualification that now was the ideal time to have a baby. Indeed, only 19 couples agreed that the timing was right for both of them.

Even when a woman has long wanted to conceive she may experience some misgiving when she actually does so, not only about the stresses and strains of pregnancy and childbearing but also about changing her role to that of principally being a mother, especially if she has never had a child before. The limitations and responsibilities of motherhood may give her pause. On the other hand women seeking a termination of pregnancy not infrequently admit in the course of abortion counselling to some positive feelings about the fetus and being pregnant. Circumstances may well make the bearing of a child at this time (or 6 months hence) unacceptable, but there is a guilt and regret about ending the existence of the baby-to-be and having to frustrate the natural culmination of the major biological event, which has been mistakenly, misguidedly, or heedlessly started. This ambivalence may well contribute to the finding by Kumar and Robson (1978b) that the 10 per cent of pregnant women in their survey who became depressed in the first trimester included a highly significant 50 per cent of those who had previously had abortions; the current pregnancy may have been reminding them painfully of the one which they had previously foregone.

The very fact of conception, when ostensibly there was not the desire to conceive, suggests ambivalence. True contraceptive failure is quite unusual. Taking a chance, being overwhelmed by passion or forgetting are far more often the causes of unwanted pregnancy; in a psychiatrist's book forgetting, except in the dementing, is usually motivated. It seems likely that the unconscious will always tend to serve the species' need to procreate by more than occasionally outwitting the conscious intention of contraception!

KEY RELATIONSHIPS

The father

Where the father of the baby to be has decamped not knowing of his part in the pregnancy or, more often, not wanting to know, the only role he has served is that of stud. The pregnant woman's anger and disillusion may extend to the pregnancy, which she will wish to terminate, especially when getting pregnant was in part an attempt to secure a shaky relationship. Otherwise she will be another single mother, who may look vaguely to the father for maintenance and to the child for the evidence of his genetic endowment, but otherwise do without him.

More often, happily, the father is to hand and is indeed the spouse. His feelings about his wife's pregnancy may be as intense as hers, and can be equally mixed and varied. If it is a first pregnancy, he may wonder how drastically their lives will be changed. The biological purpose of pair-bonding must be procreation, the male role being to protect and support mother and child and make his own contribution to rearing during the long years of childhood. However, the transition from a couple to the start of a family may be accompanied by misgiving and regret. The need to love and be loved by a woman by no means necessarily involves wanting a child or children by her, now or later. The father-to-be may miss the intimacy of an exclusive one-to-one relationship and be anxious about sharing his partner with a baby. He may fear being somewhat displaced and charged with extra responsibility. Sexual enjoyment and freedom within the marriage may seem threatened by fatherhood and domesticity.

The cynical, with some justification, see marriage in part as a battle for power, and the balance of power may be altered by pregnancy and parenthood. The wife may exploit her changed physiological state and new preoccupations by seeking to be treated as delicate and special, or even sick. She may use the baby to be less available to her partner, or to put him down. He may seek more dominance and control as the 'breadwinner' if, as is usual, his wife gives up going out to work, or he may opt out and strive to retain his freedom while she is left literally 'holding the baby'.

Paternal anxiety, rivalry and identification with the mother-to-be during pregnancy may be manifest in the Couvade syndrome (Trethowan and Conlon 1965), so named by analogy with the rituals observed by the men of primitive societies during their wives' childbearing. Fathers-to-be are apparently liable to backache, abdominal pains, weight gain, and, mysteriously, toothache!

The mother-to-be's mother

The mother of the woman who is pregnant is nearly always (for good or ill) her first model of motherhood. If she is seen as a good mother, if the feelings about her are good, if she is felt to approve and support the pregnancy, then 'a girl's best friend is (indeed) her mother'. If she is seen as imperfect or frankly bad, however, unloving, jealous, disparaging, capricious, disapproving, then the model she presents is no good, and her daughter lacks the comfort and security of feeling at one with her or that she will be of any help. She may feel bad at harbouring resentment and other unfilial feelings, and uneasy that the pregnancy cannot prosper in such an unworthy person. It is very unusual to find a very anxious pregnant woman who enjoys an uncomplicatedly close relationship with her mother. The mother herself may be dead or at a distance, but the 'mother in the head' still matters. In psychoanalytic terms she is then part of the superego and sometimes extreme fears of harm befalling the fetus can be traced to the unconscious sense of her hostility.

The baby-to-be

The third key relationship is with the baby-to-be. Pregnancy may seem at first a merely physiological event—amenorrhoea, morning nausea, altered breast sensation—and the fetus may be thought of, especially in the early weeks of an unwanted pregnancy, as a mere collection of cells, a dispensable tissue. But sooner or later—more often sooner, these days, with the use of ultrasound scans—the baby is seen or felt to be a baby, and its sex even may be known. Bonding can occur at any time during the pregnancy or not until after delivery or a good deal later, but it is facilitated by awareness of the baby as an independent being within the womb, as at quickening.

Anxiety for the fetus

This, at some stage in pregnancy, seems almost universal, and is intensified by bonding or a previous loss, such as a miscarriage or stillbirth. Usually such anxiety can be contained by the pregnant woman, though she will welcome support and reassurance at antenatal clinics and classes. Occasionally endless consultations and scans are requested, and no reassurance will last for more than a day or two. Here a special programme of support, possibly involving referral to a sympathetic psychiatrist, is needed.

While most mothers say of the prospective baby's sex 'So long as its all right I don't really mind' sometimes it matters a great deal. Sons tend to be preferred; infanticide of female babies is practised in some Chinese villages even now, because sons remain to help in tilling the land, whereas the girls grow up and go away. In some cultures the father's virility, name, and estate are all at risk if his wife fails to produce a son. A woman who feels disadvantaged by her sex may wish for a son to fulfil her ambitions. Others on the other hand may want a daughter as an ally in a man's world. On the whole, the more rigid and farfetched the pregnant woman's aspirations for her baby, the worse prognosis for their relationship, while the more flexible the better.

MOTIVATION

Planned pregnancies presumably derive largely from the biological drive to procreate on which the survival of the species depends. Children are very appealing to most people, who some time or other crave one or more of their own. They are heirs and offer the possibility of a kind of immortality. They are often seen as the ultimate consummation of pair-bonding, the fruit of love. Sometimes family and social pressures are important. Sibling rivalry may contribute, as may religion, such as Roman Catholicism. A woman may feel that she is not fully a woman until she has become a mother. Some, feeling unloved, want a baby who will bind their partner more closely or become an ideal loving love object. Some may be seeking a sort of insurance, to be cared for in later life. Some may use a pregnancy to influence or hurt parents, a lover, or a spouse. Some may seek a way out of uncongenial work or study, or even means to a council flat! Motivation, then, may be good, dubious, or mixed. Usually the better the motivation the better for mother and baby—but feelings often change in the course of pregnancy and the puerperium.

THE COURSE OF PREGNANCY

The first trimester

In the first 3 months after conception, especially in a first pregnancy, the impact and the implications of the event provide most food for thought. Unless it was wholly wanted, termination may be contemplated if only to be dismissed on moral or religious grounds or as too drastic, or actively sought. The present legislation (Abortion Act 1967) is not far off providing abortion on demand, if the demand is sufficiently desperate and insistent, and the evidence (Pare and Raven 1970) is that fewer women suffer psychological ill-effects from a badly wanted termination, than if they are somehow 'made' to have the baby—at least in the short term. Ambivalence in or over-persuasion of women apparently seeking termination are much more likely to be associated with a morbid reaction post-abortum. An important task for abortion counselling, then, is to help unmix mixed feelings and help the troubled woman to recognize and think through the consequences of her difficult decision.

Role change

Pregnancy portends a role change, most drastically from a relatively fancy free and independent young woman with a career, to a mother, tied by the cares of being the person most responsible for her infant. Even if the pregnancy is wanted she may wonder if she is up to motherhood. Is she mature, calm, intuitive, loving, and unselfish enough to bring a child into the world and rear it properly? Even if she is, is her partner? Is being a mother the best use of herself and her time? Whereas not long ago it was assumed that women should marry and have children and look after them, feminism now sometimes argues otherwise.

There are financial consequences too. In the Thomas Coram Foundation study mentioned above, many couples found that having a first child halved their income.

Even the transition from being the mother of one to the mother of two may seem fraught, with all the problems of fairness, loving equally, and balancing needs to be met. Any addition, indeed, may be critical, especially if there is a gap of some years since the last.

Teratogenesis

The risk of teratogenesis is probably now widely recognized as greatest in the early weeks of pregnancy, so there may be fears of the effects of inadvertent medication (generally groundless) or of the effects of smoking (Holcslaw and Topham 1978), or alcohol (Edwards 1983) on the baby-to-be (better justified). There may even be anxiety that sex will damage or dislodge the fetus, but that without sex the woman and her partner will be frustrated and lose their closeness. These misgivings are, of course, without foundation, but need to be aired during early antenatal care. Libido often changes during pregnancy, generally diminishing, sometimes increasing, but always liable to fluctuations (Kumar, Brandt, and Robson 1981).

Antenatal visits

By the end of the third month the first antenatal visit should have been made. Many women these days are wary of the medicalization of motherhood (Oakley 1980), and are highly ambivalent about doctors, wanting to be guided, instructed, advised, reassured and taken safely through labour, but at the same time to be consulted, and left some control of their bodies and the birth. Probably a familiar general practitioner and the midwife are more readily trusted, at first, than the consultant obstetrician who seems more remote and more committed to daunting technology. Obviously a sensitive, flexible approach in antenatal care, which recognizes different personalities and levels of anxiety and intelligence and is alert to the disguised or half-spoken question, is best suited to please most of the pregnant women most of the time.

Nausea

The nausea of pregnancy and morning sickness are physiologically, not psychologically, determined and generally well tolerated as part of pregnancy, but can sometimes be severe and distressing. *Hyperemesis gravidarum*, which appears (like hysteria) to be rarer now than formerly, is sometimes at least partly psychogenic, in that admission of the patient to hospital from the frantic anxiety of her home is often remarkable in the way it mitigates the disorder. It may sometimes represent the conversion of deep insecurity into a symbolic rejection of the pregnancy which can only be endured with the powerful support of 24-hour hospital care. Wolkind and Zajicek (1981) found an association between prolonged nausea and vomiting and a lack of family support. Perhaps, however, as obstetric units tend to be more aware and understanding of fears and feelings than once they were, the need to somatize and dramatize feelings so starkly and dangerously has been reduced.

Pica

Pica, the craving for unusual, often piquant, occasionally bizarre tastes, is, as Trethowan and Dickens (1972) have shown, not a myth but significantly associated with pregnancy. It is probably overdetermined by a physiological blunting of taste during pregnancy, an unconscious desire for symbolic fruitfulness (the food craved is often a sharp and succulent fruit) and a warrantable wish for spoiling. It rarely matters.

Overeating

A tendency to overeating may be established early in pregnancy, usually in women who have already had problems with weight control. This is often comfort eating and, after a failure to regain normal weight post partum, is likely to continue, adding to 'fat and horrible' feelings of low self-esteem during the fraught period of the puerperium, and the transitory but illusory comfort of further overeating. The rationalization of eating enough for oneself and the baby needs to be challenged, and if there is a special need for comfort, reassurance, and support it should, if possible, be met by other means.

Narcissism

Narcissism is by no means a feminine prerogative, but society ordains that beauty still matters more to the female than the male. The threat of pregnancy and breast-feeding to the figure and the bust, and the spectres of varicose veins and stretch marks, can trouble some insecure women whose sense of worth is too closely linked to how they think they look. Diet and exercises can achieve much, though stretch marks may not be avoided. It may be a compensation that some women seem to be beautified by pregnancy, while a baby may set off their looks most becomingly.

The middle trimester

The middle 3 months of pregnancy are generally the most tranquil, though still more anxious than before conception. If there have been previous miscarriages then this time is critical, and great is likely to be the grief, anger, and unjustified but still very real and painful guilt, should the loss be repeated (Pizer and Palinski 1980). Worries about the delivery, now that the pregnancy is accepted, may come to the fore. Will the baby come out the right way round? Will there be room for it to come out at all? How does one know when labour has begun? How can one be sure of being in the right place at the right time? Who will be there to help—the doctor, the midwife, surely at least the baby's father? Will it be a joyous experience or confused by interference—anaesthesia, noise, too many people giving different instructions and, above all perhaps, pain?

In the middle trimester the mother-to-be has made physiological and psychological adjustments to her gravid state, to her backache, heartburn, and swollen form, and to the rather weird condition of containing another being inside her. There is a tendency to increased introversion during pregnancy (Chapple and Furneaux 1964) and many women rather enjoy a certain passive, reflective, day dreaming broodiness, which is possibly associated with rising progesterone levels. A few feel quite euphoric and revel in what has been called the 'beatific' feeling. But a few others may resent the sense of being trapped in a slow, sluggish, swelling body with a parasitic being inside.

A pattern of support by the partner, family, and the obstetric team should by now be well established. This is often lacking where it is most needed. The unstable, young, single mother who has only lately moved into temporary accommodation, is at odds with her scattered family, is not wholly sure who fathered her child, and has a previous history of drug and alcohol abuse, delinquency, suicide gestures, debt, homelessness, abortion, battering (usually as victim), and children in care, is hard to help. She is often a late and erratic attender at antenatal clinics, but her baby is much at risk and every effort must be made, by doctors, midwives, health visitors, and social workers to give her guidance, encouragement, practical help, and steadfast support. Although such women are notoriously bad at sustaining relationships and commitments, they may prove rather more cooperative then usual during a pregnancy. Caplan (1964) has remarked that because of a relaxation of repression pregnant women in psychotherapy may make unusually rapid progress. Another likely factor is the positive feeling for the baby whose arrival is imminent and good motivation for therapy which focuses on coping with the birth and early motherhood.

The last trimester

The last trimester is somewhat dominated by the EDD (the very approximate estimated date of delivery) which is generally approached with growing impatience, changing to chagrin, misgiving, and even dismay if it is passed! By the end of pregnancy, most women have had enough of it. They are tired of being so big, of maternity clothing, of being fatigued, of backache and frequency, of finding it ever more difficult to make love, and they are very curious to meet the baby which has been wriggling or kicking inside them for what seems so long and get to grips with motherhood.

Earlier anxieties are subordinated to 'how much longer will I have to wait?' This is an adaptive reaction, a girding of the loins for labour.

By now decisions about where the baby will be born (nearly always in hospital), how long will be spent there, who will attend (nearly always these days the husband or partner), whether this will be a 'natural' childbirth, the possibility of active intervention, instrumental delivery, even caesarean section, the use of analgesia and anaesthesia, epidural or general, the position to be adopted during labour and the extent to which the principles of Leboyer or any other guru are followed will mostly have been taken, though some will have to await the course of the labour. It is also important to know by now who will be around to help at home after the birth and for how long.

Generally women are tense but reasonably cheerful as they come up to the great moment of delivery. A minority, however, become significantly depressed. This is a morbid phenomenon and may be premonitory of post-natal depression (Meares, Grimwade and Wood 1976; Tod 1964) so warrants special attention.

COPING WITH PREGNANCY

Several studies (Kumar and Robson 1978*a*; Nilsson and Almgren 1970; Pitt 1965) have shown that women are more anxious and depressed when pregnant than when not, but they are not more likely to present as 'cases' of emotional disorder when pregnant because the emotions are regarded as natural and related to the pregnancy and because pregnant women are generally well supported. Once the decision to go through with the pregnancy has been made, it seems, most women cope very well with its emotional and physical discomforts. They are less likely than at other times to seek drugs for any distress, for fear of harming the baby, and for the same reason they are readier to moderate, suspend or give up smoking and drinking alcohol. Those around them are more tolerant and helpful than usual, and less likely to ascribe any emotional vagaries to personal faults or neurotic illness than to the pregnancy, which is seen as transitory and desirable.

Even in the large hospital antenatal clinics, which are sometimes impersonal and rather regimented, there are, as well as the generally helpful staff, the other pregnant women, all in the same boat or 'club', with whom to share experiences and feelings, including scandals and superstitions as well as good advice and useful tips. This sisterly support may be one of the main strengths of antenatal care.

The exceptional women who seek medical help for extreme anxiety or depression which they cannot contain include, as has been mentioned, those with a bad previous experience of miscarriage, stillbirth, or a traumatic delivery; those under particularly severe current stress, such as marital strife, the husband's redundancy or a bereavement; a very few who are particularly afraid that they will not survive the pregnancy or that their babies are doomed; and those psychiatrically ill at the time of conception. Some women, very anxious in early pregnancy, seek termination to relieve their anxiety rather than because they are against having a baby. Temporizing, with the assurance that if the anxiety continues intolerably for more than 2 to 3 weeks an abortion can still be arranged, suffices usually to allow a spontaneous remission.

Personal regular support is paramount in the management of the emotional and psychiatric problems of pregnancy, but there is sometimes a place for medication for severe, distressing anxiety and depression or the rare psychotic symptoms. None of the established major or minor tranquillizers or antidepressants are known to be teratogenic, though as they tend not to be used in early pregnancy experience is relatively limited. Manic-depressive or recurrent bipolar depressives on lithium carbonate present a special problem. The risk of relapse off the drug is considerable, but there is a 10 per cent risk of fetal abnormality, especially for cardiovascular malformations (Weinstein and Foldfield 1975) and even in later pregnancy close monitoring of serum lithium levels is required because of changing renal function, while at parturition there are risks of lithium toxicity to mother and baby. Consequently no woman who needs lithium should have a child unless she desperately wants one and has her husband and family's full informed support. Her supervision during any pregnancy and the puerperium demands close liaison between the psychiatric and obstetric departments and the general practitioner and his team.

SUMMARY

Conception is an event of consequence and pregnancy is a time of heightened anxiety and lability and depression, yet it is a period of low psychiatric morbidity. This may partly be because pregnancy is well regarded and supported. Ambivalence characterizes wanted and unwanted pregnancies and the use of contraception. Key figures during pregnancy are the sexual partner, whose support is needed, the mother-to-be's mother, who provides a model of mothering, and the future baby, who carries diverse hopes and fears. Anxiety for the fetus is almost universal. The reasons for planning a pregnancy are diverse but generally good. In the course of pregnancy the impact and implications are felt and worked through in the first 3 months, the second trimester involves acceptance and planning with a good deal of anxiety about the quality of the delivery, while in the last 3 months there is growing impatience to be in labour. Other pregnant women help women to cope with pregnancy. Those with special emotional and psychiatric problems need special support, and there is a place for medication.

REFERENCES AND FURTHER READING

Abortion Act (1967). HMSO, London.

Caplan, G. (1964). *Principles of preventive psychiatry*, Tavistock, London.

Chapple, P. and Furneaux, W. D. (1964). Changes of personality in pregnancy and labour. *Proc. Roy. Soc. Med.* **57**, 260.

Edwards, G. (1983). Alcohol and advice to the pregnant women. *Br. Med. J.* **186**, 247.

Gould, Liz (1983). Why do you want a baby? *Parents*, **82**, 30.

Holcslaw, D. S. and Topham, A. L. (1978). The effects of smoking on fetal, neonatal and childhood development. *Paediat. Ann.* **7**, 201.

Kendell, R. E., Wainwright, S., Hailey, A., and Shannon, B. (1976). The influence of childbirth on psychiatric morbidity. *Psychol. Med.* **6**, 297.

Kumar, R. and Robson, K. (1978a). Neurotic disturbance during pregnancy and the puerperium: preliminary report of a prospective survey of 19 primiparae. In *Mental illness in pregnancy and the puerperium.* (ed. M. Sandler), p. 40, Oxford University Press, London.

Kumar, R. and Robson, K. (1978b). Previous abortion and antenatal depression in primiparae: preliminary report of a survey of mental health in pregnancy. *Psychol. Med.* **8**, 711.

Kumar, R., Brandt, H. A., and Robson, K. M. (1981). Childbirth and maternal sexuality: a prospective study of 119 primiparae. *J. Psychosom. Res.* **25**, 373.

Meares, R. and Grimwade, J. and Wood, C. (1976). A possible relationship between anxiety in pregnancy and puerperal depression. *J. Psychosom. Res.* **20**, 605.

Nilsson, A. and Almgren, P. E. (1970). Para-natal emotional adjustment: a prospective study of 165 women. *Acta Psychiatr. Scand.*, Suppl. 220.

Oakley, A. (1980). *Women confined: towards a sociology of childbirth.* Martin Robertson, Oxford.

Pare, C. M. B. and Raven, H. (1970). Follow-up of patients referred for termination. *Lancet* **1**, 653.

Pitt, B. (1965). *A study of emotional disturbance associated with childbearing, with particular reference to depression arising in the puerperium.* University of London, MD thesis.

Pizer, H. and Palinski, Christine (1980). *Coping with a miscarriage.* The Dial Press, New York.

Sim, M. (1963). Abortion and the psychiatrist. *Br. Med. J.* **2**, 45.

Tod, E. D. M. (1964). Puerperal depression: a prospective epidemiological study. *Lancet* **2**, 1264.

Trethowan, W. H. and Conlon, M. F. (1965). The Couvade syndrome *Br. J. Psychiat.* **111**, 57.

Trethowan, W. H. and Dickens, G. (1972). Cravings, aversions and pica of pregnancy. In *Modern perspective in psycho-obstetrics.* (ed. J. G. Howells). Oliver and Boyd, Edinburgh.

Weinstein, M. R. and Foldfield, M. D. (1975). Cardiovascular malformations with lithium use during pregnancy. *Am. J. Psychiatr.* **132**, 529.

Wolkind, S. and Zajicek, E. (1981). *Pregnancy—a psychological and social study.* Academic Press, London and New York.

8 A statistical view of risk factors

R. G. Newcombe

INTRODUCTION

The general practitioner who is involved in antenatal care needs to be aware of the factors that may identify a particular pregnancy as being at high risk of an adverse outcome, in order to plan intelligently the management of the pregnancy. The higher the anticipated risk is, the greater the need for involvement of a specialist obstetric team. It should always be borne in mind that there is not such a thing as a zero risk pregnancy; there is no set of maternal characteristics that would suffice to reassure the general practitioner in advance that all is certain to be well. Nevertheless he should be able to exercise informed judgement as to the most appropriate level of care, in conjunction with the pregnant woman's stated preference for general practitioner management and possible home delivery, with the personal advantages such policies would confer.

This chapter examines the predictive information contained in the various epidemiological risk factors, as illustrated by data from the Cardiff Birth Survey. It should be borne in mind that this data, along with all the most reliable data on the subject, is derived from population-based series of births, rather than hospital deliveries only. Series of hospital deliveries are necessarily less appropriate because of the selection of factors that operate to bring about hospital rather than home or general practitioner unit delivery; furthermore they tend to arise from teaching hospitals to which difficult cases are referred from elsewhere. The risk relationships that would be appropriate for a series of pregnancies under general practitioner care would be subject to selection biases in the opposite direction, namely that pregnancies with adverse risk factors would be less frequent than in a geographically defined population. We will proceed to examine the form and usefulness of the scoring system for risk assessment that have been published.

THE SURVEY DATA

Since 1965 the Cardiff Birth Survey (Andrews *et al.* 1985) has collected extensive social, obstetric, and paediatric details of all deliveries to women resident in the city. The tabulations presented here are based on singleton deliveries to Cardiff resident women during the period 1970–79. All infants with any congenital malformation or postural deformity recorded are excluded, as are deliveries in which the outcome, birth weight or gestational age is not recorded. This leaves a total of 34 891, which include 484 perinatal deaths (PND) (13.9 per 1000 deliveries), 1347 (3.9 per cent) with low birth weight under 2500 g delivered after completion of 36 weeks of gestation (LBT) and 9525 (27.3 per cent) with abnormal delivery, defined as any of the following: instrumental delivery, breech, caesarean section, total duration of labour over 24 hours, or postpartum haemorrhage. The outcomes have been selected for study as being those of which a general practitioner would particularly want to be forewarned.

These three outcomes are examined in relation to the following risk factors: age of mother, number of previous deliveries, history of perinatal death, sociomarital status, area of residence within the city, smoking, and maternal height and weight. In married women social classes I to V are defined in terms of the occupation of the husband; the group of unmarried women has not been further subdivided. Maternal weight is recorded at 20 weeks' gestation and is thus approximately 4 kg greater than the prepregnant weight. Area of residence is defined by classifying the 19 city wards into three groups according to the standard of housing. The 'good' areas consist mainly of well-maintained owner-occupied property. The 'poor' wards consist mainly of council housing or old property which is in relatively poor condition. Many of the wards are classified as 'mixed' since they contain a wide range of accommodation, and the information available to the clinician from knowledge of the particular address will be more discriminatory than this classification.

Tables 8.1, 8.2 and 8.3 show the relationship between historical, social and somatotype risk factors and the outcome of pregnancy. Each figure is a relative risk for the specified subgroup of women, compared to the whole series for which the relative risk is 100. Thus for women aged under 16 the perinatal mortality rate is 35.7 per 1000, giving a relative risk of $35.7/13.9 \times 100 = 257$.

Risk relationships applying to pregnancy are expounded in much greater detail in the publications based on the 1958 British Perinatal Mortality Survey (Butler and Bonham, 1963; Butler and Alberman, 1969) which together with the 1970 British Births Survey (Chamberlain, *et al.* 1975) have become the standard texts on the subject.

Historical factors

Table 8.1 shows the relationship of outcome to maternal age, parity, and history of perinatal death. In terms of any of the three outcomes, there is a decrease in risk from the very young to the late twenties, with a subsequent increase. (Figures for the extreme age groups and very high parity groups are subject to considerable sampling variation, being based on small numbers of cases). The risk of perinatal death or LBT is lower in the second pregnancy than in the first and steadily increases thereafter, and history of perinatal death is a highly informative indicator of such risk for the current pregnancy. Abnormal delivery is very much a feature of primiparous pregnancies.

Table 8.1   *Relative risks for perinatal death, low birth weight at term and abnormal delivery, by mother's age, previous deliveries and history of perinatal death*

	number of cases	perinatal death	Relative risk for low birth weight at term	abnormal delivery
Mother's age				
Under 16	112	257	(69)	118
16–17	1492	140	125	117
18–19	3512	105	128	113
20–24	12 043	91	111	94
25–29	10 721	77	81	100
30–34	4845	106	84	96
35–39	1678	219	122	108
40 or over	404	(196)	(64)	126
Previous deliveries				
0	14 105	104	117	159
1	11 223	72	81	67
2	5411	100	86	53
3	2357	119	109	49
4	951	167	117	52
5	432	234	120	58
6	178	243	146	58
7 or more	169	384	107	52
History of PND				
No	33 370	93	98	100
Yes	1456	248	146	101

The Cardiff Birth Survey unfortunately does not permit systematic linkage of successive pregnancies in the same woman, so it is not possible to quote here figures for the relative risks applicable when there is a history of low birth weight or preterm delivery; each of these factors is nevertheless indicative of a substantially increased risk of perinatal death or intra-uterine growth retardation in the current pregnancy. Indeed, any adverse occurrence in the past should be heeded as an indicator that a similar or related event may occur in the present pregnancy. Not only a history of perinatal death, low birth weight, or preterm delivery, but also a previous abortion whether spontaneous or therapeutic, previous breech delivery, previous multiple pregnancy, previous antepartum haemorrhage or previous preeclamptic toxaemia should be regarded as an indication of increased risk in the current pregnancy.

Pre-existing maternal conditions such as diabetes, heart disease, renal disease or epilepsy exert an unfavourable influence on the pregnancy. Since such a condition would act as a specific determinant of the management of the pregnancy, it is not appropriate to reduce it to a relative risk in the same way as for other factors. Genetically determined conditions should likewise be regarded as a specific, separate issue, and in affected kindreds genetic counselling should whenever possible take place before pregnancy is contemplated. If a multiple pregnancy is detected, the risks of perinatal death, LBT and abnormal delivery are all greatly increased, and the management of the pregnancy should be directed specifically in the light of this knowledge. The course of the pregnancy is particularly informative and attention would be paid to the occurrence or non-occurrence of antepartum haemorrhage (APH), pre-eclamptic toxaemia (PET) or urinary tract infection.

In primiparae there are two additional adverse factors to be borne in mind. Since there is no obstetric history the assessment of prognosis will necessarily be less precise than in a multipara. And the risk of pre-eclamptic toxaemia, defined as either a systolic blood pressure of 160 mmHg or a diastolic blood pressure of 100 mmHg being recorded at any stage of pregnancy, is 86 per cent higher in primiparae than in multiparae.

Social factors

Table 8.2 shows the relationship of outcome to sociomarital status, area of residence, and smoking habits during the pregnancy. There is a clear gradient in the risk of each adverse outcome according to the social class of the husband—perinatal death and LBT are low social class phenomena while abnormal delivery occurs or is resorted to more often in social classes I and II. Unmarried mothers face risks similar to those in the low social classes. Area of residence showed clear, corresponding effects.

Women who continue to smoke over five cigarettes per day are at considerably increased risk of either losing their baby or retarding its growth, and indeed in a study based on Cardiff Birth Survey data cot death was nearly five times as common in babies of heavy smokers than in those born to non-smokers (Murphy, Newcombe and Sibert 1982). Since smoking is one of the few major risk factors that is amenable to alteration, every effort should be made to persuade the pregnant woman to give up, at least for the duration of the pregnancy, even at the cost of gaining a few pounds in weight. Rather surprisingly, women who give up smoking for the whole or part of pregnancy are at lower risk that those who have never smoked, and those who smoke fewer than five cigarettes per day are also at low risk; these are small and self-selected groups of women who may well be exerting a greater than average degree of self-care during pregnancy.

Table 8.2   *Relative risks for perinatal death, low birth weight at term and abnormal delivery, by sociomarital status, area of residence and smoking habits of mother*

| | | Relative risk for | | |
	number of cases	perinatal death	low birth weight at term	abnormal delivery
Social class of husband				
I	2067	70	53	117
II	3572	77	64	118
III	16 819	90	94	98
IV	4287	101	117	89
V	2966	163	138	84
Unmarried mother	3335	128	137	112
Area of residence				
Good	3717	70	62	109
Medium or mixed	19 214	89	91	105
Poor	11 960	127	127	90
Smoking habits				
Non-smoker	18 896	88	70	108
Gave up for part or whole of pregnancy	1629	58	52	109
Under 5 cigarettes per day	1616	89	85	100
5–9	2246	119	119	95
10–19	6370	123	148	91
20 or more	3840	124	183	76

These are but three of a large set of social variables that could be considered, and are chosen because they are readily available and interpreted; the effect of smoking is mainly direct, whereas social class and area of residence are primarily indicative of outcome. It was not possible to examine ethnic groups on the Cardiff data, but clearly racial disadvantage is expected to be reflected in disadvantageous outcome. The state of nutrition of the mother is most readily examined in terms of her body weight, as shown in Table 8.3, dietary assessment being extremely difficult.

All of these variables are closely interrelated, yet each provides considerable information. For example, the relative risks of perinatal death in social classes I and V are 70 and 163 respectively. If smoking habits are held constant, the relative risks become 76 and 157—a slight narrowing of the gap, yet still a very substantial, clinically important twofold difference.

Maternal somatotype

Table 8.3 shows that there is a steady decrease in risk with increasing height, and this effect is most marked for low birth weight at term. The same applies to maternal weight, but with a particularly high relative risk of low

Table 8.3 *Relative risk for perinatal death, low birth weight at term and abnormal delivery by height and weight of mother at 20 weeks' gestation*

	number of cases	Relative risk for perinatal death	low birth weight at term	abnormal delivery
Height				
Under 147.5 cm	465	186	262	154
147.5–	788	110	201	131
150–	1785	129	186	115
152.5–	2988	128	139	105
155–	10 061	95	112	99
160–	10 434	86	77	95
165–	5448	78	55	96
170 cm or over	1960	74	49	93
Weight				
Under 45 kg	382	283	468	109
45–	6743	108	167	101
55–	13 511	87	88	100
65–	7312	86	49	104
75–	2338	64	61	104
85 kg or over	1130	115	57	112

birth weight at term and perinatal death in the lightest group—apparently short stature and thinness both contribute to risk. The perinatal mortality rate and complication rate, though not the LBT proportion, is a little higher in the heaviest group.

RISK ASSESSMENT BY SCORING SYSTEMS

The above risk factors each give certain information bearing on the risk of adverse outcome which the pregnancy faces. A scoring system based on a combination of such factors would give greater prognostic information than a single factor, and could be the basis for variations in the nature and intensity of the antenatal care offered, permitting beneficial intervention at an earlier stage of the pregnancy than would otherwise be possible. Several such risk assessment systems have been published; they aim to identify women at high risk of one adverse outcome of pregnancy or another, usually preterm labour, intrauterine growth retardation or perinatal death. It needs to be asked whether such formalized risk assessment is worthwhile: can it lead to improved management and outcome of pregnancy, and if so, would the experienced clinician using his own unformalized expertise achieve equally good results?

The risk assessment systems listed in the reference section have been examined by Newcombe (1979, 1981) and by Newcombe and Chalmers (1981). Although such risk assessment systems have been proposed for both educational and resource allocation purposes, interest in them has mainly been prompted by a desire to provide a rational basis for identifying individuals for differential prophylactic or therapeutic intervention.

A risk assessment system is useful only to the degree that it permits prospective identification of high-risk groups, and for several reasons such identification will be considerably more clear-cut on the data from which the score is derived, than it would be when used on any other series of births. Different scoring systems are designed to be applied at different stages of pregnancy. As is inevitable, the degree of predictive power improves as gestation advances and factors directly bearing on fetal wellbeing provide more direct information than the background epidemiological factors. In late pregnancy the scoring system of Adelstein and Fedrick (1978) to predict low birth weight at term has predictive performance as good as is found for any predictor applied correspondingly late in pregnancy. This scoring system is based on the mother's social class, height, weight, ABO blood group, smoking habits, the occurrence or non-occurrence of threatened abortion or pre-eclamptic toxaemia, and in multiparae history of perinatal death, low birth weight delivery or delivery of an infant weighing 4 kg or more; score components corresponding to these factors are multiplied to give a predictive score. Low birth weight at term occurred in only 2.4 per cent of the multiparae studied, so that even the fivefold increased risk in the identified high-risk group amounts to only 12 per cent of this group experiencing this outcome.

Conversely, though a scoring system can provide considerable discriminatory information, it is not possible to identify a group of women whose risk of adverse outcome would be negligible. In the above case the lowest quartile of risk scores in the population of primiparae gave rise to 8.6 per cent of the cases of LBT, a risk of 1 in 84. The lowest risk group among multiparae do rather better, with a risk of 1 in 124. In the context of a health care system presently orientated towards hospital delivery and in which the most intense levels of care are provided in the hospital, the clinician requires to assess the woman's expressed preference for delivery in a less institutional setting in the light of this fact.

REFERENCES

Adelstein, P. and Fedrick, J. (1978). Antenatal identification of women at increased risk of being delivered of a low birth weight infant at term. *Br. J. Obstet. Gynaecol.* **85**, 8.

Andrews, J., Davies, K., Chalmers, I., and Campbell, H. (1985). The Cardiff Birth Survey: development, perinatal mortality, birth weight and length of gestation. In

Genetic and population studies in Wales (ed. P. S. Harper and E. Sunderland). University of Wales Press, Cardiff.

Butler, N. R. and Bonham, D. G. (1963). *Perinatal mortality.* Livingstone, Edinburgh.

Butler, N. R. and Alberman, E. D. (1969). *Perinatal problems.* Livingstone, Edinburgh.

Chamberlain, R., Chamberlain, G., Howlett, B., and Claireaux, A. (1975). *British births 1970. Volume 1: The first week of life.* Heinemann, London.

Murphy, J. F., Newcombe, R. G., and Sibert, J. R. (1982). The epidemiology of sudden infant death syndrome. *J. Epidemiol. Commun. Health* **36**, 17–21.

Newcombe, R. G. (1979) *A critical review of risk prediction with special reference to the perinatal period.* PhD thesis, University of Wales.

Newcombe, R. G. (1981). Non-nutritional factors affecting fetal growth. *Am. J. Clin. Nutr.* **34**, 732.

Newcombe, R. G. and Chalmers, I. (1981). Assessing the risk of preterm labour. In *Preterm labour.* (ed. M. G. Elder and C. H. Hendricks), p. 47, Butterworths, London.

FURTHER READING

Aubry, R. H. and Pennington, J. C. (1973). Identification and evaluation of high risk pregnancy. *Clin. Obstet. Gynecol.* **16**, 3.

Davies, A. M. and Harlap, S. (1974). Antenatal prediction of perinatal and neonatal mortality risk. *World Health Organization*, MCH/WP/HR74, 1.

Donahue, C. L. and Wan, T. T. H. (1973). Measuring obstetric risks of prematurity. *Am. J. Obstet. Gynecol.* **116**, 911.

Fedrick, J. (1976). Antenatal identification of women at high risk of spontaneous preterm birth. *Br. J. Obstet. Gynaecol.* **83**, 351.

Feldstein, M. S. and Butler, N. R. (1965). Analysis of factors affecting perinatal mortality. *Br. J. Prevent. Soc. Med.* **19**, 128.

Goldstein, H. (1969). Predictors of birthweight and mortality risk. *Perinatal problems* (eds. N. R. Butler and E. D. Alberman), pp. 42, 56. Edinburgh, Livingstone.

Goodwin, J. W., Dunne, J. T., and Thomas, B. W. (1969). Antepartum identification of the fetus at risk. *Can. Med. Assoc. J.* **101**, 458.

Haeri, A. D., South, J., and Naldrett, J. (1974). A scoring system for identifying pregnant patients with a high risk of perinatal mortality. *J. Obstet. Gynaecol. Br. Commonw.* **81**, 535.

Hobel, C. J., Hyvarinen, M. A., Okada, D. M., and Oh, W. (1973). Prenatal and intrapartum high-risk screening. *Am. J. Obstet. Gynecol.* **117**, 1.

Kaminski, M., Goujard, J., and Rumeau-Rouquette, C. (1973). Prediction of low birthweight and prematurity by a multiple regression analysis with maternal characteristics known since the beginning of pregnancy. *Int. J. Epidemiol.* **2**, 195.

Kaminski, M. and Papiernik, E. (1974). Multifactorial study of risk of prematurity at 32 weeks. II. *J. Perinatal Med.* **2**, 37.

Lambotte, R. (1977). Epidemiology of preterm labour. In *Pre-term labour (Proceedings of the 5th study group of the Royal College of Obstetricians and Gynaecologists).* (eds. A. B. M. Anderson, R. Beard, J. M. Brudenell and P. M. Dunn), p. 40. Royal College of Obstetricians and Gynaecologists, London.

Nesbitt, R. E. L. and Aubry, R. H. (1969). High risk obstetrics II. *Am. J. Obstet. Gynecol.* **103**, 972.

Papiernik, E. and Kaminski, M. (1974). Multifactorial study of risk of prematurity at 32 weeks. I. *J. Perinatal Med.* **2**, 30.

Rantakallio, P. (1969). Groups at risk in low birth weight infants and perinatal mortality. *Acta Paediat. Scand.*, Supp. 193.

Rumeau-Rouquette, C., Kaminski, M., and Goujard, J. (1974). Prediction of perinatal mortality in early pregnancy. *J. Perinatal Med.* **2**, 196.

Rumeau-Rouquette, C., Goujard, J., Kaminski, M., Breart, G., du Mazaubrun, G., Deniel, M., and Hennequin, J. F. (1977). Risk indicators and environment—investigations in France. In *Proceedings of the 8th World congress of gynaecology and obstetrics, Mexico City, 1976* (eds. L. Castelazo-Ayala and C. MacGregor), p. 81. Excerpta Medica, Amsterdam.

Stembera, Z. K., Zezulakova, J., Dittrichova, J., and Znamenacek, K. (1975). Identification and quantification of high risk factors affecting fetus and newborn. In *4th European congress of perinatal medicine* (*Prague, 1974*), (eds. Z. K. Stembera, K. Polacek and V. Sabata), p. 400. Thieme, Stuttgart.

Thalhammer, O., Coradello, H., Pollak, A., Scheibenreiter, S., and Simbruner, G. (1976). Prospective and retrospective examination of an easily applicable score to predict the probability of premature birth defined by weight. *J. Perinatal Med.* **4**, 38.

Wilson, E. W. and Sill, H. K. (1973). Identification of the high risk pregnancy by a scoring system. *NZ Med. J.* **78**, 437.

9 Selection of patients for general practitioner care

M. J. V. Bull

The aim of selection of patients for general practitioner ('community') obstetric care is to identify women who, as far as can be determined, are at minimal risk of complications of pregnancy and may be expected to deliver spontaneously so that consequently neither they nor their babies are likely to suffer perinatal mortality or morbidity. We have already seen (in Chapter 8) that there is no such entity as the 'no-risk' pregnancy. Nevertheless women can be selected for low-risk potentiality and studies have shown (Klein *et al.* 1983; Taylor *et al.* 1980) that perinatal outcomes for such groups can be at least as good as (and perhaps better than) for similar mothers booked into specialist units.

The Hospital In-Patient Enquiry 1974–76 (HIPE 1979) sampled all maternity hospital discharges in England and Wales in 1975 and found (Fig. 9.1) that one half of all births involved one or more complications during either pregnancy or in labour. By implication, the remaining 50 per cent of women should have been suitable for community care. The problem is, how to identify them prospectively?

The seminal work for risk prediction in the United Kingdom was the British Perinatal Mortality Survey of 1958 (Butler and Bonham 1963) in which nearly 17 000 births occurring during one particular week were surveyed and outcomes in terms of perinatal mortality analysed according to a range of demographic and clinical variables. The results were expressed in the form of 'Mortality Ratios' (M); that is to say, the ratio of perinatal deaths in a given cohort of women compared to that in the total survey population and expressed as a percentage. Thus, if the mortality ratio was greater than 100 the effect of the particular variable under consideration was concluded to increase the risk of fetal loss by a similar factor in comparable cohorts. For example, a mortality ratio of 150 indicates a 50 per cent increase in the risk of perinatal death and one of 200 double that prevailing in the total survey population. This study was to a major degree responsible for the adoption of the conventional criteria for patients suitable for general practitioner obstetric care, that is:

(i) A normal medical and obstetric history.

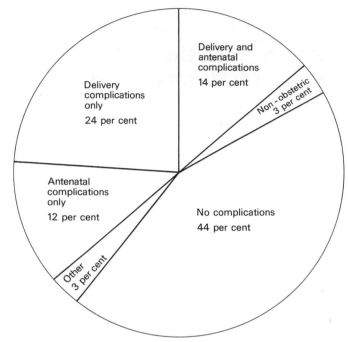

Fig. 9.1. Maternal complications—all deliveries (1975). Source: Hospital In-patient Enquiry (HIPE), 1974–76 (1979).

   (ii) If nulliparae, to be between the ages of 18 and 29 at booking; stature greater than 152 cm.

  (iii) If multiparae, parity not exceeding three previous births; age less than 35 years at booking.

Unfortunately, there are a number of illusions inherent in the application of this approach based on mortality ratios to selection of patients for general practitioner care. First, in view of improvements in both socio-economic circumstances and obstetric procedures, data adduced a quarter of a century ago may no longer be valid. Second, in terms of current national perinatal mortality rates (which in many places now approach ten per 1000 births), even if the mortality ratio were doubled ($M = 200$) in respect of a specific variable, women in that particular cohort would still have a 98 per cent probability of *not* experiencing a perinatal fetal loss. Third, risk factors often operate in combination—for example, low maternal age or high parity may be associated with low socioeconomic status, so that variables taken in isolation could be misleading. Indeed Feldstein (1966), by applying a multiple regression analysis method, confirmed that much of the observed high risk attributed to younger women in the 1958 survey was a reflection of their social class distribution and, when adjustment was made for this particular factor, youth proved to be an asset rather than a liability (see also Table 9.2).

Nevertheless, the use of the epidemiological approach in large cohorts of women to quantify the effect of certain maternal characteristics seemed an attractive basis on which to build a scoring system to apply for prospective risk prediction in individuals. A number of such systems have been described (Aubry and Pennington 1973); Haeri, South, and Naldrett 1974; Wilson and Sill 1973) but perhaps the best known (Chamberlain 1978) is reproduced in Table 9.1. As described, this method did indeed show that in groups of women with low antenatal risk scores, both perinatal mortality

Table 9.1 *The basis of the antenatal prediction score.* Source: Table 2.24 *British Births 1970*, Vol. 2

	Score
Maternal age	
20–29	0
<20 and 30–34	1
35 and over	2
Height >155 cm	1
Smokes five cigarettes or more per day	1
Parity	
1 and 2	0
0 and 3	1
4 and over	2
Social class	
I and II	0
III	1
IV, V and unemployed	2
Unsupported mothers (single, separated, divorced and widows)	2
Previous obstetric performance	
Stillbirth	4
Neonatal death	4
Abortion	4
Caesarean section	4
Antepartum haemorrhage	2
Postpartum haemorrhage	4
Immature delivery 36 weeks or less	2
Low birth weight infant (2500 g or less)	2
Medical history	
Hypertension (BP. 140/90 or more before 20 weeks gestation	4
Diabetes	4
Cardiac disease	4
Chronic respiratory disease	4
Chronic renal disease	4
Endocrine disease	4

rates and respiratory depression in the neonate were significantly better than those with higher scores. Unfortunately, as in many other epidemiological studies, the smaller the study group the greater becomes the standard error relating to measured outcomes and, when the method is applied to individuals, the sensitivity becomes very poor indeed.

A further problem concerns the weighting values allocated to particular maternal characteristics. For example (Table 9.1) a woman, para 1, aged 25, and social class II who had experienced a previous caesarean section would have the same antenatal risk score (4) as another, para 3, aged 33, social class IV with an unblemished obstetric history. Few responsible obstetricians would agree that the risk of a subsequent pregnancy in the first woman was no greater than that in the second! Risk prediction scores therefore, can at best only given an indication of broad probabilities regarding outcome when applied prospectively.

Moreover, although the perinatal mortality rate has been used for many years as the conventional index of outcome, this in itself becomes progressively less valid when applied to small populations (see Chapter 15) and, in the individual general practice, almost devoid of significance. Much more relevant to the general practitioner obstetrician therefore are prognostic indications of problems during pregnancy and difficulties during delivery. Some of the latter have been quantified in Chapter 8.

PRIMARY SELECTION FOR GENERAL PRACTITIONER CARE

Table 9.2 details some of the conventionally accepted maternal risk factors in pregnancy. It must however be obvious that many of these could be categorised as potential rather than actual and, if in practice every single one were excluded, few women would ultimately be deemed suitable for booking in GP care. A more realistic approach might therefore be to select out in the first instance patients with problems that could, with a high degree of certainty, be expected to warrant specialized care either in pregnancy or in labour. Risk classification at booking could then be presented as in Table 9.3 and the paramount importance of previous obstetric experience will be apparent. Women can then be categorized into three groups: those with actual, potential or no identified risk factors and thus may more reliably be allocated to appropriate booking systems for delivery. Women with established risks must be referred to consultant care; those with potential risk factors may in many cases (and after consultation) be booked to integrated or alongside general practitioner units (see Chapters 16 and 17) where advice or transfer of care is readily available, and only those women with no identifiable risk factor at all should be booked for home confinement or in isolated maternity units.

Table 9.2 *Risk factors in pregnancy*

General	Factors related to parity	
	Nulliparae	Multiparae
Unsupported mother	Small stature (<152 cm)	High parity (>4)
Social class IV or V	Age (<18 >30)	Age >35
Immigrant (especially Asian or West Indian)	Previous infertility	Antibodies (ABO or Rh)
Smokers (especially > ten/day)	Recurrent abortion	Previous: Stillbirth (SB) or neonatal death (NND)
Significant alcohol drinkers	Mid-trimester TOP	Forceps delivery
Obesity (>20 per cent overweight)		Retained placenta
Underweight (<5th centile)		Pospartum haemorrhage (PPH)
Diabetes (frank or chemical)		Pre-eclampsia
Hypertension		Growth retardation
Renal disease		Preterm delivery
Psychiatric disturbance		Myomectomy

Table 9.3 *Identification of pregnancy risk factors at booking*

Absolute	Relative
General: Heart disease Diabetes Hypertension Renal disease (excluding acute pyelitis) Rhesus or ABO isoimmunization Haemoglobinopathy	General: Social class IV, V or unsupported Immigrant (especially Asian or West Indian) Smoker (especially > ten/day) Significant alcohol drinkers (>2 units per day) Obesity (>20 per cent overweight) Underweight (<5th centile for height) Psychiatric disturbance Significant bacteriuria
Obstetric: Previous: Caesarean section, Myomectomy or hysterotomy Severe pre-eclampsia Rotational forceps Cervical incompetence Cervical surgery Pelvic pathology, such as fibroids, ovarian cyst or uterine deformity	Nulliparity Extremes of age (<18, >35) Small stature (<152 cm) High parity (>4) Previous: Stillbirth or neonatal death Postpartum haemorrhage Retained placenta Forceps delivery Preterm delivery (<37 weeks) Growth retardation syndrome Infant with congenital defect Spontaneous abortion or TOP Infertility (>1 year) Mild pre-eclampsia

Nulliparae present a special problem: although increasing age and small stature (Figs. 9.2 and 9.3) are generally sound predictors of abnormal delivery, many women within the conventionally accepted limits (age 18–29 years at booking; height greater than 152 cm) will nevertheless experience problems in labour, especially dystocia during the first stage. As yet there is no reliable method for predicting this complication antenatally and for this reason it is probably unwise ever to book nulliparae for delivery at home or in isolated general practitioner units unless special facilities for management are available.

SECONDARY SELECTION

So far, only criteria at booking for selection of women for general practitioner or specialist care have been considered. Numerous studies (Bull 1980; Dixon 1982; Lewis, Tipton, and Sloper 1978; Naftalin 1981; Richmond 1977) have however shown that absence of risk factors at the outset of a pregnancy is no guarantee that progress will henceforth be uncomplicated. In fact, up to one-third of low-risk mothers will require reappraisal of booking arrangements before the end of pregnancy (Chng, Hall and McGillivray 1980) and again this will be especially probable in the case of nulliparae (Bull 1983).

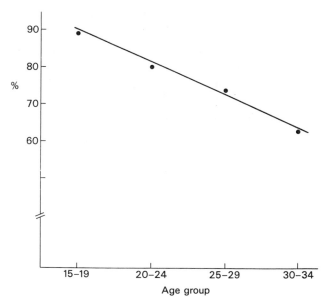

Fig. 9.2. Nulliparae: spontaneous delivery rate by age group. From Bull (1983), by courtesy of *Maternal and Child Health*.

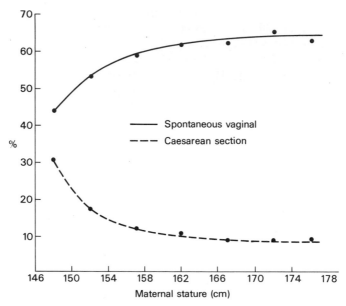

Fig. 9.3. Nulliparae: mode of delivery by maternal stature (Scotland, 1977). From Bull (1983), courtesy *Maternal and Child Health*.

Selection of women for community obstetric care must therefore be a dynamic process and any programme for antenatal examinations must be linked to the detection of new risk factors which might require modification of plans concerning the place of delivery. Table 9.4 illustrates some risk situations which can develop in pregnancy and which would not have been apparent at booking. Once more, they can be divided into an 'absolute' group, which are positive indications for transfer of care, and a 'relative' group concerning which the opinion of a consultant obstetrician may be advisable. In practice, patients in the latter group should not be delivered in isolated general practitioner maternity units or at home though bookings in integrated or alongside units may still be appropriate with specialist support (see Chapters 16 and 17). Conversely, there may be occasions later in pregnancy, when it becomes clear that anticipated complications in women booked for shared care (for example pre-eclampsia, growth retardation, preterm labour, malpresentation, etc.) have *not* occurred. In these instances it may well be justifiable to alter the booking from consultant to community care (general practitioner unit or home) and thereby achieve for the patient the ambience of continuity of care and low technology obstetrics that the latter system affords.

A progressive system linking risk detection and booking arrangements with routine antenatal care has been most succinctly described by Boddy,

Table 9.4. *Risk factors arising later in pregnancy*

Absolute	Relative
General: Gestational diabetes	Anaemia
Isoimmunization (Rh or ABO)	Glycosuria
Proteinuria (not urinary tract infection)	Vaginal infection especially beta-haemolytic strepto-coccus (BHS) or Herpes simplex virus (HSV)
	Poor weight gain
	Excess weight gain
Obstetric: Antepartum hemorrhage	Excess liquor
Pre-eclampsia	High head at term (nulliparae)
Raised serum alphafetoprotein	
Multiple pregnancy	
Preterm labour (<37 weeks)	
Malpresentation	
Unstable lie	
Small for dates	

Parboosingh and Shepherd (1980) and their charts for primary assessment and subsequent risk detection are reproduced in Figures 9.4 and 9.5. A further advantage of this system is that defined risk situations are allocated for formalize protocols for management which in most cases involve continued

NAME: .... **DOCTOR:** ....

BOOKING HISTORY
- Age less than 18 years
- Age over 38 years
- Primigravid age 30 years or more
- Parity = / more than 5.

LMP DETAILS
- LMP uncertain ± 2 weeks
- Pill stopped 1 or 2 periods before LMP
- Cycle length prior to LMP greater than 30 days
- IUCD in situ / on Pill after conception.
- Out of wedlock pregnancy
- Vaginal bleeding since LMP

PAST OBSTETRIC HISTORY
- SB / NND
- Small for dates (< 10 th centile)
- Large for dates (> 90 th centile)
- Fetal abnormality ....
- Antibodies in previous pregnancy
- Hypertension / eclampsia
- Termination of pregnancy / spontaneous abortion × 2
- Premature labour (20–37 weeks)
- Previous cervical suture
- Previous caesarean section
- PPH / MROP
- Labour of less than 4 hours

MATERNAL HEALTH
- Chronic illness / drugs ....
- Hypertension / proteinuria
- Infertility with medical advice
- Uterine anomaly including fibroids
- Smoking 10 / day at conception
- Social security benefits
- Isolated at home
- Family history of diabetes / fetal abnormality ....
- Completed by .... Date ....

BOOKING EXAMINATION
- BP = / more than 140/90
- Maternal weight = / more than 85 kg
- Maternal weight = / less than 45 kg
- Maternal height = / less than 1.5 m
- Cardiac murmur detected / referred
- Uterus large / small for dates
- Other pelvic mass detected
- Blood group rhesus negative
- Completed by .... Date ....

Fig. 9.4. Antenatal risk assessment card.

Weeks of pregnancy																	
FM not felt																	
Hb < 10 g %																	
Poor weight gain																	
Weight loss																	
Proteinuria																	
Glycosuria																	
Bacilluria																	
BP systolic >155																	
diastolic >88																	
Rhesus negative/antibodies																	
Uterus large for dates																	
Uterus small for dates																	
No increase in fundus (zone)																	
Excess liquor																	
Malpresentation																	
ECV successful																	
unsuccessful																	
Head not engaged																	
Any bleeding pV																	
Premature labour																	
Vaginal infection																	
Sign when completed																	
Insert date																	

Fig. 9.5. Risk factors arising during pregnancy.

participation by all relevant members of the primary care team. An example of the application of this approach in a socially deprived area has been described by McKee (1983). The greatly improved results in terms of perinatal mortality and other outcome indices is matched only by the approbation of the patients and the increased job satisfaction of the health care professionals involved. It seems therefore that such a system of progressive selection and monitoring is worthy of acceptance on a much wider scale and is equally appropriate to areas where there are alternative options regarding the ultimate place of delivery.

SUMMARY

The following then must be taken into account:
  (i) Normality in obstetrics is essentially a retrospective judgement.
 (ii) Formalized risk prediction systems based on perinatal mortality rates in large cohorts are of limited value in the case of individuals.
(iii) Past obstetric performance is the best predictor of future experience.

(iv) In nulliparae, small stature and advancing age increase the probability of abnormal delivery.

(v) Defined risk status should be tightly linked to planned place of delivery.

(vi) A progressive system of risk detection and problem management should be associated with routine antenatal care.

(vii) Excellent results associated with good compliance can be achieved by an appropriate community-based obstetric team approach.

REFERENCES

Aubry, R. H. and Pennington, J. C. (1973). Identification and evaluation of high risk pregnancy: the perinatal concept. *Clin. Obstet. Gynaecol.* **16**, 3–27.

Boddy, K., Parboosingh, I. J. T. and Shepherd, W. C. (1980). *A schematic approach to pre-natal care. Department of Obstetrics and Gynaecology*, Edinburgh University.

Bull, M. J. V. (1980). Ten years' experience in a general practice obstetric unit. *J. Roy. Coll. Gen. Practit.* **30**, 208–215.

Bull, M. J. V. (1983). Obstetrics: selection of patients for GP care. *Mat. Child Health* **8**, 84–90.

Butler, N. R. and Bonham, D. G. (1963). *Perinatal mortality.* E. and S. Livingstone, Edinburgh.

Chamberlain G. *et al.* (1978). In *British Births 1970. Vol. 2. Obstetric care.* William Heinemann, London, p. 40.

Chng, P. K., Hall, M. H. and MacGillivray, I. (1980). An audit of antenatal care: the value of the first visit. *Br. Med. J.* **2**, 1184–1186.

Dixon, E. A., (1982). Review of maternity patients suitable for home delivery. *Br. Med. J.* **1**, 1753–1755.

Feldstein, M. S. (1965). A binary variable multiple regression method of analysing factors affecting perinatal mortality and other outcomes of pregnancy. *J. Roy. Statistics Soc. Pt.I*, **129**, 61–73.

Haeri, A. D., South, J., and Naldrett, J. (1974). A scoring system for identifying pregnant patients with a high risk of perinatal mortality. *J. Obstet. Gynaecol. Br. Common.* **81**, 535–538.

Hospital Inpatient Enquiry (Maternity Services) 1974–76. (1979). HMSO, London.

Klein, M. *et al.* (1983). A comparison of low-risk pregnant women booked for delivery in two systems of care: shared care (consultant) and integrated general practice unit. I. Obstetrical procedure and neonatal outcome. II. Labour and delivery management and neonatal outcome. *Br. J. Obst. Gynaecol.* **90**, 118–122, 123–128.

Lewis, B. V., Tipton, R. H., and Sloper, I. M. S. (1978). Changing pattern in a general practitioner obstetric unit. *Br. Med. J.* **1**, 484–485.

McKee, I. (1983). The Sighthill Community antenatal care scheme. In *Pregnancy and its management* Macmillan, London.

Naftalin, N. J. (1981). Low risk obstetrics? *Practitioner* **225**, 209–211.

Richmond, G. A., (1977). An analysis of 3 199 patients booked for delivery in general practitioner obstetric units. *J. Roy. Coll. Gen. Practit.* **27**, 406–413.

Taylor, G. W. *et al.* (1980). How safe is general practitioner obstetrics? *Lancet* **2**, 1287–1289.

Wilson, E. W. and Sill, H. K. (1973). Identification of the high risk pregnancy by a scoring system. *NZ Med. J.* **78**, 437–440.

10 The fetal hazards in pregnancy

G. Chamberlain

Commonly the hazards of pregnancy are divided arbitrarily into those affecting the mother and those which might harm the fetus. This is an artificial dichotomy for what endangers one usually affects the other, but it is an analytical division which allows problems to be grouped into a classification. In this section we will deal with the hazards from the fetal aspect but it must be remembered that most have some effect on the mother in pregnancy and her subsequent life. Only the problems of singletons will be outlined.

The major hazards to the fetus can be judged by the principal causes of perinatal death or perinatal morbidity. In any study and in any country these stand out as:

(i)   Congenital abnormalities.
(ii) Low birthweight.
(iii) Hypoxia.

CONGENITAL ABNORMALITIES

Approximately 3 per cent of all babies born in the United Kingdom have a congenital abnormality. This proportion is irrespective of the age of the parents or any past history; it is the background figure at birth for the human species in the United Kingdom environment in this half century. Just after conception there is a much higher incidence of abnormalities but many are incompatible with development and die. Recent data from Southampton (Edmunds *et al.* 1982) indicate that about 40 per cent of pregnancies stop even before the next menstrual period (i.e. in the first 14 days of life) while 20 per cent more pregnancies are recognized to have aborted spontaneously. The vast majority of these known early pregnancy wastages were due to a congenital abnormality inconsistent with even intrauterine existence. Hence a large number of fertilized ova lead to gross abnormalities which are lost before birth.

Perhaps of more concern to the reader of this chapter is the woman who continues pregnancy with a congenital abnormality. Most common of the serious ones are those of the central nervous system; Table 10.1 shows a list

Table 10.1   *Congenital abnormalities reported from 16 994 singleton births in the British Births 1970 Survey (from Chamberlain 1976)*

Abnormality	SB	NND	Survivors	Total
Anencephaly	16	5	0	21
Spina bifida	3	3	8	14
Hydrocephaly	6	0	1	7
other CNS	1	0	1	2
Hip abnormality	1	0	140	141
Talipes	0	3	76	79
other orthopaedic	1	1	19	21
Alimentary system	1	4	46	51
Cardiorespiratory system	2	6	9	17
Urinary system	1	3	86	90
Down's syndrome	1	2	15	18
Other abnormalities	0	2	59	61
Total	33	29	460	522

of the common problems met in the United Kingdom. This table only summarizes the abnormalities diagnosed at birth.

AETIOLOGY OF CONGENITAL ABNORMALITIES

Congenital abnormalities may be structural or functional. Structural teratogenesis usually occurs before the formation of the organs and limbs is complete, that is before the 10th week of the pregnancy (Fig. 10.1). After that the same insults may still affect the fetus but cause functional problems which may be just as important as structural teratogenesis and alter the infant's way of life. A good example is rubella—in the first 10 weeks it may cause structural abnormalities. For the rest of intrauterine life, it may cause changes producing a chronic rubella syndrome with poor mental development and structural alterations in the central nervous system.

The known causes of abnormality are either genetic or environmental.

Genetic abnormalities

1. Inherited abnormalities. The tendency for this problem comes from one or other parent and is often associated with a recessive element in the other partner, for example hairlip or cleft palate.

2. Alterations may occur in the basic genetic material of one or other gamete, for example Down's syndrome which is associated with an ageing ovum (or maybe a sperm).

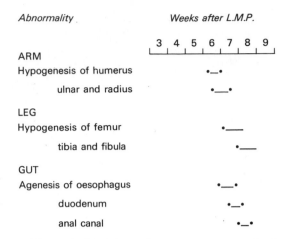

Fig. 10.1. The sensitive periods of the various organ systems of a fetus. Teratogenic insults applied during these times may cause an abnormality; outside these time periods, the organ system would probably not be effected structurally (from Chamberlain 1980).

Environmental causes

1. Infections may cause interference with the structural joining together of tubes or fusion of organ parts; for example rubella in early pregnancy may cause heart disease.

2. Drugs given at the crucial stage may be associated with abnormalities. The best example is that of thalidomide and phocomelia but there have been many other less dramatic examples since 1960 such as progestogens given in early pregnancy which may cause pseudomasculization in a female fetus. Pregnant women read in the popular press about these and are worried. They will turn to their practitioner for advice so it is as well to be ahead of the current newspapers and magazines.

In the United Kingdom the Committee on Safety of Medicines is well aware of this problem and is watching carefully. Over 500 drugs have been reported to the Committee but so far the only probable teratogens shown are:

thalidomide
aminopterine
19-alpha-progestogens
testosterone
quinine

In addition to these the following drugs may be possible teratogens:

cortisone
sulphonylurea

tetracycline
serotonin

3. Biophysical methods such as X-rays transmitted in early pregnancy may be teratogenic because of the high energy output of the radiation. Worry has been raised about the use of ultrasound but this is a very much lesser energy source and so is safe.

4. Oxygen deficit in early pregnancy to a normal woman may affect the fetus; for example an anaesthetic with a poor oxygen supply. This is exceedingly rare in normal anaesthetic practice.

5. Nutritional deficits. There has been recent work giving strong indications that there may be an association between a deficiency of some vitamins before pregnancy (Laurence *et al.* 1981; Smithells *et al.* 1981*a* and *b*) and an increased incidence of central nervous system abnormalities. Similarly, the studies published so far justify a substantial suspicion but no randomized controlled study has yet been performed. Until this is done practitioners should be cautious in offering vitamins before pregnancy as a sure prevention of central nervous system abnormalities.

When all these causes are considered, in less than 10 per cent of women who have an abnormal baby can an association be found. The other 90 per cent of cases have no obvious associated causal factor.

DIAGNOSIS OF ABNORMALITIES

Many of the abnormalities diagnosed at birth are incapable of detection before delivery. The general practitioner obstetrician may sometimes have some suspicion because the woman has polyhydramnios or oligohydramnios, both of which paradoxically are associated with an increased rate of major congenital abnormalities of different systems. By the time these shifts in amniotic fluid volume are detected, it is too late to take any useful action.

It is more practical therefore to try to diagnose abnormalities early enough in pregnancy for the woman and her partner to be offered therapeutic abortion and thus prevent them having a congenitally abnormal baby. It is allowed by law to offer termination of pregnancy up to 28 weeks' gestation but most obstetricians have a more pragmatic cutoff point at 22–24 weeks.

Termination of pregnancy is not preventing congenital abnormalities but merely stopping affected babies being born and so is a secondary defence mechanism. It is not acceptable to many Christians and those who hold other faiths in the wider world and advice should be tempered against the general practitioner's knowledge of the couple's religious beliefs.

Two major groups of abnormalities that can be detected in the antenatal period are those of the central nervous system, mainly open spina bifida and anencephaly, and major abnormalities of the chromosome system such as trisomy in the 21 position which leads to Down's syndrome.

CNS abnormalities

CNS abnormalities may be detected if the central canal of the nervous system is open to the amniotic fluid sac. A higher concentration of alpha-fetoprotein, produced in the fetus, is secreted into the liquor and from here it is absorbed into the maternal bloodstream leading to raised maternal serum levels of this fetal protein. This does not happen with closed abnormalities of the central nervous system and so the test could not detect hydrocephaly or spina bifida occulta.

Screening requires a 10 ml sample of the mother's venous blood in which the alphafetoprotein level is estimated. The upper level of normal may vary from one laboratory to another and is commonly taken as two-and-a-half times the median level. Fig. 10.2 shows how results are critically dependent upon the gestational age; hence any woman who has an alphafetoprotein test should have an ultrasound estimation of fetal gestational age. If the level is found to be elevated above the accepted normal range, a second blood test should be arranged within a week. If this too is elevated the woman should be referred for an amniocentesis under ultrasound cover. This will allow the placenta and fetus to be localized and so avoided; liquor will be removed for amniotic fluid estimations of alphafetoprotein.

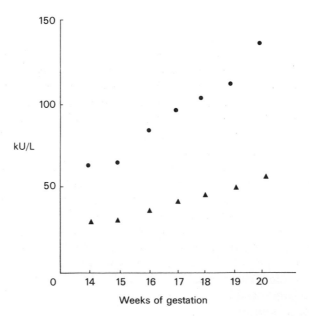

Fig. 10.2. The median ▲ + 2.5 × the median ● indicating the upper limit of normal and alphafetaprotein levels at different stages of gestation. Since the alteration is so great, the gestation must be accurately timed so that the result should be valid.

The amniotic fluid level of alphafetoprotein has a high predictive rate and a low false positive estimation rate. If it too is above the accepted levels of the normal, there is probably an open central nervous system abnormality and termination of pregnancy may be recommended to the couple with some surety, assuming that the practitioner knows the couple would wish this to be the method of coping with this pregnancy.

Raised alphafetoprotein levels are not only indicative of central nervous system abnormalities. They also are found in women who have had a threatened abortion, twin pregnancy and among those who are further on for dates than are expected. It is a non-specific guide to the baby who may later on show growth retardation in the uterus, although this association is weak.

In some centres, careful ultrasound scans made at 16–18 weeks are used to check the spine. If a good ultrasonographer examines the spine, this has as high a pickup rate as a screening test as alphafetoprotein testing.

Chromosomal changes

The other group of abnormalities which may be screened for are those associated with chromosomal changes. Most of these are Down's syndrome (mongolism). Here there is an extra chromosome in position 21—trisomy 21. The baby is born with a characteristic face and creases on the palms (which are less indicative of the condition than the facial features). The child will grow up to be mentally subnormal but often is a happy and contented member of the family, although the mental age may never rise above 4–6 years. There is a high incidence of congenital abnormality of the heart and gut in those with Down's syndrome and these may be the cause of infant death but the baby is unlikely to die of Down's syndrome itself. It is probably the commonest single cause of mental retardation found in the infant and adolescent population.

The diagnosis of Down's syndrome in the unborn fetus may be considered after an amniocentesis which extracts fetal cells. These are cultured and following about 20 days of growth are killed and exploded with colchicine which allows an examination of the individual chromosomes.

There are no external indicators that Down's syndrome may be present. The risk of this condition increases with maternal age (Table 10.2), the increased risk being mostly over the age of 40 years. This is irrespective of whether this is a first or subsequent baby. There is some evidence to suggest that maybe the age of the father has an effect also.

The problem facing the general practitioner is who to recommend for amniocentesis for potential chromosomal abnormalities. Examination of Table 10.2 shows that once 40 years of maternal age has passed, the risk of Down's syndrome is less than one in 100. Amniocentesis itself is not without some risk and in many centres the cumulative risk of abortion or fetal

Table 10.2 *Risks of having a liveborn child with Down's syndrome by maternal age* (from Hook and Chambers, 1977). *The risk of recurrence of Down's syndrome due to trisomy-21 is about one in 100 irrespective of maternal age*

Woman's age	Risk
20	1/1923
21	1/1695
22	1/1538
23	1/1408
24	1/1299
25	1/1205
26	1/1124
27	1/1053
28	1/990
29	1/935
30	1/885
31	1/826
32	1/725
33	1/592
34	1/465
35	1/365
36	1/287
37	1/225
38	1/177
39	1/139
40	1/109
41	1/85
42	1/67
43	1/53
44	1/41
45	1/32
46	1/25
47	1/20
48	1/16
49	1/12

damage is 1 per cent. This includes the chances of stimulating the uterus to contract, so causing abortion within a few days of the amniocentesis, allowing a transplacental perfusion, damage to the fetus directly by the needle and a chronic leak of liquor subsequently which may lead to flexion deformities of the fetus (hip and ankle problems), preterm labour and intrauterine growth retardation. With the incidence of all these risks about 1 per cent, it is probably wise for a practitioner to recommend that a woman over 40 years has an amniocentesis to check for Down's syndrome which itself has an incidence of about 1 per cent at that age.

Those between 35 and 40 years who request this investigation present a problem. Reference to Table 10.2 shows that at these ages the risks of

Down's syndrome are considerably less than those of performing the test itself. For example at 38 years the risk of Down's syndrome is one in 240 whereas the risks of the test itself still stay at one in 100. However sometimes the woman and her husband will consider the problems of producing a baby with Down's syndrome so enormous that the general practitioner and his consultant colleagues in hospital will be pressured to agree to amniocentesis even though they know that they have a greater chance of harming a normal child than detecting an abnormal one.

In the age group under 35 years the risks of the test now are so much greater than those of the abnormality presenting that most obstetricians advise the practitioner not to recommend patients to ask for amniocentesis.

This position may alter in the next few years as the risks of amniocentesis are reduced but it is an invasive procedure which may affect the fetus and his development in the uterus. The age of universal amniocentesis for all pregnant women is not here for two major reasons:

(i) The risks of the test are greater in most pregnant women than the risk of the condition for which they are looking.

(ii) There are not enough skilled ultrasonographers who can perform amniocentesis available in the country; to offer amniocentesis to younger women would block the service for those who have a greater need of care.

Other congenital abnormalities

Other congenital abnormalities may be detected at an antenatal scan such as renal agenesis, polycystic kidneys and ureteric obstruction; changes in the ventricles and septa of the heart; atresia of parts of the bowel. All need more than usually skilled obstetricians who are keen on ultrasound work.

Fetoscopy

Fetoscopy involves passing an endoscope into the uterine cavity under local anaesthesia. It helps detect those abnormalities which can be seen and allows sampling of fetal blood. For example hairlip and cleft palate cannot be diagnosed by ultrasound but fetoscopy, for those who had previously given birth to babies of such facial abnormalities, allows their lesions to be readily seen. Fetal blood sampling can be important for the intrauterine diagnosis of haemoglobinopathies such as thalassaemia.

LOW BIRTH WEIGHT

Probably the major problem of fetal risk in the United Kingdom at present is low birth weight. Over two-thirds of babies who die in the perinatal period have a birth weight below 2500 g. The League of Nations term *prematurity* is not now used for it grouped together two disparate populations of babies:

(i)   The baby who is born too soon but has a birth weight appropriate for the gestational age; for example, the mother may deliver a child of 32 weeks' gestation weighing 1800 g, a birth weight consistent with that stage of gestation.

(ii)   At any stage of gestation the baby might be born lighter than the 10th centile for birth weight for babies of that gestation (Figure 10.3). This baby is light for dates for he is smaller than the appropriate stage of gestation.

The two groups have entirely different prognoses: the baby who follows a preterm labour usually does well if he can be kept alive. The latter child has the worser prognosis and is harder to manage.

Low birth weight babies following preterm labour

A preterm labour is defined as one before the 37th week of gestation but the babies that really concern us are those born before the 34th week.

Aetiology

Labour may start early and usually the reason is unknown. Expulsive uterine contractions commence at an inappropriate time in an apparently normal woman. Amongst the known causes are:

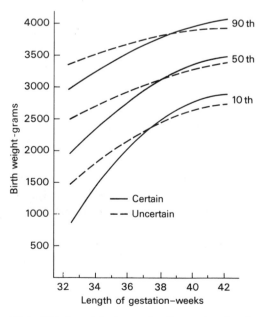

Fig. 10.3. Centiles of birth weight by week of gestation for those who were sure and those unsure of their last normal menstrual period (from Chamberlain 1976).

(i) Cervical incompetence; the cervix has been dilated previously at operation or delivery and the sphincter mechanism has not been restored.

(ii) Premature rupture of the membranes; this may be associated with cervical incompetence or may occur spontaneously with a tightly closed cervix. It might be a feature of poor nutrition causing alteration in the strength of the membranes.

(iii) Multiple pregnancy and hydramnios; these may trigger labour to start early following overdistension of the uterus.

(iv) Abruptio placentae; bleeding in the placental bed separates the placenta from the maternal blood supply. The fetus commonly dies and if not, he is at extreme hazard; labour follows the bleed very soon because of irritation of the myometrium.

(v) Iatrogenic causes; some women are induced preterm because of severe pre-eclampsia or rhesus disease, reasons which concern the practitioner.

Diagnosis

Either the preterm labour starts with a spontaneous rupture of the membranes, accompanied by a gush of amniotic fluid down the vagina or painful uterine contractions are felt. The differential diagnosis of amniotic fluid escaping from the vagina is sometimes difficult. Urine and even bath water have been confused with it. The characteristic smell of amniotic fluid should be recognized by most experienced general practitioner obstetricians. More difficult is the diagnosis of potentially expulsive uterine contractions (in other words, labour). For some women in pregnancy the Braxton Hicks contractions can be painful for such women have a greater sensitivity and notice them more, particularly in the middle of the night. There is no precise way of differentiating between painful Braxton Hicks contractions and labour contractions. A tocograph can show an increased amplitude of uterine contractions but this in itself is not diagnostic, and only if these contractions are associated with cervical dilatation can the diagnosis be fully made.

Management

The practitioner who is called to a woman who thinks she is in preterm labour needs to confirm the diagnosis. The history and examination points mentioned above must all be considered but probably the best diagnostic feature is sitting with the woman for about 20 minutes with a hand on her abdomen. Alternatively, and speedier, a vaginal examination will demonstrate the state of the os. If it is closed and unripe then it is almost certain that labour has not commenced and an alternative diagnosis must be sought for the symptoms. If after careful evaluation the practitioner is still in doubt then he should consider that she is in preterm labour and act accordingly.

Such a woman must be delivered in a centre that has good facilities to care for immature babies. It is not good practice to deliver small babies in general practitioner units and then have them transferred by the paediatric flying squad. The best incubator for a small baby is the mother's uterus and she should travel with the baby *in utero*, even in labour, to the centre where the baby can be looked after. The United Kingdom is a small country and there are very few parts where a woman could not reach such a special hospital within an hour.

In hospital, management will depend upon whether the membranes are ruptured, how far the cervix is dilated and the stage of gestation. Obstetricians may try to suppress uterine contractions if labour has not progressed too far and the membranes are intact. The individual decision would depend upon the facilities available in the special care baby unit adjacent to the obstetrical department.

Light-for-dates babies

Aetiology

Intrauterine growth retardation usually occurs with no obvious cause. There are two major types of factor under which causes are often grouped.

(i)   Decreased genetic potential for growth.

(ii)   The failure of adequate nutrients to be provided for the fetus.

Among these factors, the following causes have been identified:

(i)   Among the genetic features are the mother's and father's size which affect the size of the infant; chromosomal defects also can influence birth weight.

(ii)   The number of babies sharing the uterus will influence the weight; the mean weight of singleton babies at birth in the United Kingdom is 2920 g (7.3 lbs), that of twins is 2323 g (5.2 lbs).

(iii)   Maternal nutrition is critical if the woman is at near starvation level; otherwise, diet has very little influence on the fetal size.

(iv)   Drugs can affect fetal size, for example cigarette smoking, alcohol and heroin.

(v)   Chronic congenital infection such as rubella are associated with light-for-dates babies.

(vi)   Maternal diseases may be associated with poor placental perfusion, for example, pre-eclampsia and chronic hypertension.

Prevention

Many of the above factors contributing to intrauterine growth retardation cannot be modified (for example, parental size, or multiple pregnancy). However, for the general practitioner there are three major factors that can be modified and one or more of them apply to the majority of his antenatal women. These are smoking, alcohol and work. Because of the preventive possibilities it is worth considering these three factors in greater detail.

Smoking. More women are smoking cigarettes now than at any time since data have been collected. In the *British births survey 1970*, 59 per cent of women having babies reported having smoked cigarettes.

The effect of smoking on the unborn child is seen in a mean lower birth weight among those born to smoking mothers. This is probably due to reduced placental transfer, either by reduction in the placental bed perfusion or exchange of nutrients across the placental membranes. It may be due to substances in cigarette smoke (such as nicotine) or it may be an effect on the transport of oxygen in fetal tissues through competing chemicals, such as carboxyhaemoglobin. In addition, it is possible that the lifestyle of a woman who smokes cigarettes is different from that of other women; her appetite and eating habits may be altered or her digestive processes may be affected by cigarette smoke ingestion.

Whatever the aetiology, it is an accepted fact that babies born to smoking mothers are lighter at birth by about 7 g per cigarette smoked a day. Thus a woman who smokes one pack of cigarettes a day will probably have a baby 140 g lighter in birthweight. Unfortunately, the effect does not stop with weight alone. The maturity of the fetus is slightly reduced and follow-up studies have shown that the ability of children of smoking mothers to read and comprehend is diminished at 7 years and 11 years. These last data may relate, of course, to being brought up in a household with a smoking mother (and sometimes father) but they have a correlation with the effects in pregnancy itself.

There is no lower limit of numbers smoked a day below which it is safe. In consequence, the only theoretical advice to give a woman asking about smoking in pregnancy is to stop it completely. However, the practitioner must weigh this up against the risks that he knows the woman will undergo by deprivation and increased stress.

Alcohol. Alcohol ingestion by women in the western world is increasing. Depending upon the classification of intake, data vary but probably 70 per cent of women take some alcohol and 5 per cent are heavy imbibers just before and in pregnancy.

Heavy drinkers are more likely to produce a baby with the fetal alcohol syndrome. These have a characteristic face with squashed-up features, a low birth weight, low intelligence and an increased risk of all abnormalities of the internal organs. About 40 per cent of women who drink more than 142 ml of alcohol a week produce babies of this nature in America but the incidence in the United Kingdom is much lower. Lesser degress of alcohol intake are also unfortunately associated with an increased rate of mid-trimester abortions and low birth weight.

There is a close relationship between the amount of alcohol taken and the effect on the fetus and there is no safe limit to alcohol consumption. The ideal advice should therefore be to drink nothing in or just before pregnancy. The practitioner must, however, balance this up against the stress that such advice could cause a woman who is used to taking a little alcohol. He must come to a clinical compromise about what is best for her and her unborn child.

Work. In the western world, more women are both working in pregnancy and working later. Many couples enter marriage planning for two salaries to provide for necessities such as a mortgage. Should a pregnancy come unexpectedly, this interferes with financial planning. Further, more women are now entering professions and trades which have promotion programmes; it is an unfortunate fact of life that the years of advancement are the years of childbearing (25–35 years). For both these reasons, women are working more in pregnancy.

Certain jobs have specific hazards, such as those in the radiation industry. This does not just mean working in X-ray departments, but perhaps in the security team of an airport or in factories where X-rays examine faults in metals. Some chemicals, such as herbicides and cleaning chemicals, may have an effect on the unborn child and should be specifically excluded. If the practitioner is consulted but is uncertain about any specific job, the Health and Safety Executive will advise about the known specific hazards.

The effects of work itself are harder to assess than those of the drugs and other habits like alcohol and tobacco. It would seem obvious that heavy work and tiredness would have a deleterious effect on women but these are hard to measure. Preliminary studies in Europe show that fatigue in the first half of pregnancy relates to both an increase in preterm labours and in low birth weight babies. There is the additional problem of getting to work. In a metropolitan area this may involve an hour at each end of the day travelling in smoky, unpleasant, fatiguing conditions. This might be worse than the work itself.

Not all aspects of paid employment are deleterious. Some women may have an easier life in the workplace than at home. There may be rest rooms and meals provided. Further, a woman in paid work can take time off if she is feeling unwell, something that cannot be done in the home. In addition to paid work, all women work in the home. This should not be ignored by the practitioner, for where there is a large family this load may be enormous.

Diagnosis

The diagnosis of intrauterine growth retardation is sometimes difficult clinically. In a recent study in Aberdeen, Hall and Chng (1982) showed the deficiencies of clinical diagnosis. Among approximately 19000 women attending for antenatal care over several years, intrauterine growth retardation was overdiagnosed by about three times its true incidence of those who were born with the condition; less than half had not been diagnosed in the clinic.

Such results can be improved on by avoiding interobserver variation. Here, the service offered by the general practitioner obstetrician shows benefits, for he sees his patients for antenatal care himself more than does the hospital obstetrician who shares the load with many junior staff. In addition to the size of the fetus, the amount of amniotic fluid can be gauged clinically. If this is felt to be deficient, it is a guide for further investigation.

The diagnosis of intrauterine growth retardation is best made by a series of ultrasound readings. Since one cannot tell which women are going to produce a baby with this condition, it is wise to have a basal ultrasound measurement of biparietal diameter (BPD) made before 20 weeks of pregnancy in all women. After this, a second reading should be taken at about 30 weeks to confirm normal growth. If this is depressed (Fig. 10.4), or if the practitioner is concerned clinically, other readings can be taken to assess the condition. A more precise measure is made these days by estimating the abdominal circumference of the fetus and comparing that with the circumference of the head. Serial readings indicate poor growth.

Management

No treatment for intrauterine growth retardation is as useful as bedrest. By doing this it is hoped that a greater amount of blood perfuses through the placental bed because less is going to the limbs and back muscles. Other treatments have been tried but most have been found wanting. Abdominal decompression, intra-amniotic perfusion of glucose and protein, hyperalimentation and drugs which may influence placental bed flow have all had their advocates, but none have been shown to be significantly successful. Final treatment will be delivering the baby at the appropriate time when the risks of staying inside the uterus become greater than the risks of being outside in a good neonatal unit. In consequence, the woman should be in a hospital associated with such a competent neonatal unit for the last weeks of pregnancy.

HYPOXIA

The oxygen required for the fetus comes across the placenta, carried there in the mother's blood in red blood corpuscles. The maternal haemoglobin (HbA) gives up oxygen which disolves in the maternal plasma, passes across the placental membrane by passive difusion from a solution of higher oxygen tension to that of lower oxygen tension. It dissolves in the fetal plasma and is finally picked up in the fetal corpuscles attached to fetal haemoglobin (HbF). This has a greater affinity for oxygen than does HbA so the fetus

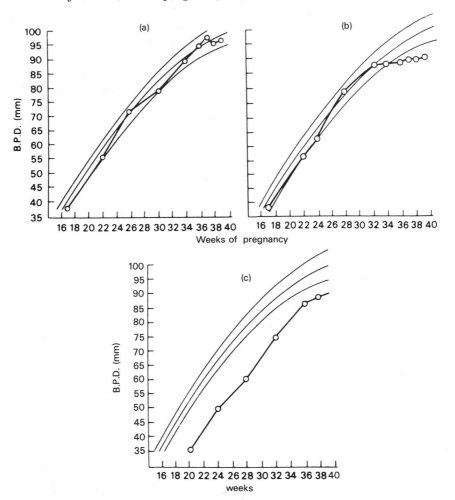

Fig. 10.4. Three women who had biparietal diameters measured with ultrasound throughout pregnancy. (a) This woman is normal and all the readings fall between the two standard deviations on either side of the mean for a normal population. (b) Fetal growth has started to slow from 31 weeks of pregnancy and there is little increase. It is doubtful if an obstetrician in the 1980s would allow this situation to go on for as long as this recording which was made in 1976, for that fetus is at grave risk from hypoxia in labour. (c) This woman was unsure of her dates. If the readings were all placed back by 4 weeks, they would fall inside two standard deviations on either side of the mean and thus show normal growth of a normal fetus (from Chamberlain 1980).

achieves reasonable oxygenation in the uterus. If there is anything wrong with the carriage of oxygen to the placental bed, the perfusion of oxygen at the central membrane or the pick up by the fetal red cell, then the fetus becomes hypoxic.

There are few conditions in pregnancy that cause this. Most of the risk of fetal hypoxia comes in labour when the uterus is contracting and pinching the blood vessels on the maternal side of the placental bed. However, any condition which causes malperfusion of nutrients in pregnancy may also lead to that of hypoxia once the uterus starts contracting, for example, maternal hypertension.

The cutoff of oxygen supply in pregnancy itself can follow a disaster such as abruptio placentae where the vessels of the placental bed go into spasm so that even the part of the placenta which is not separated from its attachment by blood clot is not perfused adequately enough to keep the fetus alive. Of the past are most of the severe conditions such as syphilis, which caused such gross pathological changes of the placenta in pregnancy that chronic antepartum hypoxia followed. Other than these, most hypoxic events are in labour (see Section C).

MATERNAL FACTORS THAT INFLUENCE FETAL HAZARD

Having described the major fetal hazards of pregnancy in some detail, one may now look at the application of these as the practitioner sees them in his surgery. Some of the higher risk factors affecting the fetus during pregnancy are shown in Table 10.3. They are grouped under biological headings.

Maternal history

These are all laid down when the practitioner first sees the woman and so cannot be altered. Age and parity have their effect on pregnancy (Chapter 8). Similarly, lower socioeconomic class and, equally important, unsupported mothers, have been known to have an association with poor fetal outcome. However, these may be added to by other features as shown in Figs. 10.5 and 10.6, where the compounding effect of poor socioeconomic class on pre-eclampsia and congenital abnormalities is shown. Thus, if a woman is of a higher socioeconomic class, it would seem that the effect of severe pre-eclampsia is much less on the fetus than if she is of class V or, worse still, an unsupported mother. With facets of unchangeable biological background like this, the practitioner should direct most of his efforts in antenatal care to prevent problems arising (see Chapter 12).

The past poor obstetrical history weights the chances of this baby greatly. Whatever caused the problems in the previous pregnancy probably still exist and may be compounded by the fact that the woman is now a little older and of higher parity.

Rhesus incompatibility is now no longer a major problem since the active use of antiD immunization after delivery. However, practitioners should

Table 10.3   *The higher risk factors affecting the fetus in pregnancy*

Maternal factors
Increasing age
Nulliparity and high multiparity
Low social class
Poor obstetric history
Rhesus incompatibility

Maternal disease
Hypertensive conditions
    Chronic hypertension
    Pre-eclampsia
Renal disease
Diabetes
Severe cardiac disease
Anaemia
Haemoglobinopathies

Fetomaternal conditions
Preterm and small-for-dates babies
Postmaturity

Fetal conditions
Multiple fetuses
Congenital abnormalities

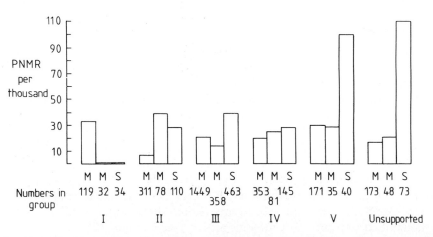

Fig. 10.5. The interacting effect of the socioeconomic class and pre-eclampsia. It will be seen in the social classes I, II, III and IV, that pre-eclampsia has little effect on the perinatal mortality rate even when it is severe (diastolic blood pressure over 100 mmHg and proteinuria). However in social class V and even more in the unsupported women, the existence of the same degree of pre-eclampsia is associated with a sharp rise in perinatal mortality. It would seem that in social classes I to IV, there is some relative buffering of the effects of pre-eclampsia.

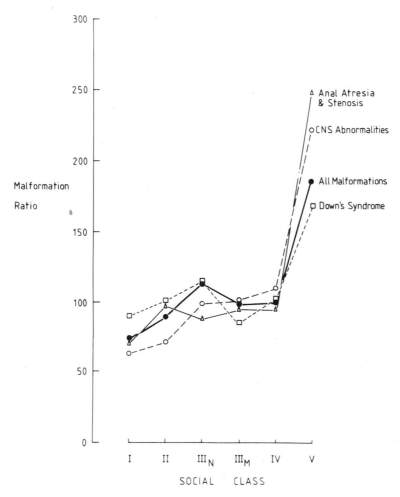

Fig. 10.6. The interacting effect of socioeconomic class and congenital abnormalities. The mortality ratio shown in this figure relates the expected number of abnormalities against the number actually found. A ratio of 100 implies that the expected number were present. Above this is an increase in congenital abnormalities and below a decreased incidence. It is seen that social classes I, II, III (both manual and non-manual) and IV, have below or about the expected number of abnormalities. Social class V, however, is grossly increased for all abnormalities and for certain specified systems as shown.

remember that occasionally women slip through the net of the hospital, particularly those delivered at weekends. They may have a pregnancy which finished early (an abortion or an ectopic) and so again might miss being given antiD gammaglobulin. All pregnancies in rhesus negative women should be carefully watched to see whether this programme has been completed.

Maternal disease

Maternal hypertension and pre-eclampsia both put the fetus at higher risk for low birth rate and hypoxia by reducing placental perfusion so that the fetus has a poorer supply of nutrients in pregnancy and a diminished oxygen reserve in labour. Renal disease affects the fetus through its effect on hypertension.

Diabetes may also cause placental malperfusion, but in addition, metabolic and carbohydrate problems to the mother can affect the fetus. An imbalanced metabolism may lead to acidaemia and even ketaemia; these metabolites cross the placenta easily and may affect fetal metabolism. There is some evidence that strict control of blood sugar levels in pregnancy diminishes the graver effects of maternal diabetes on the fetus.

Heart disease anaemia and haemoglobinopathies have to be very severe before a major fetal affect occurs. They all would affect the fetus by hypoxaemia if the disease was bad enough. Such women should be watched in labour for they might achieve low partial pressures of oxygen at this time of pregnancy.

Fetomaternal conditions

The problems of preterm and small-for-dates babies have been outlined previously in this chapter. They are different and one should not extrapolate from one group to the other merely because of a low birth weight. Postmaturity affects the fetus mostly through a diminution in placental perfusion and transfer. Placental metabolism can be readily shown to fade after 37–38 weeks and transfer probably follows this. Certainly babies of over 42 weeks stand labour less well, and the combination of a series of uterine contractions and poor placental exchange may be too much for a fetus who is a little larger than an earlier one. In consequence, any woman who is sure of her dates (or has had them checked by ultrasound), and goes past 42 weeks is probably putting her fetus at higher risk. There should be good grounds for allowing the pregnancy to proceed beyond this point and discussion with consultant colleagues is wise.

Fetal conditions

Congenital abnormalities have been outlined earlier in this chapter. The major action currently which the practitioner can take in suitable couples is abortion of those babies who have established central nervous system abnormalities or Down's syndrome or the prevention of congenital abnormalities by the avoidance of known teratogens such as infection and X-rays in early pregnancy.

CONCLUSIONS

In this chapter I have tried to outline the major hazards that affect the fetus during pregnancy. These all act through the major causes of fetal hazard and so can best be followed logically in this way. The number of women affected probably make up less than 5 per cent of the antenatal population the practitioner sees. However, it would probably be in this group that antenatal care would have its greatest benefit and it is therefore on them that the efforts of the antenatal maternity team should be most concentrated. In many cases acute episodes need to be treated in hospital, but with good and preplanned cooperation there is no reason why the practitioner should not take part in the care of such women throughout pregnancy, delivery and in the postpartum period.

Acknowledgements

I am grateful to Blackwell's Medical Publishers for allowing me to reprint Figures 10.1 and 10.4 from *Lecture Notes in Obstetrics*.

REFERENCES

Chamberlain, G. (1976). British Birth Survey 1970, Volume 1. Heinemann Medical Books, London.

Chamberlain, G. (1980). *Lecture notes in obstetrics*. Blackwell's Medical Publishers, Oxford.

Chamberlain, G., Philipp, E., Howlett, B., and Masters, K. (1978). *British births, 1970, volume 2*. Heinemann Medical Books, London.

Edmunds, D., Lindsay, K., Miller, J., Williamson, E., and Wood, P. (1982). Early embryonic mortality in women. *Fertil. Steril.* **38**, 447–453.

Hall, M. and Chng, P. (1982). Antenatal care in practice. In *Effectiveness and satisfaction in antenatal care* (ed. M. Erkin and I. Chalmers), p. 60. Heinemann Medical Books, London.

Laurence, K. M., James, N., Miller, M., Tennant, G., and Campbell, H. (1981). Double blind randomised controlled trial of folate treatment before conception to prevent recurrence of neural tube defects. *Br. Med. J.* **282**, 1509-1511.

Smithells, R. W. *et al.* [8 authors] (1981*a*). Vitamin supplementation and neural tube defects. *Lancet* **2**, 1425.

Smithells, R. W. *et al.* [8 authors] (1981*b*). Apparent prevention of neural tube defects by periconceptional vitamin supplementation. *Arch. Dis. Child.* **56**, 911–918.

11 A critical evaluation of modern techniques for fetal assessment during pregnancy

K. A. Godfrey

Pregnancy and childbirth are essentially physiological processes which should culminate in the safe delivery of a new semi-independent, healthy individual to happy parents. Sadly, this is not always the case.

The occurrence of disease associated with pregnancy and childbirth remains unacceptably high; it is reflected crudely in perinatal mortality terms (15/1000 live births or three deaths for every 200 live births in England and Wales, 1979) but also in a substantial morbidity rate amongst survivors (Chamberlain 1981). Considerable improvements continue to be evident in preventing maternal mortality and yet in the triennium 1976–78 more than 400 potential mothers died in England and Wales either as a direct result of pregnancy and childbirth or from associated causes (Report of Confidential Enquiries into Maternal Mortality 1976–78—1982).

Heightened interest in improving both fetal and maternal outcome has prompted the advent of improved techniques for assessing fetal normality, growth and health. However, a number of reservations must be expressed in their use.

One must avoid the 'blind-faith' school of non-thought which unquestioningly accepts that any new modality must improve the precision of diagnosis and must perforce reflect underlying truth. It is imperative that disciples of our specialty are first encouraged to develop clinical acumen based upon personal observation and educated discussion. Only with this background can any clinician hope to make valid judgements and utilize available investigations to best advantage. There is a risk that the modern clinician may become a dispassionate interpreter of laboratory tests and diagnostic techniques, justifying treatment solely on the basis of deviation away from an accepted range of measurements. This is particularly true of obstetrics, where one of the patients is unavailable for physical examination.

The evolution of fetal assessment during pregnancy has invoked tremendous changes in the techniques used, in the understanding of some disease processes and interpretation of results and also in the subsequent management of many pregnancy-associated disorders. Vigilance must be maintained in order that unwarranted conflict between maternal and fetal interests is not precipitated. A number of policies advocated in the genuine belief that they reduce fetal risk may well have potentially detrimental implications for the mother. The decision to expose any mother to a possible hazard must be taken on the basis of sound scientific and/or epidemiological evidence and not upon the results of unproved methods of assessment.

In this chapter, diagnostic tools currently utilized to assess fetal welfare are considered and critically appraised. Despite the reservations already expressed it is important to realize that the available techniques can prove extremely valuable if correctly employed. Furthermore, negligence may be alleged if they are not used.

The wisest counsel must be thoughtful use and interpretation of diagnostic indices in the context of the clinical disorder; not blind faith that the techniques will unmask unsuspected abnormalities or that they will unerringly reflect the true fetal condition.

In order to reduce perinatal mortality and morbidity, fetal assessment must aim to identify the three major determinants of poor perinatal outcome, namely congenital abnormalities, low birth weight and birth asphyxia. The first two are dealt with in this chapter, the third is discussed in Chapter 23.

SELECTION OF AT RISK PREGNANCIES

The major problem encountered in applying techniques of fetal assessment is knowing which pregnancies to investigate. Logistically it is not possible or efficient use of resources to monitor every pregnancy in the same detail; some method of selection is mandatory. However, it has to be accepted that whatever the method(s) of screening, the prediction and detection of problems by current antenatal procedures remain unacceptably inaccurate. Present programmes are dogged by insensitivity (for example less than half the cases of intrauterine growth retardation (<5th centile) are detected on clinical grounds), and also by non-specificity, since when suspicion and detection rates are increased, an increasing number of normal babies are included in the high-risk group.

An efficient screening procedure should separate high-risk from low-risk by its application to the non-selected population as a whole. Fig. 11.1 demonstrates a scheme for antenatal management suggested by the author.

SCREENING PROCEDURES

General application to unselected population

History and examination
A thorough history and examination at the booking clinic, may in statistical terms (Chapter 8) identify those mothers at increased risk of a complicated

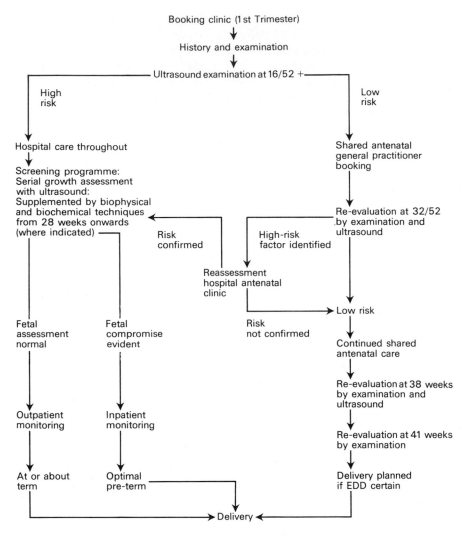

Fig. 11.1. Antenatal management.

pregnancy. Table 11.1 illustrates many of the most significant factors which may be recognized at the booking visit. Within Table 11.1 however are historical factors of grave import (such as previous caesarean section), those of trivial import (such as previous termination of pregnancy) and those whose importance wanes as the pregnancy evolves normally towards term (such as vaginal bleeding in the first trimester). Any single pointer observed in an individual cannot predict with certainty that a particular

Table 11.1 *Factors affecting perinatal mortality which may be identified by history and examination at the booking clinic*

History
    Age <18 years or >38 years
    Primigravida aged >30 years
    Illegitimate pregnancy
    Date of LMP uncertain
    Vaginal bleeding since LMP
    Parity of four or more
    Three or more successive spontaneous abortions
    History in previous pregnancy of
        Stillbirth or neonatal death
        Termination of pregnancy
        Small-for-dates or Large-for-dates fetus
        Fetal abnormality
        Premature labour
        Antibodies
    Hyptertension/eclampsia
    Caesarean section
        Postpartum haemorrhage or manual removal of placenta
    Maternal Health
        Hypertension or proteinuria
        Chronic illness such as diabetes mellitus, epilepsy

Examination
    Late booking (after 20 weeks)
    Blood pressure >140/90 mmHg
    Maternal weight <45 kg or >85 kg
    Maternal height <1.52 m
    Uterus large or small for dates

complication will occur but indicates that increased general vigilance must be exercised in the antenatal and intrapartum care of that patient if hazard is to be avoided or detected early. Too many of the risk factors simply correlate with the crudest index of pregnancy outcome, perinatal mortality, rather than a specific complication. A number of scoring systems have been devised, which attempt to add a quantitative element to the screening process (Chamberlain 1978; Goodwin, Dunn and Thomas 1969; Hobel *et al.* 1973). None, to date, has found general acceptance.

Combining a second 'assessment of risk' at 28–32 weeks increases the efficiency of screening. It allows identification of those women in whom a clinical problem has arisen since booking which may affect pregnancy outcome (Table 11.2). Combined with early sonar screening detailed below, the above scheme with slight modifications is used by a large proportion of obstetric practitioners and is applicable to the whole unselected population. It serves not only to identify the at-risk but, probably just as important, it

Table 11.2   *Complications arising during current pregnancy identified at 28–32 weeks which place the patient in the at-risk category*

Poor weight gain (<0.2 kg/week) or weight loss disparity between uterine size and gestational age (may be small or large for dates)
Vaginal bleeding (early or late)
Hypertension >140/90 and/or proteinuria
Anaemia based on mean corpuscular volume
Threatened or actual premature labour <37 weeks (including premature rupture of membranes)
Urinary tract infection on two or more occasions
Recurrent glycosuria
Polyhydramnios
Multiple pregnancy

serves to distinguish the at-least-risk group for whom the same close scrutiny is not justified. A further assessment of 36+ weeks should aim to detect malpresentation and failure of presenting part to engage in primigravidae.

Ultrasound examination

The routine screening of all pregnancies for a number of major structural defects in early pregnancy (*circa* 18 weeks) is rapidly becoming an integral part of routine antenatal care. In general this facility needs to be based in a specialist unit. Expensive and sophisticated ultrasound equipment, very experienced operating personnel and immediate access to skilled obstetric assistance are all very necessary if this procedure is to be effective. There seems little prospect at present that this type of facility could be operated efficiently on a community base. However, it should be made more readily available to all pregnant patients.

A sonar scan performed at 16–18 weeks gestational age should include detailed inspection of the fetal spine and head, as an important benefit of this examination is in the detection of major neural tube defects; anencephaly and major degrees of spina bifida should be confidently excluded at this stage. The examination also serves to verify gestational age calculated from the date of the last menstrual period; it should detect multiple pregnancy and establish fetal viability. Sonar may also on occasion identify pelvic abnormalities, such as intramural fibroids and ovarian cysts.

The role that early ultrasound plays in verification of gestational age is worthy of emphasis. Over 25 per cent of obstetric patients do not present a reliable menstrual history from which to predict the estimated delivery date and some unwittingly mislead. Sonar measurement in early pregnancy is more accurate than any other means of estimation and as such is one of the most valuable recent innovations in obstetric practice.

Ultrasound is useful later in pregnancy for screening and monitoring and will be discussed again subsequently. It is especially valuable in the management of vaginal bleeding.

Experimental and epidemiological studies to date have not revealed any evidence of physical hazard resulting from the use of ultrasound.

Alphafetoprotein in maternal serum

The estimation of alphafetoprotein in maternal serum or amniotic fluid provides an alternative or complementary screening procedure to ultrasound examination in early pregnancy.

Although a few centres advocate that maternal serum alphafetoprotein alone is useful in the detection of fetal neural tube defects it is not sensitive or specific enough to be used in isolation. Because of the physiological increase in maternal serum alphafetoprotein with advancing gestational age it is critical that the screening should be performed between 16 and 18 weeks of gestation. Gestational assessment is therefore, best verified by ultrasound examination at or about the same time. Considerable overlap exists between results in any normal population and the abnormal population whatever upper limit is chosen. As this borderline rises the number of affected fetuses which are detected decreases (sensitivity ↓); but the proportion of unaffected pregnancies included also decreases (in other words, the specificity improves). The converse is also true. As a result, the optimum range of normality must be established on a local basis, taking into account local population variability, and the precision and reproducibility of assay method used. For example, an upper cutoff level of 2.5 multiples of the normal median value which is commonly used will at 16–18 weeks of gestation detect 90 per cent of anencephaly and 80 per cent of open spina bifida but it will also include 1–3 per cent of unaffected singleton pregnancies.

An additional limitation is that a raised alphafetoprotein in maternal serum is not specific to neural tube defects, it also occurs in multiple pregnancy, following threatened or missed abortion, and also subsequent to amniocentesis. Alphafetoprotein is raised in the presence of fetal exomphalos and a number of other fetal abnormalities and in a small proportion of apparently totally normal pregnancies.

In view of the above limitations it is likely that maternal serum alphafetoprotein will prove most valuable, when the risk of neural tube defect is high, and in association with ultrasound examination to justify amniocentesis. The incidence of neural tube defects does show geographical variation being twice as common in the West of Scotland, Northern Ireland and South Wales (six to eight/1000 births) as in the South East of England (three to four/ 1000 births) (Carter and Evans 1973; Carter, David and Laurence 1968). Maternal serum alphafetoprotein will probably prove most cost-effective in these geographical areas. Cost-effectiveness must be balanced not only in terms of financial investment, but also in terms of the social implications, such as parental anxiety, and also the ethical implications of risking abortion by amniocentesis on the basis of a misleading result. The test is not diagnostic of neural tube defect but may aid determination of the high-risk group.

In those patients who have a past history of one or more affected children the recurrence rate (×10 higher after one affected child and ×20 higher after three affected children) usually warrants more accurate diagnosis by amniocentesis (Bennett 1981).

Techniques for specific application

Amniocentesis

Sampling amniotic fluid involves undisputed hazards but is occasionally justifiable. It is not a screening technique applicable to the general population. The risks of amniocentesis in early pregnancy have been extensively studied (Medical Research Council Report 1978) if not accurately translated, and are of major and minor significance. Probably the largest single excess risk is abortion precipitated by the amniocentesis; the incidence in experienced ultrasonically directed hands should be in the region of 1 per cent. This investigation should therefore be reserved for use where a particular indication exists and the likelihood of significant abnormality exceeds the complication rate of amniocentesis. For instance the recurrence risk after an affected infant with a neural tube defect is approximately 5 per cent and the incidence almost doubles to 9 per cent for a third affected child (Carter and Fraser Roberts 1967).

Neural tube defects are usually detectable by the estimation in amniotic fluid, of alphafetoprotein, acetylcholinesterase activity and rapidly adherent cells. It is anticipated that a combination of these parameters will further improve sensitivity (detection of abnormal fetuses) and also improve specificity (reduce falsely positive inferences). This remains to be substantiated statistically. In practice, combining ultrasound and amniocentesis means that very few serious neural tube defects are missed, and although it may occasionally occur it is rare to perform a therapeutic abortion in error.

The incidence of Down's syndrome in the older patient is often misunderstood. The relative incidence with age is shown in Table 10.2. (see p. 138). It is recommended that in general amniocentesis be advocated routinely after the age of 40 years although the principle may be tempered by informed parental wishes and/or previous history.

Together with the exclusion of rarer genetically determined abnormalities or diagnosable metabolic diseases in specific at-risk circumstances these comprise the main indications for early amniocentesis.

It cannot be overstated that, in the interests of maternal and fetal safety during amniocentesis, ultrasound examination should be performed immediately before or during the procedure. Contamination of the liquor amnii with maternal or fetal blood not only increases the likelihood of rhesus isoimmunization in susceptible individuals but also makes alphafetoprotein estimation and cell culture less reliable. Cell culture of a bloodstained amniotic fluid specimen is less likely to be successful and chromosomal analysis is often impossible.

Fetoscopy

Chromosomal analysis of amniotic fluid cell culture will facilitate the determination of sex and thereby double the predictability of sex-linked diseases such as haemophilia and Duchenne muscular dystrophy. Fetoscopy may take the screening process a step further allowing distinction of the affected male from the unaffected male. The investigation relies upon the direct sampling of fetal blood from the umbilical cord but it is not as dangerous as it may sound. As yet the technique is practised routinely in only a small number of centres but the facility is available. Evaluation of the procedure in terms of sensitivity, specificity and safety is currently underway.

Utilizing amniocentesis with or without fetoscopy the potential number of unusual conditions which may be diagnosed before birth is enormous and include genetic, metabolic and haematological disorders. The investigations are carried out on amniotic fluid or amniotic fluid cells uncultured or cultured or on fetal blood, pure or mixed with amniotic fluid.

[*Comment*: Using the aforementioned methods it is possible to divide the obstetric population into higher than average and lower than average general risk. A number of major structural abnormalities can also be detected or excluded. The exclusion of congenital abnormalities is important in the strategy to reduce perinatal mortality and morbidity as almost half the perinatal deaths (six out of 15) are due to lethal congenital anomalies. They constitute 32 per cent of all stillbirths and 18 per cent of first week neonatal deaths. However, having once made the diagnosis, a problem that was previously experienced as a perinatal dilemma becomes one of abortion. While the impact of present screening programmes on reducing the population frequency of all genetic disorders and birth defects is modest, the greatest benefit derives in preventing various genetic diseases in families with previously affected members.]

Once the higher-risk pregnancies have been identified the next requirement is to maintain regular surveillance over them.

MONITORING PROCEDURES

There is considerable overlap between the range of results of any monitoring method when normal and abnormal groups are compared. Due largely to this deficiency inherent in all current methods of fetal health assessment a number of different investigations are often utilized concurrently without necessarily proving complementary. No method is particularly competent in making the diagnosis of incipient fetal deterioration or predicting the length of fetal survival. The ideal test needs to be accurate in this respect but also to be sufficiently prospective to allow for intervention to prevent death or major morbidity.

Some of the investigations devised for surveillance may in fact be of more value when used as screening procedures.

Fetal growth

The assessment of growth requires accurate measurement of reproducible fetal or closely related parameters. The earlier in pregnancy that monitoring begins the more precise is the gestational assessment and the better is the impression of intrinsic growth potential. All too often, as a result of delayed recognition, attention is addressed in late pregnancy to the already stunted fetus resulting from established gross deficiencies of maternal or placental support.

Clinical examination

Serial abdominal palpation throughout pregnancy is the most widely used method of fetal growth assessment. Gauging fetal size in this way has been shown to be subjective, indirect and imprecise. Variations in the length of the maternal abdomen, the tone of the uterus, presentation and position of the fetus, thickness of maternal tissues and the volume of liquor amnii all contribute to make the method inaccurate.

Because the distances between the symphysis pubis, umbilicus and xiphisternum demonstrate wide variation from individual to individual, the height of the uterine fundus above the symphysis pubis is measured more objectively using a tape measure. However even when this procedure is combined with maternal abdominal circumference measurement it produces considerable discrepancies within and between patients.

Clinical assessment, at best, has an accuracy of ± 2 weeks yet it remains the monitoring method of most clinicians. A number of studies have illustrated the fallibility of simple palpation of fetal growth (Beazley and Underhill 1970; Leoffler 1967). Westin (1977) in Sweden has however described an impressive improvement in the detection of growth retardation and perinatal mortality as a result of abdominal measurement in conjunction with a gravidogram.

Ultrasound

The application of ultrasound to obstetrics since the late 1950s has proved revolutionary and almost wholly beneficial especially as a monitoring device. Its biggest single advantage is in its proven safety, which makes it applicable to large numbers of pregnancies of varied gestational age and also secure for repetitive examination. Sonar can be useful in confirming fetal viability following early pregnancy bleeding and in verifying gestational age assessment from LMP as already demonstrated in the screening programme.

In early pregnancy (up to 14 weeks) fetal crown–rump length (CRL) measurement may permit accurate age assessment to ± 5 or 6 days (in 95 per cent of pregnancies) (Drumm, Clinch and McKenzie 1976; Robinson and Fleming 1975). The exponential rate of CRL growth at this time facilitates this precision and minimizes the significance of measurement errors. Biparietal diameter (BPD) measurement in the first 18 weeks of pregnancy allows gestational ageing on average to ± 7 days (95 per cent); but rapidly becomes less useful and a single measurement made after 30 weeks has a predictive value of ± 3/52 or more, which is little better than an experienced clinician's subjective impression (Kurtz *et al.* 1980).

Once gestational age has been determined by early ultrasound examination, subsequent serial measurements facilitate growth estimation. The most widely used and conventional sonar measurement is fetal biparietal diameter (BPD), taken at a precise cephalic plane which includes the third ventricle. It is possible using this parameter to identify severe states of intrauterine growth retardation and also to detect a number of 'abnormal' growth patterns (Table 11.3). The 'low growth profile' often associated with genetic abnormalities demonstrates small BPD measurement and low normal growth rate throughout pregnancy; the growth rate may fall further in the last trimester. One difficulty in interpreting this type of growth retardation is that although it is associated with genetic anomalies in over 50 per cent of cases it is also the pattern of growth demonstrated by a number of genetically normal but constitutionally small infants and the overlap between the two is considerable. The normal fetuses do not generally demonstrate the same degree of growth rate compromise in the last trimester.

The second growth pattern described by BPD measurement is the 'late flattening pattern'. Here characteristically growth rate and BPD measurement are within the normal range until after 30 weeks of pregnancy when the growth rate slows or stops. This is likely to be the situation seen with uteroplacental insufficiency, for instance as a result of pregnancy-associated hyptertensive disease.

There are several deficiencies in the use of biparietal diameter measurement in assessment of fetal growth. The biggest is the phenomenon of

Table 11.3

Type	Aetiology	Ultrasound appearance	Comments and prognosis
1. Physiological	Normal, small infant Genetically determined Constitutional intra-uterine growth retardation	Consistent biparietal diameter growth Normal to low	Most common type of intrauterine growth retardation 70–80 per cent
		Growth rate normal Head/abdominal circumference ratio normal Symmetrical growth retardation	Maternal/paternal height and weight may indicate likelihood
2. Pathological A. Inherent IUGR	Genetic abnormality or early embryonic/fetal insult, e.g. Potter's syndrome, rubella	Poor biparietal diameter growth Low growth profile Reduced growth rate (often more marked in last trimester) H/A ratio normal	10 per cent intrauterine growth retardation Associated anomalies common (>50 per cent) Very poor prognosis
		Symmetrical growth retardation	
B. Extrinsic IUGR	Acquired disease, e.g. mid-trimester infection, or pre-eclampsia producing uteroplacental insufficiency	Initial biparietal diameter growth normal Late flattening pattern Growth rate reduced after insult Increased H/A ratio	10–20 per cent of intra-uterine growth retardation Maternal factors common Prognosis improved by early delivery
		Reduced amniotic fluid volume	

'brain sparing' whereby during intrauterine malnutrition blood is preferentially redistributed to the brain; as a result brain weight is relatively least affected by growth retardation and BPD measurement is not therefore the most sensitive index of growth restraint. It is frequently difficult to measure BPD especially in late pregnancy when the fetal head may be deeply engaged in the pelvis. Normal variations in head shape such as scaphocephaly may produce misleading measurements. As a result of these deficiencies a wide variety of fetal parameters have been measured by ultrasound in order to improve the detection of growth retardation. Head circumference and abdominal circumference and area measurements combined as a ratio can identify up to 80 per cent of intrauterine growth retardation (Varma, Taylor and Bridges 1979) and characterize it into symmetrical and asymmetrical forms. Until the recent application of microprocessor units to ultrasound measurement, circumference and area measurements have proved too inaccurate and time-consuming for routine use (Godfrey *et al.* 1981). It seems likely that as microcomputers become increasingly available for such measurement, abdominal area measurement will become more widely used in detecting intrauterine growth retardation. Abdominal area measurement provides an index of liver size and skin thickness both of which are most affected by poor intrauterine nutrition.

More accurate trunk measurement should also improve the precision of fetal weight prediction which is currently around ± 15 per cent (Deter *et al.* 1981). This limits the usefulness of weight estimation to the severely growth retarded and premature babies, as accuracy is not so good in the bigger babies. Work is currently in progress to evaluate the possibilities of more accurate abdominal measurements.

Despite providing more insight into fetal growth than any other technique, ultrasound has not yet achieved its full potential. Because, there is enormous biological variation in all fetal parameters as evidenced by birthweight (at term overall mean = 3.42 kg, 2 SD = 800 g), unless longitudinal studies are undertaken to determine individual growth profiles in specific populations the sensitivity to detect growth aberrations will continue to be blunted. It is impossible for instance to determine whether a baby born weighing 3 kg has achieved its inherent growth potential. Babies of 'average' birth weight may have been affected by malnutrition and therefore be prone to the same complications as their smaller brethren. Improved programmes of ultrasound assessment are needed to identify the affected baby before severe irreversible compromise has taken place. The best discriminator will be at least a two-stage screening programme, the parameters need to be quickly, easily and reproducibly measured for general application, but details remain contentious at present (Neilson, Whitfield and Aitchison 1980).

Fetal wellbeing

Maternal appreciation

The maternal perception of fetal movements has been suggested as a crude but useful screening exercise in fetal surveillance. The mother is asked to count fetal movements in a specified period of time. A 50 per cent reduction in fetal movement, less than ten movements in 12 hours, or complete cessation of movements for 12 hours in the last 10 weeks of pregnancy are variously quoted as adverse signs (Pearson and Weaver 1976). However, maternal appreciation of fetal movements has been shown to be poor by concurrent ultrasound visualization (Gettinger, Roberts and Campbell 1978) and huge variations occur in fetal movement from hour to hour, day to day and mother to mother. If normal it may prove reassuring but if abnormal may engender unwarranted emotional upset.

Placental function tests

Although placental function tests are of very limited value in monitoring fetal wellbeing they are widely used. The overlap between the results in the normal population and those pregnancies complicated by disease is large, such that isolated results serve no useful purpose. Wide fluctuations occur in most of the biochemical tests both within and between subjects with time, unrelated to fetal condition. Sustained trends of serial measurements can be the only justification for use, although single measurements at or around 32 weeks have been suggested as a screening device.

Plasma progesterone and urinary pregnanediol demonstrated the least correlation with fetal welfare and have therefore been superseded by plasma and urinary oestrogens and human placental lactogen which have only marginally better reputations.

Because the maternal excretion of oestriol in part depends upon the function of the fetal adrenal and liver and placental enzymes it was thought to reflect the function of the 'fetoplacental unit' which is an attractive concept. However the wide normal range of values, diurnal variation and collection difficulties in the case of urine have made results unreliable as an index of fetal wellbeing. With accurate knowledge of gestational length oestrogens may permit the detection of abnormal trends in late pregnancy, but will often add little to the appreciation of fetal compromise, which is often severe, by the time they become persistently abnormal. Oestrogen surveillance is not applicable to all the different types of pathophysiology encountered in pregnancy; for example maternal renal function largely determines excretion in urine and may if compromised occasion misleading low levels of urinary oestriols as may intrahepatic cholestasis. Plasma estimation of oestriol has few advantages; fetal death has been recorded in the presence of apparently normal maternal plasma oestriol levels; conversely, falling oestrogen levels may be innocent on 20 per cent of occasions (Duenhoelter, Whalley and Macdonald 1976). Thus the incidence of misleading low oestrogen levels during pregnancy is substantial. However normal levels are less likely to mislead hence the value of oestrogen assay in selected high risk conditions is to support the decision to postpone delivery until the fetus is more mature.

Human placental lactogen (hPL) levels in maternal serum below 4 μg/ml after 30–32 weeks of pregnancy suggest impaired placental function and so may be of value as a screening procedure at this gestation (Spellacy 1979). However, the use of hPL values serially are disappointingly poor in detecting or monitoring fetal compromise due to the wide range of normal values and poor identification of trends (Hull and Chard 1976).

The measurement of such placental products as oestrogens and hPL do not really reflect 'fetoplacental–maternal' integrity or placental transport functions. Many maternal factors affect them and fetal compromise is often severe by the time they are appreciably abnormal. Fetal death or vitality are unpredictable using such methods.

The pregnancy-associated plasma proteins (PAPPs)—Schwangerschaft's protein 1 (SP1), PAPP-A and placental protein 5 (PP5) are newly identified proteins produced by the placenta and measured in maternal blood. Although currently being evaluated the preliminary correlation with fetal wellbeing is poor, for all but one, and it is unlikely that they will be other than general non-specific indicators of placental activity.

The optimum role for this group of investigations may be in screening for a higher than average pregnancy risk. They are all of extremely limited value for fetal surveillance once vitality is threatened.

Specific biochemical investigations

The bilirubin content of amniotic fluid continues to be the most popular and valuable of investigations in the management of the isoimmunized pregnancy. The degree of fetal disease can also be measured directly using fetoscopy to obtain fetal blood and inferred from hydropic features which can be visualized by ultrasound examination. The severity and response to treatment can also be monitored in this way. Further discussion on the management of haemolytic disease is outside the remit of this chapter (but see Whitfield 1982).

Maternal serum uric acid levels have been correlated to perinatal outcome in hypertensive diseases of pregnancy (Redman *et al.* 1976) and used in conjunction with maternal serum creatinine to predict optimal time for delivery (Wood 1977). Unfortunately sensitivity and specificity are crude even in these quite specific circumstances and further refinement is required.

Biophysical assessment

This group of observations includes both fetal heart rate monitoring and fetal body and breathing movements. Fetal heart rate (FHR) monitoring has been widely used antenatally for the last 5–10 years. In this situation it investigates the relation of fetal heart rate reactivity to spontaneous fetal movements or spontaneous uterine activity (Braxton-Hicks contractions); less commonly it is used to relate fetal heart rate changes to induced contractions (stress test).

As with intrapartum monitoring (Chapter 23) the presence of heart rate accelerations with fetal movements or uterine contractions indicates a normal or reactive trace, associated in general with a healthy fetus and favourable prognostic significance. The absence of fetal heart rate accelerations, an increase in the baseline fetal heart rate and/or a reduction in baseline variability (normally >10 beats/min) are intermediate signs of fetal hypoxia. Late and variable decelerations of the fetal heart rate in response to fetal movements or uterine contractions are signs of serious fetal asphyxia. Although the reactive trace is generally a favourable prognostic index (Flynn and Kelly 1977), it is not infallible and babies can die shortly after apparently normal traces. The non-reactive or abnormal trace is much more difficult to interpret. The risk of fetal death increases fourfold in the presence of an abnormal trace (Evertson *et al.* 1979), but up to 97 per cent of fetuses with a single non-reactive trace will still be alive 1 week later. In addition 95 per cent of non-reactive traces obtained in the conventional 40-minute period will become reactive when the observation period is extended to 80 minutes (Brown and Patrick 1981). A number of scoring systems based upon the above characteristics have been devised (Myer-Menk *et al.* 1976; Pearson and Weaver 1978), their worth in predicting fetal compromise is not yet established and because fetal welfare may change exceedingly quickly the optimal interval of repetition remains uncertain. In the absence of continuous antenatal monitoring by this method it seems unlikely that intermittent assessment will significantly affect perinatal mortality or morbidity. Clinical deterioration necessitating intervention often precedes heart rate changes; additionally by the time significant heart rate changes are detected and confirmed, neonatal survival is often prejudiced.

The use of the contraction stress test, still employed in North America, is little used in this country. The infusion of an oxytocic agent is frequently required to induce contractions and this carries the risk of membrane rupture, labour and uterine hypertonus. Both the sensitivity and specificity of the test are poor.

Fetal chest and body movements have been studied in detail relatively recently using ultrasound visualization. Both are intermittent exercises practised by the fetus in the last few weeks of pregnancy (Roberts, Little and

Campbell, 1977). The frequency of the two types of movement varies widely throughout the day such that even when the two are combined and fetal activity is expected to occupy up to 40 per cent of the time studied, a lower limit of 10 per cent total activity would allow the erroneous diagnosis of fetal compromise to be made. Many factors influence the respiratory and trunk movements including maternal blood glucose levels and drugs, so complicating their use for routine assessment of the fetus. Biophysical profiles currently topical in America (Manning, Platt and Sipos 1980) combine a number of the above parameters on the assumption that several assessments are better than any one due to the limitations of each. This may not be a bad hypothesis, but remains to be substantiated. Large-scale epidemiological studies will be needed to demonstrate any significant benefit in terms of perinatal outcome.

Maturity assessment

Radiology

The real and theoretical hazards to the fetus of X-ray examination make it impractical for serial measurements. Very few centres now use radiological assessment of epiphyseal calcification to estimate gestational maturity. Because calcification is often delayed in intrauterine growth retardation it would be of little value in this situation even if considered safe.

There are a small number of specific indications for this technique: for pelvimetric assessment, where a small pelvis may be suspected or exclusion is required in preparation for vaginal breech delivery. Multiple pregnancy and breech presentation are the other obstetric indications for radiological examination where fetal abnormality may be suspected.

Amniotic fluid

Fetal lung maturity can be estimated by the measurement of lecithin and sphyngomyelin in amniotic fluid. A ratio of the two lecithin: sphyngomyelin (L:S ratio) obviates the need to consider amniotic fluid volume. The normally excellent predictive accuracy of the L:S ratio may be overturned if the liquor is contaminated with meconium, chlorhexidine or blood. Maternal diabetes mellitus may also make the prediction unreliable if there is significant delay (>48 hours) before delivery. A lecithin–sphyngomyelin ratio greater than 2:1, less than 48 hours prior to delivery, implies that the risk of hyaline membrane disease will be less than 1 per cent. Improved neonatal intensive care with better respiratory support has however reduced the importance and frequency of surfactant estimation. The limitations of thin layer chromatography used to estimate L:S ratio have resulted in the cutoff level of 2:1 being biased towards safety; up to 60 per cent of infants with a L:S ratio between 1.5:1 and 2:1 will not develop respiratory distress syndrome (Harvey, Parkinson, and Campbell 1975). Phosphatidyl-glycerol may be a better index of pulmonary maturity in diabetics and when the amniotic fluid sample is contaminated by blood or meconium.

A number of other constituents of amniotic fluid may be used to estimate functional maturity. The maturing fetal skin sheds increasing numbers of cornified cells and anucleate squames into the amniotic fluid. If these cells contain or are coated with lipid as a result of fetal sebaceous gland activity, they will stain orange with Nile Blue sulphate. A proportion of 10 per cent or more of these cells correlates with a gestation of 38 weeks or more (Brosens and Gordon 1966). However it is not uncommon for a significant number of patients at or past term to have very few or no orange staining cells.

Urea and creatinine concentrations in amniotic fluid are thought to reflect maturation of fetal renal function. Estimations with (Lind and Billewicz 1971) and without cytological information (Pitkin and Zwirek 1967) have been used to estimate functional maturity. True creatinine is not the standard biochemical measurement performed in most hospitals and therefore not always readily available. The false negative rate is relatively high; between 5 and 20 per cent of infants with low amniotic fluid creatinine levels will be mature (Doran, Bjerre and Porter 1970). The combination of creatinine, urea and cytological parameters was directed at improving gestational assessment from amniotic fluid; few if any studies have tested this premise. Pre-eclampsia and Rh-isoimmunization adversely affect the validity of amniotic fluid creatinine values.

CONCLUSIONS

The comments in this chapter are intended as constructive criticism of the philosophy that any objective measurement must be valid in fetal assessment. A large number of investigative techniques, genetic, biochemical and biophysical, have now evolved which can be applied to fetal surveillance. Few have yet withstood the test of time. Often the investigations are based on tenuous scientific foundations and have undergone insufficient and uncontrolled evaluation. Yet they are accepted along with deficiencies and iatrogenic hazards, which may well not be justifiable.

A number of the methods are largely outmoded such as human placental lactogen. Many are currently developing and are under evaluation—antenatal cardiotocography for instance. Ultrasound and genetic studies are undergoing an active phase of growth and expansion into an increasing number of applications. Fetoscopy is on the horizon and shows potential for the next obstetric revolution—intrauterine fetal therapy. But none of the techniques described is a universal panacea in all high-risk obstetric situations. The aim must be, by the various screening procedures, to identify the high-risk situation and then concentrate attention on fetal growth assessment and monitoring fetal wellbeing, intervening only when justified in maternal and fetal interests.

A number of the methods of fetal assessment will need to be employed concurrently. The value of the sum of information will only be substantiated if interpreted with good obstetric judgement and in the light of sound clinical experience and intelligence.

REFERENCES

Beazley, J. M. and Underhill, R. A. (1970). Fallacy of the fundal height. *Br. Med. J.* **4**, 404–406.

Bennett, M. J. (1981). The value of alpha-fetoprotein screening programmes. In *Progress in obstetrics and gynaecology.* (ed. J. Studd). Churchill Livingstone, Edinburgh. pp. 18–29.

Brosens, I. and Gordon, H. (1966). The estimation of maturity by cytological examination of the liquor amnii. *J. Obstet. Gynaecol. Br. Commonw.* **73**, 88–90.

Brown, R. and Patrick, J. E. (1981). The non-stress test. How long is enough? *Am. J. Obstet. Gynecol* **141**, 646–651.

Carter, C. O. and Fraser Roberts, J. A. (1967). The risk of recurrence after two children with central nervous system malformations. *Lancet* **1**, 306–308.

Carter, C. O., David, P. A., and Laurence, K. M. (1968). A family study of major central nervous system malformations in South Wales. *J. Genet.* **5**, 81–92.

Carter, C. O. and Evans, K. (1973). Spina bifida and anencephalus in Greater London. *J. Med. Genet.* **10**, 209–234.

Chamberlain, G. V. P. (Ed) (1978). *British Births 1970 Vol. 2,* Ch. 2, 39–53. Heinemann, London.

Chamberlain, G. V. P. (1981). The epidemiology of perinatal loss. In *Progress in obstetrics and gynaecology.* (ed. J. Studd). Churchill Livingstone, Edinburgh, Vol 1, pp. 3–17.

Deter, R. L., Hadlock, F. P., Harrist, R. B., and Carpenter, R. J. (1981). Evaluation of three methods for obtaining fetal weight estimates using dynamic image ultrasound. *J. Clin. Ultrasound* **9**, 421–425.

Duenhoelter, J. H., Whalley, P. J., and Macdonald, P. C. (1976). An analysis of the utility of plasma immunoreactive oestrogen measurements in determining the delivery time of gravidae with a fetus considered at high risk. *Am. J. Obstet. Gynecol.* **125**, 889–898.

Doran, T. A., Bjerre, S., and Porter, C. J. (1970). Creatinine, uric acid and electrolytes in amniotic fluid. *Am. J. Obstet. Gynecol.* **106**, 325–332.

Drumm, J. E., Clinch, J. and McKenzie, G. (1976). The ultrasonic measurement of fetal crown–rump length as a method of assessing gestational age. *Br. J. Obstet. Gynaecol.* **83**, 417–421.

Evertson, L. R., Gauthier, R. J., Schifrin, B. S., and Paul, R. H. (1979). Antepartum fetal heart rate testing. 1. Evolution and the non-stress test. *Am. J. Obstet. Gynecol.* **133**, 29–33.

Flynn, A. M. and Kelly, J. (1977). Evaluation of fetal wellbeing by antepartum fetal heart rate monitoring. *Br. Med. J.* **1**, 936–939.

Gettinger, A., Roberts, A. B., and Campbell, S. (1978). Comparison between subjective and ultrasound assessments of fetal movement. *Br. Med. J.* **2**, 88–90.

Godfrey, K. A., Flanagan, G. J., Gerrard, J., and Lind, T. (1981). A microcomputer measuring system applied to real-time ultrasound video imaging. *J. Clin. Ultrasound* **9**, 309–313.

Goodwin, J. W., Dunn, J. T., and Thomas, B.W. (1969). Antepartum identification of the fetus at risk. *Can. Med. Assoc. J.* **101**, 458–464.

Harvey, D., Parkinson, D. C., and Campbell, S. (1975). Risk of respiratory distress syndrome. *Lancet* **1**, 42.

Hobel, C. J., Hyvarinen, M. A., Okada, D. M., and Oh, W. (1973). Prenatal and intrapartum high-risk screening. 1. Prediction of the high risk neonate. *Am. J. Obstet. Gynecol.* **117**, 1–9.

Hull, M. G. R. and Chard, T. (1976). Hormonal aspects of feto-placental function. In *Fetal physiology and medicine.* (eds.) R. W. Beard and P. W. Nathanielsz Saunders, London, **19**, 371–394.

Kurtz, A. B., Wagner, R. J., Kurtz, R. J., Dershaw, D. D., Rubin, C. S., Cove-Beuglet, C., and Goldberg, B. B. (1980). Analysis of biparietal diameter as an accurate indicator of gestational age. *J. Clin. Ultrasound* **8**, 319–326.

Lind, T. and Billewicz, W. Z. (1971). A point-scoring system for estimating gestational age from examination fluid. *Br. J. Hosp. Med.* **5**, 681–685.

Loeffler, F. E. (1967). Clinical foetal weight prediction. *J. Obstet. Gynaecol. Br. Commonw.* **74**, 675–677.

Manning, F. A., Platt, L. D., and Sipos, L. (1980). Antepartum fetal evaluation: development of a fetal biophysical profile score. *Am. J Obstet. Gynecol.* **6**, 787–795.

Myer-Menk, W., Ruttgers, H., Boos, R., Würth, G., Adis, B., and Kubli, F. (1976). A proposal for a new method of CTG evaluation. In *5th European congress of perinatal medicine.* (eds. G. Rooth and L. B. Bratteby) Almquist and Wiksell, Stockholm, p. 138.

Medical Research Council Report (1978). An assessment of the hazards of amniocentesis. *Br. J. Obstet. Gynaecol.* **85**, Suppl. 2.

Neilson, J. P., Whitfield, C. R., and Aitchison, T. C. (1980). Screening for the small-for-dates fetus: a two stage ultrasonic examination schedule. *Br. Med. J.* **280**, 1203–1206.

Pearson, J. F. and Weaver, J. B. (1976). Fetal activity and fetal wellbeing—an evaluation. *Br. Med. J.* **1**, 1305–1307.

Pearson, J. F. and Weaver, J. B. (1978). A six-point scoring system for antenatal cardiotocographs. *Br. J. Obstet. Gynaecol.* **85**, 321–327.

Pitkin, R. M. and Zwirek, S. J. (1967). Amniotic fluid creatinine. *Am. J. Obstet. Gynecol.* **98**, 1135–1138.

Redman, C. W. G., Beilin, L. J., Bonnar, J., and Wilkinson, R. H. (1976). Plasma urate measurement in predicting fetal death in hypertensive pregnancy. *Lancet* **1**, 1370–1373.

Report on confidential enquiries into Maternal Deaths in England and Wales 1976–1978. (1982), HMSO.

Roberts, A. B., Little, D., and Campbell, S. (1977). In *Current status of fetal heart rate monitoring and ultrasound in obstetrics.* (eds. R. W. Beard and S. Campbell) RCOG, London. pp. 209–220.

Robinson, H. P. and Fleming, D. E. E. (1975). A critical evaluation of sonar 'crown-rump length' measurements. *Br. J. Obstet. Gynaecol.* **82**, 702–710.

Spellacy, W. N. (1979). The use of human placental lactogen in the antepartum monitoring of pregnancy. *Clin. Obstet. Gynaecol.,* **7**, 245–251.

Varma, T. R., Taylor, H., and Bridges, C. (1979). Ultrasound assessment of fetal growth. *Br. J. Obstet. Gynaecol.,* **86**, 623–632.

Westin, B. (1977). Gravidogram and fetal growth, comparison with biochemical supervision. *Acta Obstet. Gynaecolog. Scand.* **56**, 275–282.

Whitfield, C. R. (1982). Future changes in the management of rhesus disease. In *Progress in Obstetrics and Gynaecology,* (ed. J. Studd) Vol. 2, 48–59.

Wood, S. M. (1977). Assessment of renal functions in hypertensive pregnancies. Clin. Obstet. Gynaecol., **4**, 747–758.

Further reading

Report of the UK Collaborative Study of alpha-fetoprotein in relation to neural tube defects (1977) Maternal serum alpha-fetoprotein measurement in antenatal screening for anencephaly and spina bifida in early pregnancy. *Lancet* **1**, 1323–1332.

12 The primary health care team in obstetrics

G. N. Marsh

EVOLUTION OF THE TEAM SYSTEM

In the years prior to the mid-1960s the general practitioner commonly saw his antenatal patients during his normal surgery sessions and the midwife saw them in her local authority antenatal clinic; thus general practitioner and midwife antenatal care was separated and to a large extent duplicated. The general practitioner and midwife often met at the delivery, however, although midwives at that time were a fiercely independent group proud of their professional status and were more than happy to conduct deliveries at home on their own. Nevertheless when the midwife had problems during labour, or some dramatic event occurred, it was to the general practitioner that she usually turned. Concomitant with the development of health centres and group practices in the 1960s general practitioner and midwife began to work together; the midwife was either attached and seeing only women from the practice, or at least one particular midwife would attend clinics regularly even though she would have antenatal patients in other practices. They would still meet around home deliveries, but with more and more deliveries taking place in hospital the number of deliveries carried out by district midwives fell markedly. Similarly the general practitioner's home delivery workload fell, although in a small number of areas he would work with the midwife in his own general practitioner unit. But the major switch of deliveries to hospital in no way equated with the provision of general practitioner intranatal facilities. Accordingly it was hospital midwives working with hospital specialists who became responsible for an increasing proportion of deliveries, and the number of district midwives was allowed to fall.

With the increasing provision of statistics on the outcome of obstetric care and more particularly the ability to localize perinatal mortality rates to region, district and even hospital, specialists became increasingly anxious about the results. Since good antenatal care was considered to be an important factor in achieving a satisfactory outcome many obstetricians tried to provide this and it has resulted in huge antenatal clinics at centralized, and sometimes remote, large hospitals of which there has been much criticism by consumer groups. The 'cattle market atmosphere', the 'conveyor belt' style of care, the lack of appreciation of the psychosocial aspects of care and its emotional content has been vigorously criticized. There was certainly no hope of anything resembling a dignified and leisurely system. Increasingly hospital specialists have recognized this and are attempting to release themselves from this huge burden of work and hand antenatal care largely back to the general practitioner and the community midwife associated with him in his primary health care team.

THE DEVELOPMENT OF GROUP PRACTICE

Following the Family Doctor Charter (1966) there was a great increase in the proportion of doctors working in groups and the number of single-handed doctors began to fall. This has proceeded steadily until the present day. A very high proportion of young doctors entering practice have gone into the larger groups. This has been furthered by DHSS encouragement of the building of group practice centres and also by the provision of local authority-owned health centres. Approximately 25 per cent of general practitioners now work in such health centres. The DHSS not only established a General Practitioner Finance Corporation prepared to lend money for private building, but also allowances were payable to groups, rent was payable for doctor-owned premises, rates were reimbursed and improvement grants up to 30 per cent of capital costs were made available. In addition design guides for the construction of both group practices and health centres were published. In these specially designed buildings provision was frequently made for antenatal clinics. In parallel with the development of premises came the attachment of local authority nursing staff to group practices and health centres. For obstetrics this meant particularly the attachment of midwives and health visitors. Following the development of a separate social services structure in the local authority in the mid-1970s some social services department thought it appropriate to have liaison schemes whereby particular social workers associated themselves with group practices. This however remains comparatively uncommon.

As far as lay staff were concerned—receptionists, secretaries etc.—70 per cent of such staff employed by doctors were reimbursed up to a ceiling of two staff per doctor.

GROWTH AND COMPOSITION OF A MODERN PRIMARY HEALTH CARE TEAM

In the late 1960s a primary health care team could well consist of nothing more than three or four doctors, three or four receptionists and perhaps one attached nurse and one attached health visitor. Attachment of midwives came later, but like all the attachment schemes once started the concept grew rapidly. Currently over 80 per cent of midwives are attached to general practice. Today a fully developed primary health care team will consist of a group of doctors plus possibly a trainee doctor and one or two medical students as the medical component (Marsh and Kaim Caudle 1976). There will be approximately twice as many receptionists, filing clerks and secretaries as there are doctors. Attached will be health visitors, midwives, SRNs (one of whom may be trained as a family planning nurse) and SENs. Several of the nursing staff could be fieldwork trainers and have students. A social worker will probably liaise with the practice and visit it weekly. The numbers of these staff in proportion to the number of women served will vary enormously. Some of the variation will be due to cognisance of the demography of the population, for example, more health visitors and midwives if there are a lot of young families; more SRNs and SENs if the population is heavily geriatric. It will also have some relationship to the ease of recruitment of nursing staff in the particular area and also some relationship to DHSS guidelines. Nevertheless probably the major influence on the extent of nurse attachment to and involvement in primary health care teams is the enthusiasm (or otherwise) for this concept by the local area nursing administrators. The primary health care team can also develop informal liaisons with various groups, the commoner ones being marriage guidance counsellors, the local ministers, Samaritans, National Childbirth Trust, etc.

One successful way of implementing liaisons of this type is the organization of joint meetings, lunches etc. between the practice staff and members of the agency concerned (Marsh and Barr 1975). Once attachment or liaison is operative it is also important to have progress meetings from time to time with management or administration in order to ensure harmonious continuity.

ROLES OF TEAM MEMBERS

Clerical staff

The filing clerk's major role is to ensure that the correct record is available at the correct time for the correct person. They are frequently the youngest members of the team and their job is useful for familiarizing themselves with practice routine prior to development into the more senior role of receptionist, secretary etc.

The receptionists are responsible for the receiving of patients, the smooth running of clinics and the organization of the appointment system. The general happiness, efficiency and tone of the antenatal clinic depends very much upon them. In practices with a large number of antenatal patients one particular receptionist can be assigned to the clinic for these women. As a result the receptionist can learn and implement many of the more routine procedures of the antenatal clinic—providing packages of literature, weighing, completing forms, telephoning, testing urine, providing specimen containers, ensuring that waiting room facilities are adequate, and occasionally entertaining the remaining children of the family.

The secretary's task is the general one of correspondence—typing, dictaphone, shorthand, etc.—as well as the more specific one of completing the claim forms for the obstetric care provided. More sophisticated work such as the auditing of records according to preordained protocols, the provision of simple statistical data on process and outcome in obstetrics, can all be undertaken by competent secretaries. As a background to the obstetric care the total record can be improved—date ordered, rubbish removed etc.—and even clinical summaries can be compiled by an appropriately trained person (Marsh and Thornham 1980).

Nurses

When midwives are present and receptionists are efficient and well trained there is no major role for the state registered or state enrolled nurse in obstetric care. However if she has a family planning certificate she can relieve the midwife and doctor of this task by carrying out family planning interviews during the pregnancy and at the postnatal examination. This could well be part of other family planning care which she provides routinely for the entire practice. By having a family planning clinic at the practice early attendance in pregnancy, as just one of many preconception counselling measures, can be encouraged (see Chapter 4).

The midwife

Although an independent professional in her own right the midwife seems perfectly happy to work alongside the general practitioner in his premises. The quality of her work and the need for it is of paramount importance. She it is who carries out the standard protocols laid down in modern antenatal care (Chapter 6). She sees the women at every attendance whereas the doctor may only see the women at set times (Chapter 31). She can visit women at home when necessary. She carries out the various technical routines of pregnancy—venepunctures, cervical smears, vaginal swabs etc. In more recent years the development of the 48 hour discharge from hospital, and the 'domino' system of even earlier discharge within a few hours of the birth has expanded the puerperal role of the midwife (see Chapter 25). In many areas community midwives are now delivering women booked for early discharge and even for 48 hour discharge from hospital in order to maintain their intranatal care skills. In the puerperium she carries out twice daily and later daily care. The general practitioner formerly visited the mother and baby on alternate days for about 10 days. However, as the relationship between general practitioner and midwife has become closer and they have had more frequent contact, the need for him to visit has decreased (see Chapter 31). Currently general practitioners may visit women discharged early on possibly only one or two occasions, and only once those that were in hospital for 6 or 7 days. An overview of the domestic scene and more particularly a comprehensive well-baby check are the major reasons for the visit (see Chapter 28).

The health visitor

The health visitor has a statutory obligation to visit all newborn babies after discharge from hospital. Ideally she should see all pregnant women antenatally and especially primigravidae. Frequently, however, she finds herself having to ration her time to certain groups of pregnant women particularly those who are unsupported and in danger of becoming isolated. Single women and teenagers are part of her high-risk group and they often have special physical and emotional needs. She is able to offer counselling not only to the woman herself, but also to her entire 'family'. She aims for an informed effective working relationship with the pregnant woman and tries to ensure that her health needs and those of her 'family' are met. She tries to imbue her clients with a realistic concept of parenthood and to accept and adjust to their individual changes in lifestyle. She advises regarding some physical problems such as diet, alcohol, smoking, rest, and exercise. She can make appropriate home visits during the antenatal period. Her role expands considerably in the puerperium (see Chapter 26).

The social worker

There is considerable overlap in the work of the health visitor and the social worker. When meeting frequently in the setting of the primary health care team, however, duplication can be avoided. In general the social worker orientates on the material and social needs of the pregnant woman rather than on her health. Nevertheless her clientele is very similar to the health visitor's, particularly including the 'deprived' women. In early pregnancy the social worker can be involved in various alternatives for the pregnancy, including adoption and termination. She can also concern herself with the provision of appropriate accommodation or lodging for the expectant mother as well as housing after the baby has come home. She can provide advice on maternity grants and benefits that may be of particular relevance to certain people. She can contact voluntary bodies for help with the provision of prams, cots, baby clothes, and other material assets. In large, or badly supported families she can arrange for short-term fostering of older children while the mother is in hospital. Many young, single-parent women owe a great deal of their later happiness and stability in life to the efforts of a well-informed and enthusiastic social worker.

Marriage counsellors, ministers etc.

These members of the team are rarely found in general practice although a recent study found that 10 per cent of teaching practices have a marriage counsellor working with them (Rhodes 1983).

When present they can, for the very occasional patient, play an important part in the pregnancy. Marital unhappiness, or even breakdown is not uncommon in pregnancy and the puerperium and support and advice is much appreciated. The birth of a handicapped child or even perinatal death can provide an important role for a minister. Informal liaisons and occasional face-to-face contacts with people of this type who work in the community are of great benefit to the team.

Breast-feeding counsellor

The National Childbirth Trust, an almost universally present organization in Great Britain, usually has available trained voluntary personnel interested in instructing pregnant women about breast-feeding and encouraging this in the puerperium. In very occasional practices the counsellors attend the antenatal clinic and also pay home visits. Their work partly overlaps that of the midwife, but with good interpersonal relationships and a democratic team spirit prevailing (see below), 'job competition' and 'job rivalry' can be avoided.

The doctor

The doctor has the major responsibility for the pregnant woman. She is registered as his patient, and he has contracted to provide obstetric care for her. She is effectively paying him for it, albeit indirectly. By working in a team general practitioners are finding that they are increasingly able to provide high quality comprehensive clinical care. They are able to delegate a great deal of work to lay people which previously they did themselves. Smaller list sizes, less and more accessible home visiting, often the result of defined practice boundaries, use of deputizing services, health education aimed at demedicating the population and persuading people to look after their own minor illnesses, have all decreased the total workload thus permitting time for expanded and better obstetric care (Marsh and Kaim Caudle 1976).

The sharing of clinical care with fellow professionals has also reduced the doctor's workload considerably. Nurses can now follow up chronic illness, treat minor illness and minor injuries and carry out much of the preventive care in a practice (Marsh 1976). By having a personal list of patients that the doctor knows well and who in turn know him also reduces workload and particularly reduces duplication of work (Marsh 1972; Pereira Gray 1979). The volume of antenatal care given by the doctor can be reduced by sharing care with the midwife. In a large patient satisfaction survey the majority of women who had had antenatal care at a particular group practice considered that at antenatal clinics the midwife did the same job as the doctor (Marsh and Kaim Caudle 1976). However a substantial minority of women who had had antenatal care from that practice would have been 'unhappy' or 'very unhappy' if the midwife always provided routine care with the doctor only seeing them fairly occasionally or in case of any abnormality. There does seem to be something special about the general practitioner himself seeing his patients.

THE FUNCTIONING OF THE TEAM

Consulting the same women at the same clinic and sharing the responsibility certainly enhances the functioning of the team. In a well-organized practice there can be day-to-day and even hour-by-hour contact. Each member of the team knows how to reach any other member virtually at any time. Each morning the team will meet together preferably sitting round a table, good coffee available, and in a degree of comfort. These small tangible evidences of care of fellow workers, as well as pleasant in themselves, promote happiness within the team. The meetings should be short, no longer than 20 minutes, completely informal, and very much concerned with day-to-day problems of individual patients. Large teams with many liaising members will obviously not *all* meet *every* day, but the inner core of doctors, nurses, health visitor, and midwife should meet almost daily. It is advantageous if social workers, marriage counsellors etc. have regular days when they are known to attend and relevant problems can be kept until then. Other more formal meetings can be arranged to discuss operational or clinical topics when health visitors, midwives, nurses, and doctors can formulate policies on various aspects of obstetric care—breast-feeding, cigarette smoking, alcohol, preconception counselling etc. It is as a result of these meetings that the general aims of the team can be developed and its overall philosophy can emerge. As a sequel when a woman meets several different 'carers' during her pregnancy there should be no contradictions in what she hears them say.

A regular, say monthly, house committee consisting of the senior representative of all the disciplines within the team can meet to finalize and implement policies and serve as a forum for discussion of matters relevant to all team members. Problems of accommodation, timing of clinics, numbers of staff would be matters relevant to these meetings.

Business meetings, when the financial return from obstetric care can be examined, can take place twice a year as part of a formal 'accounts' meeting (Medeconomics 1982). An accountant well versed in the details of general practitioner finance and particularly the 'fee for service' system for contraception, cervical cytology, antenatal, intranatal and postnatal care, and immunization schedules, can be of inordinate value. Although attended usually by those bearing responsibility for the financial success of the business—usually the doctors and the practice manager, or secretary—the profitability (or otherwise) of the obstetric care can be related in general terms to those members of the team that have contributed towards it.

The team should function democratically not hierarchically. It would be invidious of the general practitioner to assume that he is the leader of the team when he may be working with independent professional colleagues such as social workers, health visitors, and ministers of the church. It is better if general practitioners look upon themselves as coordinators rather than leaders of the team. It is the problem that the patient presents that leads the team, and those primarily responsible for that problem will for a period lead the team in dealing with it. Hence leadership can change from week to week as problems come and go. Certainly many teams have foundered and many more never become established, because of an automatic assumption by the doctors in them that they lead, and that they will organize their colleagues according to their own preference.

A comprehensive date-ordered communal record in which each team member can write can be of enormous benefit in coordinating team effort and encouraging a team spirit. The DHSS A4 folder is excellent for team obstetric care, containing as it does separate records for contraception, antenatal care, preventive health procedures and nursing and health visitor notes as well as day-to-day notes of general practitioner clinical care (Marsh and Thornham 1980). Any missing data can be identified by lay staff, working to a protocol, and pencilled on the front of the folder for appropriate members of the team to note and rectify whenever the patient presents.

THE ROUTINE OF THE PRIMARY HEALTH CARE OBSTETRIC TEAM

The numbers attending antenatal clinics in general practice are usually fairly small. Fathers, accompanying friends, children and grandmothers can and should be made welcome. Fathers in particular should be encouraged to attend antenatal clinics with their wives. The filing clerks will have available the appropriate records and the receptionists will have organized a smooth fairly leisurely appointment system. Women can be weighed and urine tested by the receptionist, and literature packs provided for new attenders. The midwife will carry out the usual obstetric protocols of history, examination and recording. New bookings and women in the last six weeks of pregnancy will usually also see the general practitioner but a differential system of care for each woman can be worked out so that though work is not duplicated, adequate care is provided. Pathology specimens will be collected shortly after the clinic, taken to the laboratory, and most results should be available next day. There should be access to all diagnostic laboratory and X-ray services (including ultrasound). Consultant opinion should be available within 48 hours for 'semi-urgent' cases not actually requiring immediate admission or domiciliary visit. Maternal anxiety regarding the need for referral (for example, for possible fetal abnormality) should be included as a reason for 'semi-urgency'. Health visitor, social worker and family planning nurse should all be available either at the clinic or by appointment within a day or two. Women who fail to keep their appointment should be sent another one or if at high risk for any reason the midwife should visit her at home.

DIFFERENTIAL TEAM CARE

The doctor can provide continuity of care from preconception, through pregnancy, ideally through labour, and certainly through the puerperium to the postnatal period and thereafter. With such continuity the woman's pregnancy becomes merely one part of her normal life-cycle. However, in a team setting the general practitioner will not necessarily see the woman at every consultation in the antenatal period. He will see her at the first ante-natal consultation, take a detailed history (often a rapid procedure when dealing with someone he knows), carry out an individually appropriate examination and decide to which particular risk group this woman belongs. If she is social class I, II, or III—assessed for the most part on the registrar general's classification based on husband's occupation, but with his own allowances being made from personal knowledge of the family, and particularly if she is having a second, or third baby after normal previous pregnancies and deliveries—he could well allocate the care of such a woman to the midwife until much later in pregnancy. From that stage he and the midwife will carry out joint care, partly as a double check on clinical findings, but more importantly to fortify the all important rapport prior to the onset of labour.

By contrast there are other women that he himself will wish to see each time and often more frequently than the normal monthly routine. In parti-cular unmarried women, those under 18, women considering adoption, cer-tain ethnic groups, women with certain illnesses (for example, diabetics) and women from social classes IV and V (MacVicar 1983; Russell 1982). These women also need to be seen automatically by social worker and health visitor and often on a continuing basis. Certainly the smaller stature, the larger families, the inadequate diet, the lower haemoglobin, the heavier smoking, and the infrequency of breast-feeding apparent in the lower social classes indicate that these groups are most in need of comprehensive and intensive team care and support (OHE Briefing No 10 1979). In this way the two or three-fold difference in perinatal mortality between high and low social classes, which is such an unfortunate feature of obstetric outcome in

Britain today, can be reduced. This principle of giving more care where it is needed, with positive discrimination in favour of high-risk groups and concomitant lessening of care for lower-risk groups must be a major aim of the primary health care obstetric team in the future (Marsh 1977).

TEAM CARE IN LABOUR

The midwifery staff of a general practitioner unit should be very closely associated with and aware of the care given by the primary health care obstetric team. From time to time midwives from the unit should attend antenatal clinics of general practitioners who use the unit frequently. By the same token pregnant women should visit the general practitioner unit, be shown around the various facilities, and meet members of the unit who may well be involved in their delivery. It should be an aim of the primary health care obstetric team to bring personal and continuing care into the labour room. The answer to 'will you be there'—frequently posed and more frequently thought but unspoken—should if possible be 'yes'. This is patently more probable if the general practitioner offers 24 hour cover for his obstetric care, in contradistinction to other patients for whom a practice rota may operate. Although uncommon some practices do this. The alternative of the partnership rota at least reassures the doctor that his patient will be cared for by someone with whom she is at least slightly familiar. Some practices run antenatal clinics for the whole practice at one session, in order that the woman gets to know several of the general practitioners in the group so the chances of having a known medical face in labour increase (McKenrick, M., personal communication). The unknown deputy from a commercial deputizing service seems singularly inappropriate for care during a delivery which has been preceded by so much personal antenatal care. Unfortunately the current prolonged rota systems of community midwives around a specific number of hours each week preclude the promise of intranatal care by the midwife who may have given the majority of the antenatal care. However, women are usually passed back after delivery to their 'usual' antenatal midwife so continuity into the puerperium at least can be assured.

The question needs answering as to what role the woman's family doctor has in a normal labour when it is conduced by a well-trained and experienced midwife not infrequently accompanied by a pupil.

(1) He provides continuity of care and may be the only person in the labour room to have met and have knowledge of the women prior to her going into labour—as a result he can instill greater confidence in her.

(2) He can confirm the normality of the labour.

(3) He can support the midwife in her plan of management.

(4) He can deal with, or take responsiblility for, minor abnormalities

which the midwife will detect—for example, a meconium-stained liquor, mild elevation of diastolic blood pressure, rather long first stage, slight ketonuria etc. Midwives are taught to detect abnormalities and report them, but in the main they do not deal with them. The level to which they need report is not necessarily that of the specialist obstetrician, and many abnormalities are comparatively minor and can be dealt with by a general practitioner.

(5) The general practitioner can decide when any detected abnormality is of such a degree that specialist help is needed.

(6) He can support and encourage any relatives or friends who are with the mother in labour. Usually this means the father of the child who is probably known to the family doctor too.

(7) He can 'score' the bonding between mother and baby, and father and baby, and can even predict future nurturing problems with which he may have to deal in the future. There is some evidence that 'baby-battering' can be predicted.

(8) He can enjoy the climax of all his work with the woman over many months or even years; bringing considerable job satisfaction.

(9) He can provide a second pair of skilled hands should abnormalities occur in the second or third stage, particularly the unexpectedly non-breathing baby, or severe haemorrhage.

With this impressive list of reasons it seems almost negligent for general practitioners who have delivery facilities not to attend their patients in labour.

The primary health care obstetric team aims for a physiological pregnancy and a physiological labour. The temptation to use 'technology', and particularly unnecessary technology, or technology which although valuable to high risk cases may in fact make low-risk cases worse, should be strenuously avoided. The general practitioner should feel a greater sense of satisfaction in achieving a normal outcome following normal labour and normal delivery than he would from a forceps delivery with a drip running.

THE TEAM IN THE PUERPERIUM

The midwife plays the major role in the puerperium, and carries out day-to-day nursing of the mother and routine care of the baby (Chapter 25). She supervises the breast-feeding or bottle-feeding. The doctor has a smaller role, mainly concerned with checking the baby's general physical state at birth and customarily more comprehensively during the first week of life (see Chapter 28). For all women discharged early from either specialist or general practitioner unit the family doctor should pay a home visit to assess the home situation and carry out the baby's 6th day' examination. With the level of communication possible in a team setting between midwife and doctor, the need for the latter to do as many routine home visits has disappeared (see Chapter 31).

The health visitor has a statutory obligation to visit babies at home usually between the 10th and 14th day of life. Hence she will see all new babies in the practice, and can report any problems of bonding, breast-feeding etc. to the doctor (Chapter 26). Similarly he can draw the health visitor's attention to specific mothers and babies where he feels that either may be at high risk. Again health visitors could well restrict their care of low-risk women in the higher social classes in order to spend more time with the disadvantaged groups.

HOSPITAL LINKS

Primary health care obstetric teams have a great deal to offer not only the women booked for the general practitioner unit, but also the higher-risk women booked for specialist delivery. They too will have their multiple medicopsychosocial problems and have preventive health needs that are the prerogative of the primary health care team—and which can only be effectively provided by that team. Increasingly as hospitals become more confident in the care given by the primary health care team women booked for specialist unit delivery may need only one or at the most two attendances at the specialist unit. In some areas such collaboration has reduced the number of specialist appointments significantly (McKee 1982). If more specialist teams had confidence in the primary health care team care in pregnancy and encouraged the use of general practitioner units, or integrated intranatal facilities, then the consultant workload would fall considerably. More time could then be alotted to the significantly problematic women who are referred to them. One of the major condemnatory criticisms of consultant care has been the delegation of severely at-risk patients to inadequately trained juniors (Chamberlain *et al.* 1975; Department of Health and Social Security 1975). This has presumably resulted from the excessive workload associated with the supervision of so many normal cases.

REFERENCES AND FURTHER READING

Chamberlain, R. *et al.* (1975). *British births, 1970 Vol 1*, Heinemann Medical, London.
Department of Health and Social Security (1975). *Report on confidential enquiries into maternal deaths in England and Wales 1970–2* HMSO, London.
MacVicar, J. (1983). Cutting Asian death toll at birth. *Curr. Pract.* **April 29**, 16–17.
Marsh, G. N. (1972). Controversial view: 'back to single-handed'. *North East Faculty Newsletter.* Royal College of General Practitioners, London.
Marsh, G. N. (1976). Further nursing care in general practice. *Br. Med. J.* **2**, 626–7.
Marsh, G. N. (1977). Obstetric audit in general practice. *Br. Med. J.* **2**, 1004–6.

Marsh, G. N. and Barr, J. (1975). Marriage guidance counselling at a group practice centre. *J. R. Coll. Gen. Practit.* **25**, 73–5.

Marsh, G. N. and Kaim Caudle, P. (1976). *Team care in general practice.* Croom Helm, London.

Marsh, G. N. and Thornham, J. R. (1980). Changing to A4 folders and updating records in a 'busy' general practice. *Br. Med. J.* **2**, 215.

McKee, I. H. (1982). Community antenatal care—the way forward. *Scot. Med.* **2**, 5–9 (Sighthill Health Centre Scheme, shared care, started in 1975).

Medeconomics (1982). Maternity care is well worth organising properly. **July**, 48–53.

OHE Briefing No. 10 (1979). Perinatal mortality in Britian—a question of class. Office of Health Economics, London.

Pereira Gray, D. J. (1979). The key to personal care. *J. Roy. Coll. Gen. Practit.* **29**, 666–78.

Rhodes, P. (1983). Teaching. *Br. Med. J.* **286(6375)**, 1426–7.

Russell, J. K. (1982). Early teenage pregnancy *Current reviews in obstetrics and gynaecology 3.* Churchill Livingstone, Edinburgh, p. 108.

13 Obstetric records

L. I. Zander

INTRODUCTION

Although it is generally accepted that a good data system is a prerequisite for the effective delivery of health care, record-keeping has tended to generate comparatively little general interest. This should be a cause for concern because, in view of the very considerable amount of medical, administrative, and financial resources devoted to medical recording, it is an activity that warrants critical attention.

Obstetrics has, for a long time, given a lead in the development and utilization of appropriate forms of record-keeping and shown an example to others in their utilization both for clinical care and for the monitoring of maternity services. The importance of an appropriate record system has been stressed by the recent working party of the Royal College of Obstetricians and Gynaecologists (1982) and the Maternity Services Advisory Committee (1982) engaged in discussions about standards in obstetric care, and a review of the information required for national maternity statistics is being undertaken by a steering group on health services information (Korner Committee 1982).

The management of pregnancy is a form of clinical care characterized by a number of factors which are highly relevant to its method of recording:

(i) Pregnancy care can be well defined and consists largely of monitoring certain specific and predictable parameters regularly and systematically, the process of care is continuous, not episodic.

(ii) Pregnancy care for any individual is frequently provided by members of different professional groups.

(iii) The care may be undertaken in different settings.

(iv) The outcome of care can be readily standardized and therefore is well suited for clinical audit.

When considering the design of a record system, it is necessary to give attention to both its content and structure, and its utilization, and to judge its effectiveness by the degree to which it satisfies the requirements that are to be made of it.

FUNCTIONS OF THE OBSTETRIC RECORD

The many different functions of a record system can be considered under the following headings:

Provision of clinical care

The principal function of a record, and the one which inevitably will be of greatest concern to the clinician, is to assist in the provision of medical care for the individual patient. It should therefore contain all relevant past medical, obstetric and social history and give details of the ongoing clinical care.

The record should however not just be considered as serving solely a passive function of containing details of the care provided, but should be viewed as having an active role in stimulating the clinician to undertake aspects of care which might otherwise have been neglected or overlooked. Its effectiveness should therefore not be judged just by the degree to which it is complete, but by the extent to which it has itself contributed to an improvement in patient care.

The obstetric health care team

The record should enhance the working of the health care team. All members of the team should have the relevant information available to them irrespective of the setting in which the patient is seen, and each should be able to contribute to the total data source.

Clinical audit

Audit is a necessary stimulus for the improvement of clinical care. A form of assessment should ideally be part of every programme of patient management, so that information concerning its delivery is readily available and readily fed back to those responsible for its provision. The characteristics of many aspects of maternity care are ideally suited to clinical audit and it is important that this opportunity is fully realized.

Patient education

An important component of patient care involves the giving of information. As part of the communication process between the mothers and the providers of pregnancy care, the record can serve a useful function in this activity.

THE COMPOSITION OF THE OBSTETRIC RECORD

No other information-gathering process in medicine involves collecting so much data on so large a proportion of the population as that routinely obtained during antenatal care. The major component of the antenatal record consists of two parts: information (*a*) collected at the booking clinic, and (*b*) relating to the ongoing clinical care.

Information collected at the booking clinic

This consists primarily of basic background obstetric, medical and social history. Although there is general agreement amongst most obstetricians about the areas to be covered, there is considerable variation in the details of the questions asked. In a study analysing case records used in antenatal booking clinics of 41 teaching hospitals, it was shown that there was an average of 80 items per hospital, but in order to include all items considered important by at least one major teaching centre, case-notes with well over 500 items of medical and social history would be required (Fawdry and Mutch 1984). Whereas in Norway agreement has been reached on a standardized antenatal record, such a situation seems far off in the United Kingdom.

Information relating to the ongoing clinical care

The nature of the care and the parameters to be measured are predetermined and to a large extent will be similar wherever and by whoever the care is to be provided. The significance of the findings at each visit is greatly dependent on their relationship to previous findings. They will therefore almost always be recorded in the form of a flowchart so as to allow for the easy and rapid appreciation of any deviations from the normal (Fig. 13.1) (Bergsf, P., personal communication).

The design of the record can have a considerable influence on the quality of the care provided. If there are certain items of information that are important to know about, it is relevant that they should be asked, and

| Date | Weeks | Weight (kg) | Urine | | BP | Fundus (.cm) / Girth | Pres. | Level | FHH | Hb | Problems, investigations, treatments, etc. | Return visit | | GP Copy sent |
			P	S								Date	Place	
											AFP 16 weeks Yes/No			

Fig. 13.1. Flowchart.

subsequently recorded in a place where they will be noticed. In the management of certain chronic conditions, it has been shown that a structured record format increases the clinical activity undertaken by the physician by providing him with an *aide-mémoire* (Watkins 1981). Thus in recording past medical history, individual conditions may be listed as follows:

Allergies	☐	Hypertension	☐	Venereal disease	☐
Rheumatic fever	☐	Diabetes	☐	Depression	☐
TB contact	☐	Kidney problems	☐	Blood transfusion	☐
Cardiac disease	☐	Epilepsy	☐		

Another example is the recording of dietary intake. This is frequently omitted as part of the history-taking at the booking clinic, although it is known that for cultural, social and economic reasons, the mother's diet may be quite inappropriate or inadequate. Some records not only include the topic, but itemize the principal components; such as:

Dairy products	☐	Eggs	☐
Protein	☐	Fruit and vegetables	☐
Meat/fish	☐	Cereals	☐
Cheese	☐		

Alcohol and smoking are now well recognized as being of potential danger to the fetus and are often listed as separate items.

Non-clinical aspects of care

A highly important component of antenatal care is that of patient education. This may often be overlooked during the antenatal visit partly because of the clinician's preoccupation with the physical components of care and partly as a result of the 'team approach', with the same patient being seen by a large number of different individuals, with no one being quite certain what areas have been covered by others. If important issues are not to 'slip through the net', they need to be itemized and included as part of the structured record. In the MacMaster obstetric record the following items are listed:

Parent classes	☐	Pelvic floor exercises	☐
Maternity benefits	☐	Vitamins	☐
Diet sheet	☐	Birth requirements	☐
Breast preparation	☐	Postnatal back-up	☐

As soon as any of the above are dealt with satisfactorily, by any member of the obstetric team, the appropriate box is ticked.

Many different forms of obstetric records have been developed. The RCGP have produced an obstetric card with a structured format very suitable for the provision of pregnancy care in general practice (Figs. 13.2

BREAST. FEED YES/NO
OBSTETRIC CARD
The Royal College of
General Practitioners

SOCIAL CLASS
OR
OCCUPATION

Doctor

| Name | | Age | NHS No. |

Address

Midwife

Booked for delivery at

Previous Pregnancies

	S	M
MSC		
MSD		

General Health

RECORD OF____ PREGNANCY (Excluding____non-viable deliveries)

L.M.P.		Quickening		E.D.D.	
Blood Group		Hb	date	WR/Kahn	Height

Date	Durat-ion wks	Hght of Fundus	B.P.	Urine	Wght		Notes and Special Investigations
							Rh.

Smoking during pregnancy   YES [ ]   NO [ ]

Estimation of pelvic capacity

Fig. 13.2. RCGP obstetric card, side A.

and 13.3). It has a distinctive green colour and is of a size suitable for the standard NHS EC5/6 envelopes. Information contained on such cards can be further amplified as has been done by Marsh (personal communication), by use of a number of specially produced stamps or labels such as:

Social class or occupation	

Marital status at conception (MSC)
Marital status at delivery (MSD)

Smoking during pregnancy
Yes   No

General practitioner	Stages		
Present	1	2	3

Type of labour	Type of delivery	Perineum
Spontaneous, no drip Induced ARM and/or Synt. Spontaneous and accelerated Spontaneous & intravenous fluid	Spontaneous vertex Forceps Breech Caesarean section Other	Intact perineum Sutures to laceration Episiotomy

Postnatal
Breast feeding:
None
1–5 weeks
6 weeks

IDENTIFICATION OF THE AT-RISK PATIENT

When a large amount of data is collected, there is always the danger that important details may be overlooked in the overwhelming mass of negative information—the 'quantity–quality dilemma'. The limitations of doctors as information processors, even when well trained and motivated, is well recognized. In one study 23 per cent of serious medical conditions recorded by midwives at the antenatal clinic were overlooked by the senior medical staff (Chng, Hall, and MacGillivray 1980). One of the most important characteristics of a record system is to ensure that important facts are not neglected and that the 'at risk' patient can be easily identified. In Sighthill a special risk card has been designed for this purpose (Figs. 13.4 and 13.5) (Boddy, Parboosingh, and Shepherd 1982). The factors on the risk card are placed under six headings:

(i)   Factors relating to age and parity.

(ii) Factors indicating that the gestational age may be uncertain.

(iii) Factors in the past obstetric history which relate to the main causes of fetal mortality and morbidity including malformation, prematurity and fetoplacental dysfunction.

(iv) Factors relating to those maternal health problems which have an adverse effect on pregnancy outcome.

CONFINEMENT

G. P. PRESENT	STAGES
	1	2	3

Date	Place

Length of Stages:	1st	2nd	3rd

Spont., no drip
Induced ARM &/or synt.
Spont. & accelerated
Spont. & IV Fluid

Spont. Vx
Forceps
Breech
C.S.
Other

Intact Perineum
Sutures to Lacn.
Episiotomy

Birth Weight	Sex	Apgar	OTHER NOTES

POSTNATAL ATTENDANCES

Date	Notes

FINAL POSTNATAL EXAMINATION   Date

Symptoms

General Health   **Weight**

                                            B.P.

Abdomen

Pelvis

Breasts

Lactation

Breast feeding
None
1-5 weeks
6 weeks

CONCLUSION CONCERNING FUTURE PREGNANCY

Fig. 13.3. RCGP obstetric card, side B.

(v) Factors noted at the first antenatal examination.

(vi) Factors arising during pregnancy.

Side A (Fig. 13.4) is completed at the time of booking and side B (Fig. 13.5) at subsequent antenatal visits when any of the identified risk factors such as proteinuria, raised blood pressure, etc. are detected. For each of these a structured protocol has been developed which indicates the course of action to be followed by the different members of the health care team. Thus when the blood pressure is raised, it is agreed that the midwife should make a home visit the following day. If the pressure remains high, a second home visit is made before any decisions concerning treatment are taken.

The introduction of the 'at risk' card and the establishment of such plans of management enables each member of the health care team to contribute maximally to the care of the patient. It encourages the use of planned protocols for the management of pregnancy complications and lays the foundation for the evaluation of regimes of treatment. It provides a mechanism whereby innovations in management may be instituted in an orderly manner, thus ensuring that all pregnant women receive the benefit.

Fetal movement charts

Intrauterine movement has long been known to be an indicator of fetal wellbeing. In cases of chronic placental insufficiency it has been shown that fetal activity decreases and finally ceases 12–48 hours before the heart stops (Sadouski and Yaffe 1973)—a period of time which clearly provides for the possibility of medical intervention to take place.

For many years a number of obstetricians have used the fetal kick chart as one component of their antenatal care (Neldon 1980). The benefits to be derived from this procedure have recently been underlined by a large Danish study which showed that women who were instructed to count fetal movements had a statistically significant reduction in stillbirths as compared to a matched control group (*Danish Medical Bulletin* 1983).

In Cardiff, Dr Pearson has developed a more precise system based on a 'count to ten' chart, in which each day is divided into half-hour periods (Fig. 13.6). Mothers are asked to enter the time at which they notice the tenth movement, following which no further entry is made for that day. If fewer than ten movements are felt on two consecutive days, or no movements on any one day, women are asked to come immediately to the hospital for further investigations to be undertaken (Pearson 1979).

As a screening procedure the use of fetal kick charts would seem to have an important role to play and, because it is a simple low technology test, it is of particular value in the field of general practitioner obstetrics (but see Chapter 11).

NAME: .... DOCTOR: ....

BOOKING HISTORY (completed by midwife)

☐ Age less than 18 years
☐ Age over 38 years
☐ Primigravid age 30 years or more
☐ Parity = / more than 5.
■ **LMP DETAILS**
☐ LMP uncertain ± 2 weeks
☐ Pill stopped 1 or 2 periods before LMP
☐ Cycle length prior to LMP greater than 30 days
☐ IUCD in situ / on Pill after conception.
☐ Out of wedlock pregnancy
☐ Vaginal bleeding since LMP
■ **PAST OBSTETRIC HISTORY**
☐ SB / NND
☐ Small for dates (< 10 th centile)
☐ Large for dates (> 90 th centile)
☐ Fetal abnormality ....
☐ Antibodies in previous pregnancy
☐ Hypertension / eclampsia
☐ Termination of pregnancy / spontaneous abortion × 2
☐ Premature labour (20–37 weeks)
☐ Previous cervical suture
☐ Previous caesarean section
☐ PPH / MROP
☐ Labour of less than 4 hours
■ **MATERNAL HEALTH**
☐ Chronic illness / drugs ....
☐ Hypertension / proteinuria
☐ Infertility with medical advice
☐ Uterine anomaly including fibroids
☐ Smoking 10 / day at conception
☐ Social security benefits
☐ Isolated at home
☐ Family history of diabetes / fetal abnormality ....
☐ Completed by .... Date ....
■ **BOOKING EXAMINATION** (completed by doctor)
☐ BP = / more than 140/90
☐ Maternal weight = / more than 85 kg
☐ Maternal weight = / less than 45 kg
☐ Maternal height = / less than 1.5 m
☐ Cardiac murmur detected / referred
☐ Uterus large / small for dates
☐ Other pelvic mass detected
☐ Blood group rhesus negative
☐ Completed by .... Date ....

Fig. 13.4. Special risk card, side A.

Weeks of pregnancy																		
FM not felt																		
Hb < 10 g %																		
Poor weight gain																		
Weight loss																		
Proteinuria																		
Glycosuria																		
Bacilluria																		
BP systolic >155																		
diastolic >88																		
Rhesus negative/antibodies																		
Uterus large for dates																		
Uterus small for dates																		
No increase in fundus (zone)																		
Excess liquor																		
Malpresentation																		
ECV successful																		
unsuccessful																		
Head not engaged																		
Any bleeding pV																		
Premature labour																		
Vaginal infection																		
Sign when completed																		
Insert date																		

Fig. 13.5. Special risk card, side B: factors arising during pregnancy.

A BIRTH PLAN

A birth plan is a written form which indicates a mother's/couple's stated preferences about many of the different aspects of her coming labour and postpartum care. If a woman is to take part in the decision-making process concerning her own labour, she requires appropriate information about the available options. Similarly, if those providing obstetric care are to take account of the wishes and emotional needs of their patients, they require to know what these needs are.

Birth plans should not be seen as a fixed contract, but as representing provisional management plans which can be modified at any time in response to changing views and circumstances. They are usually filled in by the mother/couple and then discussed with those responsible for her management. Thus, besides indicating the views and hopes of the parents, they also provide a valuable opportunity and focus for discussion.

While there will inevitably be marked variation in the format of different birth plans there is likely to be much in common between them as regards the areas covered. In Adelaide, MacLellan (personal communication) uses

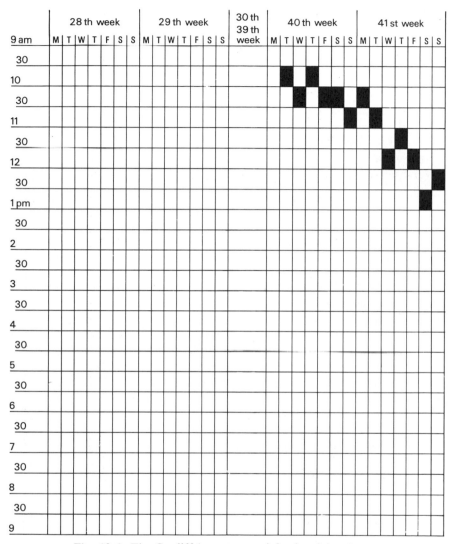

Fig. 13.6. The Cardiff 'count-to-ten' fetal activity chart.

a patient preference form which is headed: 'The management of this hospital is anxious to make your visit here as pleasing as possible to you and your family. It is therefore anxious to know of any special requirements you may have and in particular any desire you have in regard to the conduct of your labour'.

The woman is then asked to indicate her preferences beside a number of stated alternatives such as:

I would like my partner to be present:
   (a) during the early part of labour ☐
   (b) during the whole of labour ☐
   (c) even if forceps are needed for delivery ☐
During early labour I would like:
   (a) freedom to move around as I wish ☐
   (b) to spend most of the time lying down ☐
I would like alternative style delivery:
   (a) lights dimmed ☐
   (b) music which my partner will bring ☐
   (c) the baby delivered on to my abdomen ☐
   (d) to hold the baby (if all is well) immediately ☐

At the end of a fairly long list there is space for extra requests.
In MacMaster University Medical Centre, Murray Enken (personal communication) uses a more unstructured format.

Pregnancy: are you (or have you taken):
   (a) Any childbirth education classes? If not, do you plan to take any?
   (b) The hospital maternity tour?
Labour and birth
   (a) *If all goes normally*: Please make note of anything that may be important to you, such as who you might wish to have with you, your plans in regard to medication, epidural, place or position for birth, etc.
   (b) *Contingency plans*: Please note your thoughts about what you might want done if things don't go the way you planned; if, for example, you have a long or difficult labour, require more pain relief than you had anticipated, need forceps, episiotomy, or a caesarean; if the baby is premature or ill. It is often valuable to think about things like this in advance.
   (c) *Personal plans*: Do you wish to take photos, bring in a tape recorder for music, or do you have any special requests to bring to our attention?
Post partum: Any special plans about baby feeding, or baby care?

The completed form is then discussed with the obstetrician and an agreed plan of management arrived at.

Although written birth plans are a comparatively new innovation, particularly in the United Kingdom, they represent, in reality, only a further step in the generally developing change towards a more patient-centred approach to maternity care.

THE COOPERATION CARD

The antenatal care provided to a mother is frequently undertaken by clinicians working in different settings. Shared care between the general practitioner and his hospital-based obstetric colleagues has become widely practised and if this form of management is to be successful, it is essential that an appropriate mechanism for sharing information between those involved is established. The most usual method by which this is achieved is a patient-held cooperation card. This is usually designed to contain solely the basic information of the ongoing antenatal care, together with details of the relevant past medical and obstetric history. It is intended that the card will be completed at each visit by whoever undertakes the antenatal care and then retained by the patient.

In practice however, the system frequently works rather less than perfectly. The general practitioner is likely to be motivated to enter his findings regularly partly because it is the only obstetric record available to him, and also because he will be concerned that the data is available to those ultimately responsible for his patient's management in labour. In the hospital setting, however, the situation is somewhat different in that the obstetrician will record his findings in the hospital-held obstetric file which will be the data source for all subsequent decision-making. He is likely to make use of the information on the cooperation card only if he considers it essential for his assessment of the ongoing care. Also, the specialist's entries on the card will frequently be incomplete if they are not considered to be of critical importance to his management of the pregnancy, as they necessitate him duplicating what he enters into his own record. A further factor is that the card will not contain the details of investigations carried out in the hospital unless the results have been specially transferred to them.

This situation has important implications. At a psychological level there is a danger that it will lead to some intraprofessional tension if members of a team do not feel that there is adequate cooperation and an equal sharing of information between them. At a clinical level the importance of the cooperation card depends, in large measure, on the role that the general practitioner is to play in the overall care (House of Commons Social Services Committee 1980; Maternity Services Advisory Committee 1982; RCOG Working Party 1982). If it is really intended that the majority of antenatal care can most appropriately be carried out by the general practitioner, it is essential that a high quality of recording the clinical data of shared care is achieved. One way in which this might be achieved is to allow patients to retain their full obstetric record (see below), which will avoid any duplication of entries, and also ensure maximal motivation of those providing care to enter all relevant details.

PATIENT-HELD RECORDS

A characteristic of much clinical care is the reluctance of the health care profession to share clinical information with the patient. Not only is the record seen as belonging to the providers of care, but very strenuous efforts are usually made to prevent the patient having any access to its contents. Thus, it is very common for hospital folders to have NOT TO BE GIVEN TO THE PATIENT stamped boldly across the front.

Such an approach is clearly based on the principle that the record might contain certain items of information that would be inappropriate or even dangerous for the patient to be aware of, and it is the responsibility of the profession to protect her from such a situation in her own best interests. This is not to mention those situations in which the clinician may be reluctant for the patient to have access to information that might lead to criticism or even litigation.

The question of information sharing between doctor and patient needs, however, to be seen in the wider context of the doctor/patient relationship. Much evidence has now been collected which indicates the inadequacy of doctor–patient communication and the high level of dissatisfaction felt by many patients over the difficulty they have experienced in obtaining the information they seek (Byrne and Long 1976). Patient satisfaction with the care provided, compliance with the advice given and appropriate uptake of medical services are all related to patients' knowledge and attitudes. Reading (*et al*. 1982) showed that when patients were given a high level of feedback about the findings of an ultrasound examination, they were much more likely to report that they had followed the advice concerning the need to reduce their smoking and drinking given to them during their first antenatal visit than a control group to whom no such feedback had been given. Rather than being considered as solely of use to the clinician, the record should be viewed as providing a valuable contribution to the doctor–patient interaction.

The possibility and advisability of allowing patients to have access to their clinical records is being increasingly suggested. In the St Thomas' district, a system of obstetric care has been developed in which many mothers receive all their care in the community. In order to have their records available in the labour ward it was necessary for them to be given to the mothers to retain throughout their pregnancy (Zander *et al*. 1978). Initially, considerable doubts were expressed about the advisability of this decision, partly because it was felt that the notes would be mislaid and secondly because it was thought unwise to allow patients to have access to the clinical information concerning their own pregnancies. On both accounts these fears have been shown to be unfounded. The mothers, as might have been expected, were exceedingly reliable in producing their records whenever required and they were in fact more often available at the time of labour than those actually filed in the hospital. The psychological benefits derived from this procedure has, however, been more important. The mothers clearly enjoy having access to their records and it increases their interest and involvement in the process of care. It was found that the record was often used as the basis for discussion and explanation and when advice was to be given, it was often more effective to write in large letters—SHOULD STOP SMOKING—knowing that within a matter of hours, the message was likely to be read, not only by her husband, but more importantly perhaps by her mother-in-law!—than if the advice were to be given orally during the antenatal visit without the possibility of reinforcement. The full benefits to be derived from giving patients their own records are yet to be evaluated.

REFERENCES

Boddy, K., Parboosingh, I. J. J., and Shepherd, W. C. (1982). Schematic approach to prenatal care. *Appendix to report of RCOG working party on antenatal and intrapartum Care.* RCOG, London.

Byrne, R. S. and Long, E. L. (1976). *Doctors talking to patients.* HMSO, London.

Chng, P. K., Hall, M. H., and MacGillvray, I. (1980). An audit of antenatal care—The value of the first antenatal visit. *Br. Med. J.* **2**, 184.

Danish Medical Bulletin (1983) **30**, 274.

Fawdry, R. D. S. and Mutch, L. M. M. (1984). *Antenatal History Taking—What Are We Asking?* National Perinatal Epidemiology Unit (Oxon). (In preparation).

Korner Committee—Steering Committee on Health Services Information (1982). *Report of joint group maternity.* HMSO, London.

House of Commons Social Services Committee (1980). *Second report on perinatal and neonatal mortality. HMSO, London.*

Maternity Services Advisory Committee (1982). First report: maternity care in action HMSO, London.

Neldon, S. (1980). Fetal movement as an indicator of fetal wellbeing. *Lancet* **1**, 1222–4.

Pearson, J. F. (1979). Fetal movement recording. *Nurs. Times* **1**, 639.

Reading, A. E. *et al.* (1982). Ultrasound scanning in pregnancy. Short-term psychological effects of early real live scans. *J. Psychosom. Obstet. Gynaecol.* **1**, 57.

Royal College of Obstetricians and Gynaecologists working party on antenatal and intrapartum care (McNaughton Committee) (1982). RCOG, London.

Sadowski, E. and Yaffe, H. (1973). *Obstet. Gynaecol.* **1**, 845.

Watkins, C. J. (1981). Medical audit in general practice—fact or fantasy? *J. Roy. Coll. Gen. Practit.* **25**, 520.

Zander, L. I., Watson, M., Taylor, R. W., and Morrell, D. C. (1978). Integration of general practitioner and specialist care. *J. Roy. Coll. Gen. Practit.* **28**, 455.

Section C
Intranatal care

14 Safety in intranatal care— the statistics

Marjorie Tew

INTRODUCTION—THE CONFLICTING THEORIES

There is no disagreement that the primary objective of the maternity services should be to provide facilities to make birth as safe as possible for mother and child. But there is fundamental disagreement about the best way to achieve this objective. Opposing views are based on conflicting theories.

The theory which in modern times has had fewest proponents is clearly described by a Dutch Professor of Obstetrics: 'giving birth is mostly a normal physiological event which does not require any form of medical intervention . . . a natural phenomenon that only requires medical interference in pathological and rather exceptional situations' (Kloosterman 1978). 'Spontaneous labour in a normal woman is an event marked by a number of processes so complicated and so perfectly attuned to each other that any interference with them only detract from their optimal character . . . the danger will arise that the physiological part of obstetrics will be threatened by doctors who all too often will change true physiological aspects of human reproduction into pathology' (Kloosterman 1982). In this country hospital reports consistently record over 80 per cent of births as being 'without complication or anomaly' (Maternity Statistics 1981). Thus in the majority of births obstetric intervention is, according to this theory, disadvantageous.

The alternative theory, that nature unassisted is a poor obstetrician, has come to be accepted, not only by most of those who determine and carry out policy for the maternity services, doctors and midwives, administrators and politicians, but also by parents and the general public. The natural process, it is claimed, is always fraught with dangers which obstetric interventions can in most cases reduce and in no case increase. Therefore birth is usually safer, never less safe, when it takes place in a consultant hospital under obstetric management.

On this premise provision has been made for all births to take place in obstetric hospitals and ever more stringent conditions have been laid down to restrict the cases where general practitioners, working with community midwives, may carry out intrapartum care, whether in general practitioner maternity units (GPMUs) or in the mother's home. The policy has been carried out with such thoroughness that one assumes there must be unequivocal evidence to justify it. The purpose of this chapter is to review this evidence and to trace briefly how the present situation developed.

INTRANATAL CARE 1920–58

Between 1870 and 1925 the national death rate fell dramatically. The decline was caused almost entirely by improvements in diet and the environment and hardly at all by medical care since medical science had few life-saving treatments to offer. Nevertheless, the public were disposed to give doctors the credit for the improvement.

In contrast to the general picture, mortality of mothers and newborn babies fell very little and by the 1920s this was causing public concern. So naturally appeals were made to doctors to remedy the situation. In 1929 a group of surgeons founded what was to become the Royal College of Obstetricians and Gynaecologists (RCOG). More resources were made available for maternity care and for the training of obstetricians.

Traditionally nearly all births took place at home under the care of midwives, who called in a doctor only when complications developed and interventions, usually surgical, were considered necessary. Only those who could afford to pay booked the attendance of a general practitioner (Cookson 1967). Increasingly, however, these middle-class women came to espouse the doctrine that treatment which seemed beneficial in pathological cases would be beneficial also in normal cases. They led the fashion away from birth at home and into private institutions to be delivered under the care of a general practitioner or specialist obstetrician. Confinements increased also in the public hospitals, staffed by obstetricians, which had been made much safer as stricter attention to hygiene reduced the incidence of infection, formerly the cause of the frightening total of maternal and infant deaths there. By 1946 only 42 per cent of births took place at home (Chamberlain *et al.* 1975).

The expectation that the increased input of obstetric care would be immediately reflected in reduced mortality was not born out by early results, for both the maternal and early neonatal mortality rates were actually higher in 1935 than they had been in 1921. Then the sulphonamide drugs became available and this weapon against infection started a remarkable decline in the maternal mortality rate which continued, influenced also by other factors, to reach a very low level by the 1970s. By 1950 perinatal mortality had become the more urgent problem. During the war fewer medical facilities were available to the maternity services, but pregnant mothers were given priority in food rations, together with dietary supplements. The perinatal mortality rate (PNMR), which had fallen by only 6 per cent between

1931 and 1939, fell by 33 per cent between 1940 and 1948, a rate of decline not repeated until the 1970s, despite increasing hospitalization (Registrar General, annual).

However, these early results did not shake obstetricians' belief that the quickest way to reduce perinatal mortality was by increasing the use of obstetric interventions. The belief appeared to be confirmed by the Aberdeen experience where, with a very high rate of hospitalization, the PNMR was brought down by 38 per cent between 1946 and 1958 (Baird 1960). The death rate from all causes fell and this was attributed to the generally high standard of care the obstetric teams were inspired to provide. But the decrease was much the greatest in those causes most amenable to obstetric intervention—'placental insufficiency' and 'mechanical'. This success was attributed to the increased use of induction of labour and caesarean section to avoid prolonged pregnancy and difficult labour and to forestall fetal distress in high risk cases, though no clinical trial was mounted to verify the assumed causal relationship.

In contrast to the Aberdeen achievement, the PNMR in England and Wales fell by only 6 per cent in the first 10 years of the National Health Service despite the increase in obstetric provisions. It was felt that a survey of perinatal mortality was needed 'to provide information of value upon a number of aspects relating to the safety and health of mother and infant, including the possible effects of place of confinement' (Butler and Bonham 1963). A nationwide survey was carried out in 1958 under the auspices of the RCOG and the first report was published in 1963 (Butler and Bonham 1963).

WHAT THE PERINATAL MORTALITY SURVEY 1958 WAS THOUGHT TO SHOW

Place of confinement might affect perinatal mortality for two reasons: first, since the natural process of delivery functions most successfully when the mother feels relaxed and confident, she might find one place more conducive to this state than another. But the survey offers no information on this aspect for no questions were asked about the mothers' views. Second, the methods of delivery used in one place might be safer than in another. By the time the survey was analysed, however, it had apparently become accepted as an unassailable fact that the methods used in obstetric hospitals were safer; it was no longer a theory which still had to be tested against actual evidence. No attempt was made to submit the data collected to logical, impartial analysis.

The crude PNMRs per 1000 births were found to be 50 for deliveries in hospital and 20 for deliveries under general practitioner care, the results in GPMUs and at home being very similar. Two explanations were offered for the discrepancy. First, since the PNMR in hospital was inflated by cases transferred there after a complication had developed, the proper comparison should be between the PNMR for births booked and delivered in hospital (36) and those booked for general practitioner care, including those transferred to hospital for delivery (31). The excess mortality in hospital, however, remained highly significant ($P < 0.001$), so the further explanation was invoked that this was due to the excess among hospital bookings of cases at high predicted risk.

Comparing PNMRs by place of booking would be a logical method of analysis if the objective were to compare the total risk of mothers booking for hospital with the total risk of mothers booking for general practitioner care, including the risk of being transferred. It is *not* a logical method for comparing the 'possible effects of place of confinement'—the objective of the survey. If different techniques of managing labour used in different places are to be compared, only the results of actual, not intended, delivery by each technique are relevant. The widespread acceptance of this logical fallacy has confused the issue and bedevilled understanding of the problems of intranatal care ever since.

As for the excess of high risk births booked for hospital, no attempt was made to confirm that this was arithmetically sufficient to explain the excess mortality. A risk score, combining risk from several factors, was constructed (Butler and Alberman 1969), but it was never used as an instrument in quantifying the relative risks of delivery in each place, either overall or at specific levels of risk. Nevertheless, though supporting evidence was totally lacking, allusions to the greater safety of hospital delivery were repeatedly made in the two reports.

These unfounded assertions were to have great influence on the medical profession and the public in persuading them, not simply that the intervention techniques of obstetricians were beneficial, but also that the low intervention techniques of general practitioner accoucheurs and midwives were totally inadequate and so positively dangerous. Because of its critical importance in the development of the maternity services, it is important to consider the findings of the survey in some detail.

WHAT THE PERINATAL MORTALITY SURVEY 1958
ACTUALLY SHOWED

Though one of its original objectives was to 'provide information about the effects of place of confinement', details of perinatal mortality in each place were published only in respect of three predelivery risk factors—parity, social class and toxaemia. These revealed that in fact hospital births included only a modest excess at high risk on account of parity and toxaemia and no excess on account of social class. If each place had had the same proportion of births at each level of risk, the disparity between their crude PNMRs would hardly have been reduced: for example, the PNMRs, standardized to allow for the unequal distribution of toxaemia, were 49 in hospital and 20 under general practitioner care.

Hospital births probably included a relatively greater proportion at high risk on account of more than one factor. But the risk factors are all to a greater or lesser degree interdependent. Allowing for the risk attaching to any one accounts for a large part of the risk attaching to others, so standardizing PNMRs to allow for the combined effect of several factors explains very little more of the disparity between crude PNMRs in different places than does standardizing for one single factor (see p. 210 for example).

That standardizing for unequal risk should explain so little of the hospitals' excess mortality is inevitable, for the PNMR specific to each grade of risk was in every case much higher for hospital deliveries. The picture is exactly the same if the comparison is between births booked and delivered in hospital and births booked and delivered under general practitioner care; that is, if transferred and unbooked cases, which inflate the PNMR for hospital deliveries and do not measure general practitioner intranatal care, are completely excluded.

But the group booked and delivered under general practitioner care does not include those cases transferred after an unpredicted complication developed for which hospital treatment was judged necessary. Similar unpredicted complications probably also develop among hospital-booked births. It would be more accurate to compare the actual general practitioner deliveries with hospital-booked deliveries excluding such complications. Actual data are not available for these, but they can be estimated if it is assumed that they developed in the same proportion of hospital-booked cases as the transfers were of general practitioner booked cases and that they had the same high PNMR as the transfers. Hospital births without such complications would then be the same proportion of all hospital bookings as the births under general practitioner care were of all general practitioner bookings, and similarly for associated deaths. This estimation can be calculated for births in total and separately for each grade of risk. The resultant PNMRs are set out in Table 14.1.

In the case of first births, the PNMR in the estimated hospital group is slightly the lower, but in every other subgroup and in total the PNMR is lower in the actual general practitioner group and in several cases very significantly lower. Corresponding analysis by length of gestation and infant birth weight tells the same story (Table 14.2); in fact, even babies under 1500 g who had to be transferred had lower PNMRs that those booked for hospital delivery, despite immediate access to resuscitation facilities.

However, since the whole point of advocating specialist obstetric antenatal and intranatal care is precisely to prevent complications arising or

Table 14.1   *Perinatal mortality rates per 1000 booked births 'without complication' (as defined in the text) (Source: Butler and Bonham 1963)*

Risk group	Hospital (estimated)	General practitioner care (actual)
All deliveries	21	18***
Parity 0	21	22
1–2	18	14***
3	26	17***
4 and over	36	26***
Social class I–II	17	13*
III–IV	20	18
V	25	21
Toxaemia: none and mild	20	16***
moderate	29	28
severe	41	37

Levels of significance *P<0.05; ***P<0.001

Table 14.2   *Perinatal mortality rates per 1000 booked births 'without complication' (as defined in the text) (Source: Butler and Bonham 1963)*

Risk group	Hospital (estimated)	General practitioner care (actual)
Gestation <32 weeks	608	390***
32–37 weeks	72	63*
38–41 weeks	12	11
>41 weeks	18	17
Birthweight <1500 g	754	518***
1501–2500 g	108	103
2501–3000 g	19	18
>3000 g	9	8

Level of significance *P<0.05; ***P<0.001

mitigate their consequences, obstetricians would surely expect them to arise less often and to result in lower mortality than in the cases developing under general practitioner care and requiring transfer. In which case the PNMRs for hospital births without complications would be higher than those shown and so their excess over general practitioner PNMRs would be even greater.

These results cannot possibly be interpreted as demonstrating that the births under general practitioner care, even those in groups at high predicted risk, would have been safer in hospital. On the contrary they give very convincing support to the theory that delivery is safer without intervention for births without complication, estimated on the definition used here at 80 per cent of all births in the survey. If this is not so, then births with complication must be safer without intervention—a conclusion equally confounding to obstetricians. Yet the survey was accepted without proper analysis as sufficient authority for intensifying the policy of hospitalization. In particular, though PNMRs were actually lowest at home where 36 per cent of births had taken place (Table 14.3), the survey was declared to have demonstrated that the danger there was greatest. So the first objective was to contract provision for home delivery, but initially more beds were provided in general practitioner maternity units as a more palatable alternative for mothers unwilling to go into hospital.

Table 14.3 *Percentage of births and perinatal mortality rates (PNMRs) per 1000 births by place of delivery (Sources: Butler and Bonham 1963; Chamberlain et al. 1978)*

Place	Percentage		PNMR	
	1958	1970*	1958	1970
Hospital	49	66	50.1	27.8
General practitioner maternity unit	12	19	20.3	6.1
Home	36	12	19.8	4.3

* The official percentages for the whole year 1970 are hospital 73, general practitioner maternity unit 12, home 13. Classification of some hospitals may have been different.

THE SURVEY OF BRITISH BIRTHS 1970

The successful pursuit of these policies was measured in the RCOG's next survey in 1970, of which the analysis of mortality was not published until 1978 (Chamberlain *et al.* 1978). As Table 14.3 shows, the proportion of births at home had been reduced by two-thirds. The proportion in hospital had greatly increased but so also had the disparity in mortality. There was now a five-fold difference between the PNMRs in hospital (27.8) and under general practitioner care (5.4), a difference that surely required careful investigation, though none was reported.

Certainly hospital births included a greater proportion at high predicted risk. They included relatively more births to mothers in the higher-risk age groups, but standardizing PNMRs to allow for the unequal age distribution reduces the difference hardly at all (Table 14.4). In this survey an antenatal prediction score (APS) was constructed to incorporate all the risks known in early pregnancy—maternal age, parity, social class, obstetric history, and relevant coexisting disease—and every birth was classified according to this score. Hospital births included relatively more at high and moderate risk, but standardizing for this inequality reduces the difference between the

Table 14.4   *Standardized PNMRs by type of care and risk factors, British Births 1970 survey* (*Source: Chamberlain* et al. *1978*)

PNMR/1000 births	Hospital	General practitioner care
Crude	27.8	5.4
Standardized for age	27.3	5.7
Standardized for antenatal prediction score (APS)	26.6	6.0
Standardized for toxaemia	27.6	5.4

crude PNMRs by very little more than does standardizing for one single factor. This illustrates the point made earlier (p. 207) about the small arithmetical effect of combining interdependent variables. That the excess in hospital of births at high predicted risk explains so little of their excess mortality is inevitable, for the PNMR for the low-risk group in hospital was itself much higher than for the high-risk group under general practitioner care (Tew 1984).

The APS did not include complications which develop in pregnancy, of which the most frequently occurring and the cause of many transfers are toxaemia and antepartum haemorrhage (APH). Both of these were found to be strongly correlated with the APS, so most of the risk attaching to them has already been allowed for in standardizing for the APS. Standardizing for toxaemia by itself, the only complication for which the necessary data were published, again explains only a trivial part of the difference in PNMRs. The effect of APH would probably be similar. It is highly implausible that postmaturity, disproportion, malpresentation and other complications identified before the start of labour, which together affect such a small proportion of all births, could possibly account for the large unexplained excess PNMR in hospital. If the explanation does not lie in an excess of risk before delivery, it can only lie in an excess of risk during or after delivery.

The survey's analysts actually constructed a labour prediction score which incorporated all the conditions, including those in the first stage of labour, 'known to affect perinatal mortality and morbidity adversely', the overall score being 'the ultimate indicator of the type of care which a mother should receive' (Chamberlain *et al.* 1978). All births in the survey were classified according to this score also, but the distribution of these, with associated deaths, by place of delivery was not made available until 1983 (Golding 1983, personal communication).

The results are summarized in Table 14.5, from which it is clear that, in accordance with policy, the hospitals' share of births increased as the level of risk increased. But it is equally clear that the PNMR at every level of risk was higher in hospital. The margin was two-fold for births at very low risk,

Table 14.5   *Percentage of births and perinatal mortality rates by labour prediction score and place of delivery. (Source: British births 1970 Survey, unpublished data)*

Level of risk on labour prediction score	All births		Percentage at each score		PNMR/1000 births	
	Number	Percent	Hospital	General practitioner care	Hospital	General practitioner care
Very low	7488	45.9	58.7	41.3	8.0	3.9*
Low	3723	22.8	68.8	31.2	17.9	5.2**
Moderate	2273	13.9	76.6	23.4	32.2	3.8***
High	2417	14.8	84.0	16.0	53.2	15.5**
Very high	427	2.6	96.5	3.5	162.6	133.3
All risks	16328	100.0	68.2	31.8	27.8	5.4

Levels of significance $*P<0.05$; $**P<0.005$; $***P<0.001$.

but considerably wider for births at low, moderate and high risk. Only in the small group at highest risk, where only fifteen deliveries (3.5 per cent) were not in hospital, was this excess not statistically significant. To the extent that general practitioners transferred cases where the fetus had died or was moribund before the second stage of labour, hospital deliveries would include an excess of cases where predicted risk had already become certainty. But this factor could not nearly explain their excess PNMR, for their mortality rate for live births was by itself more than twice the PNMR for all births, live and still in general practitioner care. Thus, except perhaps at levels of very high risk experienced by a very small proportion of the total, the obstetricians' evidence is at total variance with their generally accepted claim that the benefits of obstetric care increase as the risk status of mother and fetus increases.

A prediction score which stopped short of first stage conditions would have given a more exact evaluation of the different systems of managing labour. Lacking this, but using data supplied privately (Golding 1982, personal communication), an attempt has been made to quantify the PNMRs for normal births without complication (defined as before) booked for hospital and general practitioner care respectively. Assuming, as was done in the corresponding analysis of 1958 data (p. 207), that complications developed among hospital-booked births in the same proportion and carried the same PNMR as among general practitioner bookings who required transfer, then hospital bookings without such complications would have had a PNMR about 2.4 times the PNMR for actual deliveries under general practitioner care (Tew 1984). This margin would be larger if complications arise less often and carry less risk in cases booked initially for hospital, as obstetricians surely believe they should. The margin would be rather smaller if obstetric care throughout does not reduce the PNMR associated with complications, as the now-released evidence implies. The 1970 survey, therefore, repeated the true findings of the 1958 survey, only more strongly, and challenged orthodox beliefs more disconcertingly.

TRENDS SINCE 1970

In the same year as the survey, but without waiting for its results, the Peel Report (1970) recommended that provision should be made for all births to take place in obstetric hospitals. It was apparently influenced by obstetricians' interpretations of the 1958 survey and by the observation that the national PNMR had decreased over the same period when the proportion of births in hospital had increased. As was later demonstrated, however, the former trend was not caused by the latter (Tew 1978) and this fact is now generally accepted except by wistful obstetricians (Booth 1981; Philipps 1982; Russell 1981). Nevertheless, though the recommendation had no evidence to support it, it has been given effect to with great thoroughness.

First, the domiciliary midwifery service was all but dismantled. Next, despite protests from general practitioners and mothers, a programme of closing 'unattached' general practitioner maternity units has been carried out, some being replaced by units attached to obstetric hospitals or general practitioner beds in these. By 1980 only 4 per cent of births took place in general practitioner maternity units, regardless of the fact that mortality there was consistently about one-quarter of that in hospital, where the high risk cases were increasingly being outnumbered by low-risk cases and so explaining even less of the excess PNMR there (*Birth Statistics*, annual).

The risk to the few of complications developing in places without facilities to deal with them was emphasized; the risk to the many of exposing normal births to obstetric interventions was not recognized. General practitioners were persuaded that an attached unit would be optimal. The only data known to this author where mortality in attached and unattached units can be compared show the reverse. In the 1970 survey the PNMR was 9.5 in attached units compared with 5.4 in unattached units; this difference is not statistically significant, but it certainly does not confirm the supposed advantage of the attached units. In 1978 the stillbirth rates (SBRs), calculated from official data, were 7.4 in attached and 1.6 in unattached units—a highly significant difference ($P<0.001$). Indeed the SBR in attached units was not significantly lower than the SBR of 8.9 in hospital. In their mortality experience attached units have apparently become more like obstetric hospitals than like their unattached counterparts (Tew 1981). Perhaps a surgical milieu tends to reduce restraint.

After 1970 more and more births became subject to obstetric interventions and the national PNMR continued to fall steeply. However, as the graph in Fig. 14.1 shows, this decrease was not dependent on the increase in births in hospital. On the contrary, the correlation coefficient between the variables is significantly negative ($P<0.01$): the years with the smaller increases in the percentage of births in hospital were the years with the larger decreases in the PNMR. The line, drawn from the estimating equation which best represents the underlying relationship between the variables, indicates that, if there had been no increase in hospitalization, the decrease in the PNMR could have been greater than it actually was.

In this period the only national data distinguishing place of birth and risk factors are the official stillbirths statistics by maternal age and parity (*Birth Statistics*, annual). Analysis of these has shown that while the SBR in hospital continued to fall as the proportion of births there increased, some 30 per cent of this decrease was due simply to dilution with low risk births which formerly would have taken place in general practitioner maternity units or at home with low mortality (Tew 1981). Despite this boost the SBR in hospital, where interventions were widely used, fell proportionally less

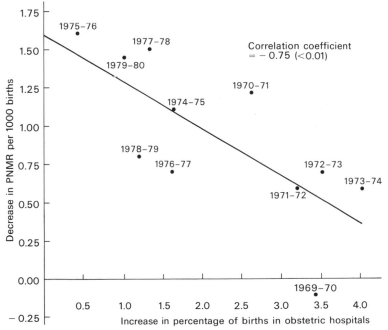

Fig. 14.1. Increases from one year to the next in the percentage of births in obstetric hospitals and concomitant decreases in the perinatal mortality rate, England and Wales, 1969–80.

than did the SBR in general practitioner maternity units, where interventions were little used and which could not have benefited so much from dilution with low-risk births. The SBR at home, once the lowest, rose as the number of births there was drastically reduced, leaving the subgroups whose mortality is high for social rather than medical reasons to form an increasing proportion of the whole. Increasingly reflecting the mortality experience of these, the SBR at home ceased to be an indicator of the safety of planned domiciliary confinements, though even in 1979–80 the SBR for legitimate births after the first, the subgroup least prejudiced by social factors, was significantly lower than the SBR for the corresponding group in hospital.

Since the falling PNMR cannot be attributed to the increase in obstetric management, to what can it more probably be attributed? By far the most important determinant of the PNMR is the health status of mothers and there are many indications that this has improved greatly over the century. Though the overall death rate began to fall after 1870, it was not until after 1900, a generation later, that the infant mortality rate began to fall, and when it did, most of the decline was among postneonatal infants. It was not until the 1940s, another generation later—probably lengthened by the economic depression of the 1930s—that perinatal mortality began to fall substantially and it took another generation to achieve the rapid decline of the 1970s. It would seem that the healthiest babies are born to mothers who were themselves the healthy babies of healthy mothers. It has taken at least three generations of improvement to reach the present low levels of perinatal mortality.

THE EVIDENCE FROM GENERAL PRACTICE

What did general practitioners think of the changes that were taking place and of the theories on which they were based? A survey of practices before 1955 had found that only 30 per cent of general practitioners interviewed were anxious to do midwifery (Annis Gillie 1956), so presumably the majority viewed with some relief a policy which would justify on ostensibly scientific grounds their relinquishing this responsibility, at least as regards intranatal care. Their influence on pregnant women to accept the policy has been very strong, sometimes going beyond persuasion. But the interested minority, who had practised conscientiously and who had coped with a fair range of complications with considerable success, must have been puzzled, to say the least, to be assured that they were competent to deal with only straightforward deliveries and, as no delivery can be guaranteed to remain straightforward, really unfit to be responsible for intranatal care.

Some of those who were least convinced by the dogma and who had kept careful records found time to write up their results. It is uncertain how representative their reports are since they are inevitably based on small numbers, cover different periods and do not always measure the same variables in the same way. Generally they confirm that the risk of booking for general practitioner care, including the risk of complication and transfer, is less than the national average and hence less than booking for hospital. Some of them demonstrate that the low PNMRs under general practitioner care are not obtained simply by identifying and transferring all deviations from normal and also that general practitioners are capable of providing a high level of safety for the large majority of births arising in the community.

General practitioners book some pregnancies from the start for delivery in hospital; of the remainder booked for home or a general practitioner maternity unit, some are transferred to hospital during pregnancy, some in labour, and a few in the puerperium. The booking and transfer decisions depend on various factors: the proximity of an obstetric hospital and the availability of beds there, obstetricians' guidelines for selection, the general practitioner's judgement regarding clinical indications, social reasons, and the wishes of the mother if strongly expressed. The importance of each of these factors varies from place to place and from time to time. Consequently the proportion of pregnancies in each of the categories of booking and transfer varies correspondingly.

In the 1950s and 1960s in areas where hospital beds were scarce or considered to be too far away, the majority of bookings had to be for general practitioner care. They had to include some at high predicted risk and some who were to develop complications whatever their predicted risk. As the following examples show, by no means all of the latter were transferred, so that general practitioners were accustomed to managing abnormal deliveries and they did so with PNMRs below, often much below, the national average.

Of 1000 cases between 1957 and 1964 in a rural practice in Wales, 245 shared 'a wide variety of abnormalities as challenging as the 23 referrals to a consultant' (Cavenagh 1966). Only twelve out of 411 deliveries between 1948 and 1959 in a rural practice in Scotland took place in a specialist hospital; the general practitioner concluded that 'where there are adequate facilities, 95 per cent of an obstetric practice can be conducted unaided by experienced general practitioners with satisfactory results' (McGregor and Martin 1961). In a rural practice in Kent between 1946 and 1970 there was 'a low rate of booking and delivery in hospital, a relatively large proportion of high risk cases under sole practitioner care, a low rate of transfer from GP to consultant care at all stages, a majority of complicated cases managed by GPs', and a PNMR, including transfers, about two-thirds of the national average (Wood 1981). In an Essex practice about 5 km (3 miles) from an obstetric unit between 1955 and 1961, 67 per cent of cases were booked for and 60 per cent achieved home delivery; in the event more than half of those booked for hospital were uncomplicated, so that over 75 per cent were by any standards suitable for general practitioner care. General practitioners dealt with 60 per cent of the complications arising in home bookings, clearly with success since their PNMR was less than half the national average, so they could probably have dealt as successfully with similar complications arising in hospital booked cases. It can be estimated from their evidence that they could have cared safely for 80–85 per cent of cases in the practice, compared with the 30 per cent recommended in the Cranbrooke Report on the advice of the RCOG (Maternity Services Committee 1959). 'Obstetric indications for booking . . . appear to be based on the assumption that general practitioners should never be placed in the position that they should have to exercise their judgement on an obstetric matter' (Bury and Garson 1963).

THE RISKS OF TRANSFER

As more hospital beds became available, general practitioners were under pressure to use them. They observed the continuing decline in perinatal deaths and they had no evidence to contradict the claim that this was due to increased hospitalization. So gradually most of them, even the sceptical ones, modified their practices and applied the more strict criteria advocated for selecting the cases they could book and retain for intranatal care. Mothers in certain categories of high predicted risk, who must formerly have fared quite well under general practioner care given the overall results, were no longer booked and, though one would have expected the opposite, a greater proportion of this more select low-risk group was found to need transfer in pregnancy or labour. This increase in diagnosed abnormality was surprising at a time when the general fitness of mothers was improving; it surely reflected a change in criteria rather than in condition. The evidence is, however, that transfers as a whole, whether on more strict or less strict criteria, did not benefit from the change of management.

For example, a study (by obstetricians) of home and hospital confinement in Newcastle-upon-Tyne (Barron, Thomson, and Philips 1977) found that the proportion of births booked for hospital increased from 48.7 per cent in 1960–62 to 76.8 per cent in 1966–69, while of those births booked for home the proportion transferred increased from 12.9 to 20.9 per cent (Table 14.6, columns 5 and 2). On the hypothesis that in 1966–69 births in each subgroup had remained in the same proportion as in 1960–62 but experienced the actual PNMRs of 1966–69, the PNMRs overall and for home bookings in 1966–69 would have been considerably less than they actually were: 19.8 as against 24.1 and 14.2 as against 18.0 respectively (columns 7 and 6). Similarly, in an attached general practitioner maternity unit in Oxford, the PNMR for all booked births, which was 9.2 in 1975–77, would have been

Table 14.6 *The composition of PNMRs, Newcastle 1966–69. (Source: Barron et al.* 1977; *estimated from Fig. 2 of the article)

Deliveries	Actual			Hypothetical		
	Proportion of births 1966–69	Rate/1000 in 1966–69	Product	Proportion of births 1960–62	Rate/1000 1966–69	Product
Home	0.184	7.9*	1.5	0.447	7.9*	3.5
Transfers	0.048	56.4*	2.7	0.066	56.4*	3.7
Hospital	0.768	25.9	19.9	0.487	25.9	12.6
All	1.000	24.1 =	24.1	1.000	24.1	19.8
Home bookings						
Home	0.791	7.9*	6.2	0.871	7.9*	6.9
Transfers	0.209	56.4*	11.8	0.129	56.4*	7.3
All	1.000	18.0 =	18.0	1.000	18.0	14.2

Note. This table illustrates a necessary arithmetical relationship which is essential to understanding how the overall (average) PNMR for a group reflects the experience of subgroups with different degrees of risk, weighted according to the relative number (proportion) of births in each; the average PNMR is equal to the sum of the products of the proportion of births multiplied by the specific PNMR in each subgroup. The relationship is the same if the proportions are multiplied by 100 and expressed as percentages, as is more familiar, and the products which would then result are divided by 100 to relate them again to unity.

only 8.1 if the proportion transferred had remained at 33 per cent, as it was in 1968–70, instead of increasing to 36 per cent (Bull 1980).

When only a small proportion of bookings is transferred, it is likely to be made up of cases with very serious complications and its PNMR is likely to be much higher than that for the general practitioner deliveries. The greater the proportion of transfers—figures over 40 or 50 per cent have been reported (Richmond 1977; Taylor *et al.* 1980), the more the average risk for the group is decreased by the inclusion of less serious cases, so that one would expect the PNMR for a larger transfer group to exceed that for the retained general practitioner deliveries by a smaller margin. Reported differentials, however, remain wide. In the Newcastle study the PNMRs were seven to eight times as high for transfers as for home deliveries; in the Oxford study the ratios were 22 and 35. It is popularly said that this disparity reflects the general practitioner's skill in segregating high-risk cases. Is this rationalization sufficient?

The reasons for transfer in pregnancy include most frequently toxaemia and postmaturity and much less frequently antepartum haemorrhage (APH), disproportion and malpresentation. The PNMR associated with severe toxaemia has been quantified as just over twice that associated with no toxaemia; the PNMR at over 42 weeks' gestation as just over twice that at 39–41 weeks; the PNMR associated with APH as less than four times that associated with no bleeding. If malpresentation, disproportion or the conditions which lead to transfer in labour result in caesarean section, then a PNMR about 2.5 times that for spontaneous cephalic presentation would be expected (Chamberlain *et al.* 1978). Even if the other reasons for transfer carry a high fatality rate, they make up such a small proportion of all transfers that they have little effect on their overall average. Thus a generous forecast of the PNMR of a group made up of such high-risk cases would be higher than that of a low-risk group drawn from the same area by a factor of 3 or 4, but not by a factor of 7 or 8, and certainly not by a factor of 22 or 35, unless the transfer itself (and only a minority were emergency transfers) and the subsequent treatment added to the risk.

These findings lead to the same conclusion as did the 1970 survey: however beneficial the new treatment may have been in a few pathological cases, it was not beneficial for the transferred group as a whole (Tew 1984). This leads to the further speculation: if obstetric methods are not beneficial for most of the conditions which caused transfer, are they beneficial for the same conditions when they develop in hospital-booked cases? This question will be further discussed below.

CONTROLLED TRIALS

The ideal way to evaluate alternative methods of treatment is by conducting a properly designed randomized controlled trial. No such trial to evaluate the effects of place of confinement has ever taken place and it is extremely doubtful that one could be set up prospectively since this is an issue where the attitudes of all who would take part, doctors, midwives, and mothers, would probably be already strongly prejudiced one way or the other.

As a very modest substitute a study was carried out comparing a series of pregnancies booked for delivery in four Berkshire general practitioner maternity units with a matched series booked on the same criteria for delivery in two obstetric hospitals in Rochdale and the Isle of Wight. Comparison of various parameters favoured the general practitioner maternity units and it was concluded conservatively that 'booking into a GPMU was as safe for low risk women' and 'booking into a consultant unit did not reduce perinatal mortality' (Taylor *et al.* 1980). Of the general practitioner maternity unit bookings 56 per cent were transferred to consultant care in pregnancy or labour (plus a further 10 per cent in the puerperium). Since the results related to bookings and the transfers were not separately distinguished, the study did not contribute to an evaluation of the effect on birth of the actual place of confinement. The PNMR for the general practitioner maternity unit bookings, an average which inevitably reflected the experience of the transfers more than that of the general practitioner maternity unit deliveries, was much higher than the national PNMR for general practitioner maternity unit deliveries.

Using computerized records which enabled very accurate matching, a comparison was made between two groups of low-risk women booked respectively for delivery in 1978 in a consultant unit (CU) and the attached general practitioner maternity unit of the same Oxford hospital (Klein *et al.* 1983). Of the general practitioner maternity unit bookings 31 per cent were transferred (confirming the trend noted on p. 216), but their results were included with the general practitioner maternity unit deliveries; the consultant unit group included no transfers. Various obstetric procedures were found to have been carried out significantly more often in the consultant unit. As most of the interventions in the general practitioner maternity unit group related to the transfers, their actual usage in the consultant unit must have exceeded that in the general practitioner maternity unit by an even wider margin. The proportion of infants needing intubation or care in a special care baby unit was significantly greater for the consultant booked group. (This repeated the finding of the *British Births 1970* survey (Tew 1980)). A further refinement of the groups was made to exclude induced labours and their possible consequences. In this second comparison significant differences were found: in women booked for the general practitioner maternity unit 'both first and second stage labours were longer' but 'they received less electronic fetal monitoring, augmentation and forceps delivery and fetal distress was diagnosed less often'; more than twice as many of them received 'nothing' for pain; their infants were three times less likely to have low Apgar scores.

In this study every step was taken to exclude from the consultant unit group any condition or circumstance which might have increased their risk status preferentially or biased the interpretation of results in their disfavour: 'Infants weighing under 2500 g were excluded after the fact because they confounded the results. The few low birthweight infants booked in the GPMU were between 2000 and 2500 g and did well while a number of small sick infants appeared in the CU group.' Thus though given the benefit of every doubt, the consultant unit emerged unfavourably from the comparisons which demonstrated 'the simplicity and safety of delivery of low-risk women' in this attached general practitioner maternity unit. The interventions inflicted on similar women in the consultant unit were shown to be unnecessary and on the whole harmful.

THE EFFECT OF OBSTETRIC INTERVENTIONS

The fact is that 'scientific' interventions have been universally adopted without prior 'scientific' evaluation to establish that they were indeed the cause of the reduced mortality which happened to follow their introduction. Nor have retrospective studies been able to demonstrate this causal relationship either for interventions in general (Chalmers *et al.* 1976) or in particular for caesarean section (Francome and Huntingford 1980) or electronic fetal monitoring (Banta and Thacker 1979).

All studies confirm the finding of the *British Births 1970* survey (Chamberlain *et al.* 1978) that PNMRs are higher where interventions have been used than where they have not. The argument that the interventions were used only in cases where the PNMR would otherwise have been even higher cannot be sustained. Throughout the 1970s well over one-third of labours were induced, compared with 13 per cent in 1964; the proportion was nearly as great in births without as in births with 'complication or anomaly' (*Maternity Statistics* 1981). Induction may be beneficial in the small proportion of cases where the mother has certain life-threatening conditions, though a caesarean section is more likely to produce a live child (Llewellyn-Jones 1969), or in cases of 'placental insufficiency' resulting in intrauterine growth retardation (IUGR) which, however, cannot yet be reliably diagnosed and induction has produced many babies immature but not growth retarded (Hall, Chng and MacGillivray 1980).

One of the most frequent reasons for induction (and transfer) is postmaturity. Baird attributed the rise in PNMR after 40 weeks' gestation to a decline in placental function (Baird, 1960). More recent studies dispute that this commonly happens. A comparison of 2000 induced and spontaneous labours otherwise matched led to the conclusion that 'a pregnancy prolonged after 42 confirmed weeks of gestation may affect perinatal outcome but induction of labour does not improve this and that uncomplicated postmaturity is not an indication for induction of labour' (Gibbs *et al.* 1982). Other studies by obstetricians have found that the PNMR would not have been reduced by an induction rate above 9.5 per cent (O'Driscoll, Carroll and Coughlan 1975) or 8 per cent (Williams and Studd 1980).

Induction by shortening gestation and disrupting the natural process, brings its own risks and it leads to significantly higher levels of further interventions—analgesia, including epidural, and anaesthesia; electronic fetal monitoring; forceps delivery and caesarean section—all of which make their own contribution to increasing the risk of fetal distress and neonatal difficulties in breathing and sucking (Chamberlain *et al.* 1975). The extent of these consequential interventions was measured in a study of 400 deliveries with no medical or obstetric complications, in half of which labour started spontaneously and in the other closely matched half was induced; 99 per cent of the spontaneous group, compared with 68 per cent of the induced, went on to have a spontaneous delivery. 'Our findings are that healthy women, with no medical or obstetric abnormality, who are allowed to come into labour spontaneously will nearly all experience an uncomplicated labour and delivery' (Yudkin *et al.* 1979).

The experience of the French obstetrician, Michel Odent, leads him to go further. The conditions most conducive to a successful outcome in labours without problems—watchful support while the mother, without drugs of any kind, adopts the positions that seem most natural to her—are even more essential in labours with problems, most of which will then solve themselves successfully. No time limits are set for the stages of labour. (In Britain, delay at any stage, relative to set criteria, is the commonest reason for transfer in labour.) Only a small minority, under 10 per cent, are ultimately found for individual reasons to need intervention and then a caesarean section is performed. The rates of mortality and morbidity of body and mind achieved by this system are very low (Odent 1984).

Odent's hypothesis finds support in the newly available analysis of the *British Births 1970* data, which shows obstetric care to be no more effective in benefiting births at moderate and high risk than those at low risk (see Table 14.5).

CONCLUSION

It is clear which of the conflicting theories, described in the introduction to this chapter, the evidence unanimously and unambiguously supports and why. There is no doubt that intrapartum care without intervention is safest for births to mothers at low predicted risk and without complication; but the evidence is strong that such methods are safest also for most births at high predicted risk or with certain complications. Such births probably make up over 80 per cent of all births. From the point of view of physical safety it matters little in which place or by which accoucheur delivery takes place, provided that the panoply of intervention techniques is reserved strictly for the small proportion of mothers whom they will benefit. From the point of view of satisfaction, which safety in the wider sense embraces, mothers should be free to choose the place where and the accoucheur with whom they will feel most confident, and that will often mean general practitioner care. These findings have fundamental implications for the training of obstetricians as well as general practitioners and midwives.

In a book for general practitioners it is appropriate to end this chapter by reporting the outstanding record of one of them who, in 30 years' practice in the North-East, has cared for 5010 births, excluding fifteen transferred to consultant care but including 186 transferred by the mother's wish from consultant care and many from outside his own group practice. He accepts women in all risk categories but attaches great importance to antenatal care. Deliveries have been in the mother's home, in nursing homes and in general practitioner beds in hospital. His careful records show a forceps rate of 2 per cent and six caesarean sections. There have been ten perinatal deaths (five in the transfers to consultant care), giving a PNMR of two. Confinement in his care has been a very safe procedure (Richardson, J. 1983, personal communication).

REFERENCES

Annis Gillie, K. (1956). In *Proceedings of a conference on general practitioner obstetrics.* College of General Practitioners, London, 2–3.

Baird, D. (1960). The evolution of modern obstetrics. *Lancet* **2**, 557–64 and 609–14.

Banta, D. and Thacker, S. (1979). Electronic fetal monitoring: is it of benefit? *Birth and the family J.* **6.4**, 237–49.

Barron, S. L., Thomson, A. M., and Philips, P. R. (1977). Home and hospital confinement in Newcastle-upon-Tyne 1960–1969. *Br. J. Obstet. Gynaecol.* **84**, 401–11.

Birth statistics (Annual 1974–80) Office of Population Censuses and Surveys, HMSO, London.

Booth, R. T. (1981). Never at home. *J. Mat. Child Health* **6.6**, 228–32.

Bull, M. J. V. (1980). Ten years' experience in a general practice obstetric unit. *J. Roy. Coll. Gen. Practit.* **30**, 208–15.

Bury, J. D. and Garson, J. Z. (1963). Home or hospital confinement? *J. Coll. Gen. Practit.* **6**, 590–605.

Butler, N. R. and Alberman, E. D. (1969). *Perinatal problems.* Churchill Livingstone, Edinburgh.

Butler, N. R. and Bonham, D. G. (1963). *Perinatal mortality.* Churchill Livingstone, Edinburgh.

Cavenagh, A. J. M. (1966). Role of the general practitioner maternity unit—1000 deliveries analysed. *Br. Med. J.* **1**, 533–4.

Chalmers, I., Zlosnik, J. E., Johns, K. A., and Campbell, H. (1976). Obstetric practice and outcome of pregnancy in Cardiff residents 1965–73. *Br. Med. J.* **1**, 735–9.

Chamberlain, R., Chamberlain, G., Howlett, B, and Claireaux, A. (1975). *British Births 1970, vol 1*, Heinemann, London.

Chamberlain, G., Philipps, E., Howlett, B., and Masters, K. (1978). *British Births 1970, vol 2*, Heinemann, London.

Cookson, I. (1967). The past and future of the maternity services. *J. Coll. Gen. Practit.* **13**, 143–62.

Francome, C. and Huntingford, P. J. (1980). Birth by caesarean section in the United States of America and in Britain. *J. Biol. Sci.* **12**, 353–62.

Gibbs, D. M. F., Cardozo, L. D., Studd, J. W. W., and Cooper, D. J. (1982). Prolonged pregnancy: is induction of labour indicated? *Br. J. Obstet. Gynaecol.* **89**, 292–5.

Hall, M. H., Chng, P. K., and MacGillivray, I. (1980). Is routine antenatal care worthwhile? *Lancet* **2**, 78–80.

Klein, M. Lloyd, I., Redman, C., Bull, M., and Turnbull, A. C. (1983). A comparison of low-risk pregnant women booked for delivery in two systems of care: shared care (consultant) and integrated general practice unit. I. Obstetrical procedures and newborn outcomes and II. Labour and delivery management and neonatal outcome. *Br. J. Obstet. Gynaecol.* **90**, 118–22 and 123–8.

Kloosterman, G. J. (1978). Organization of obstetric care in the Netherlands. *Ned. Tijdschr. Genieskunde*, 1161–71.

Kloosterman, G. J. (1982). The universal aspects of childbirth: human birth as a socio-psychosomatic paradigm. *J. Psychosomat. Obstet. Gynaecol.* **1**, 35–41.

Llewellyn-Jones, D. (1969). Quoted in *Birthrights* by S. Inch. Hutchinson, London (1982).

McGregor, R. M. and Martin, L. V. H. (1961). Obstetrics in a general practice. *J. Coll. Gen. Practit.* **4**, 542–51.

Maternity Statistics 1978 (1981). Office of Population Censuses and Surveys, Monitor MB4 81/1. HMSO, London.

Maternity Services Committee (1959). *The Cranbrooke Report*. HMSO, London.

Odent M. (1984). How to help women in labour. In *Pregnancy care for the 1980s* (eds. L. Zander and G. Chamberlain). The Royal Society of Medicine and Macmillan Press, London.

O'Driscoll, K., Carroll, C. J., and Coughlan, M. (1975). Selective induction of labour. *Br. Med. J.* **2**, 727–9.

Philipps, E. (1982). Skilled process of delivery. Letter to the *Daily Telegraph*, **30 August**.

Registrar General, *Statistical reviews of England and Wales (annual to 1973)* HMSO, London.

Richmond, G. A. (1977). An analysis of 3199 patients booked for delivery in general practitioner maternity units. *J. Roy. Coll. Gen. Practit.* **27**, 406–13.

Russell, J. K. (1981). Should home births be ruled out? *The Times* 21 January. Standing Maternity and Midwifery Advisory Committee (1970). *Report on domiciliary midwifery and maternity bed needs* (The Peel Report) HMSO, London.

Taylor, G. W., Edgar, W., Taylor, B. A. and Neal, D. G. (1980). How safe is general practitioner obstetrics? *Lancet* **2**, 1287–9.

Tew, M. (1978). The case against hospital deliveries: the statistical evidence. In *The place of birth*. (eds. S. Kitzinger and J. A. Davis) Oxford University Press, Oxford.

Tew, M. (1980). Facts, not assertions of belief. *Health and Soc. Ser. J.* **September 12**, 1194–7.

Tew, M. (1981). Effects of scientific obstetrics on perinatal mortality. *Health and Soc. Serv. J.* **April 17**, 444–6.

Tew, M. (1984). Understanding intranatal care through mortality statistics. In *Pregnancy care for the 1980s* (eds. L. Zander and G. Chamberlain). The Royal Society of Medicine and Macmillan Press, London.

Williams, R. and Studd, J. (1980). Induction of labour. *J. Mat. Child Health* **5.1**, 16–21.

Wood, L. A. C. (1981). Obstetric retrospect. *J. Roy. Coll. Gen. Practit.* **31**, 80–90.

Yudkin, P., Frumar, A. M., Anderson, A. M. B, and Turnbull, A. C. (1979). A retrospective study of induction of labour. *Br. J. Obstet. Gynaecol.* **86**, 257–65.

15 Audit in obstetric care

M. J. V. Bull

INTRODUCTION

Audit in medicine has been succinctly defined as the planned examination of patient care. It may variously be utilized (Mourin 1976) for:

- (i)   setting professional standards;
- (ii) assessing clinical performance;
- (iii) modifying clinical behaviour.

It can therefore provide a powerful tool not only for the examination of quality of care but also for continuing education in medical practice. Simplistically, audit may be portrayed (Fig. 15.1) as a continuous process of measurement, evaluation and modification—in other words, learning by experience.

Obstetrics has for long been an attractive target for audit and one of consuming interest from national down to individual level. Pregnancy is still a

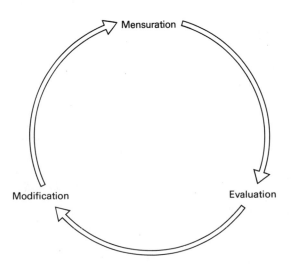

Fig. 15.1. The mechanism of audit.

relatively frequent occurrence: its course is reasonably predictable, complications are well documented and outcome variables generally amenable to objective scrutiny. Most women (in the United Kingdom at any rate) suspecting pregnancy will consult a general practitioner in the first instance and to this primary care professional falls the task of making appropriate decisions for subsequent management. It is the testing of the validity of these decisions by means of audit that quality of care can be maintained and advanced.

It is customary to examine medical care at three levels (Donabedian 1966):

Structure — the prerequisite skills, equipment and facilities necessary for the work under examination
Process — the manner in which the structure is utilized
Outcome — the end results of the process applied.

In obstetrics, perhaps a little manipulation of this classification is permissible. While skills, equipment and facilities are of obvious importance, there are also particular maternal characteristics which could be included under 'structure' since they are well established factors in influencing decisions regarding 'process' and (ultimately) 'outcome'. This concept is shown in Table 15.1.

DATA COLLECTION

The fundamental basis for any system of audit must of course be data collection. Methods are available at varying levels of sophistication but the essential features of any system must be that the information recorded is reliable, complete and easily accessible. A number of methods of data collection appropriate to the general practitioner obstetrician will now be described.

The log book

Patients can be listed as deliveries occur in an obstetric casebook ruled in columns to record:

(i) basic maternal characteristics (age, parity, marital status, social class, etc.)
(ii) notes concerning the pregnancy (complications, transfer of care, etc.)
(iii) details of the birth (mode of delivery, analgesia, complications, etc.)
(iv) details of the baby (sex, birth weight, etc.)

While this system is simple to set up subsequent analysis of data can be time-consuming and laborious. Simple counts of number of patients by mode of delivery is of course, straightforward but if cross-tabulation is required by (say) maternal parity, difficulties are immediately encountered unless the number of cases is very small.

Table 15.1   *Variables in obstetric audit*

Structure	Process	Outcome	
		Maternal	Neonatal
Facilities available, e.g.	Styles of care	Mode of delivery	Outcome
Specialist opinion	Specialist care	Spontaneous	Live birth
Ultrasound	Shared care	Forceps	Stillbirth
Cardiotocography	Community care	Breech	Neonatal death (1–7 days)
Fetal monitoring		Caesarean	(8–28 days)
Special care baby unit	Complications	Other	
Blood bank	Antenatal		
	Labour	Perineum	Other variables
	Puerperium	Intact	Birth weight
		Laceration	Apgar score
Maternal factors, e.g.	Interventive procedures	Episiotomy	Perinatal morbidity
Age	See Table 15.2		Congenital malformation
Parity		Other events, e.g.	Feeding method
Stature		Retained placenta	
Social class		Postpartum	
Ethnic origin		haemorrhage	
Basal body weight			
Smoking			
Intended place of delivery	Transfer of care	Final place of delivery	Transfer of baby to:
			NICU
			SCBU

Punched card system

Edge-notched cards

A simple, yet much more flexible system, is that of using edge-punched (Cope-Chat)* cards, one for each patient. Each hole represents a particular variable which is identified by notching out. The cards can be overprinted to specification (Fig. 15.2) but a much less expensive system is to use standard-sized blank cards laid on a template (Fig. 15.3). The potential number of identifiable variables depend on the number of available holes and thus on the size of the card. Sorting is achieved by passing a knitting needle through the pack of cards at the required location whereupon cards for all patients with that particular attribute will fall out and can be counted manually. Quite complicated analyses can be performed utilizing this method, although sorting becomes unwieldly if applied to a series of more than 100 cases.

Feature cards

Whereas in the edge-notched card system each card represents a particular patient, in the feature card method one card represents a given feature or attribute. The cards are overprinted (Fig. 15.4) with a numbered grid and each small square represents a patient with that particular serial number. Punching a given location thus indicates that the patient with that serial number has the feature or attribute that the card represents. Analysis of data can be achieved by straight counts of punch holes for given features or, by means of stacking, to count the number of patients with multiple attributes since in these instances the holes will pass clear through the stack. For example, if one card represents nulliparity, another pre-eclampsia, and a third delivery by caesarean section, when these three cards are stacked, the number of positions punched clear will identify all the nulliparae suffering from pre-eclampsia who were delivered by caesarean section. Each card carries up to 2500 patient locations and the method has been described in detail by Harden, Harden and Reekie (1974).

Hollerith cards

A more sophisticated system yet is that using standard business machine cards (Fig. 15.5) which are both punched and sorted mechanically. Data for each patient delivered are recorded on a coding sheet (Fig. 15.6) and are subsequently transferred by key punch operators to the Hollerith cards. Each card permits ten items for each of 80 columns and so has a potential capacity for up to 800 variables for each patient. Ultimately the cards are machine-sorted selectively to provide counts and cross-tabulations or can be

* Copeland-Chatterson Co. Ltd., Station House, Darkes Lane, Potters Bar, Herts EN6 1AW.

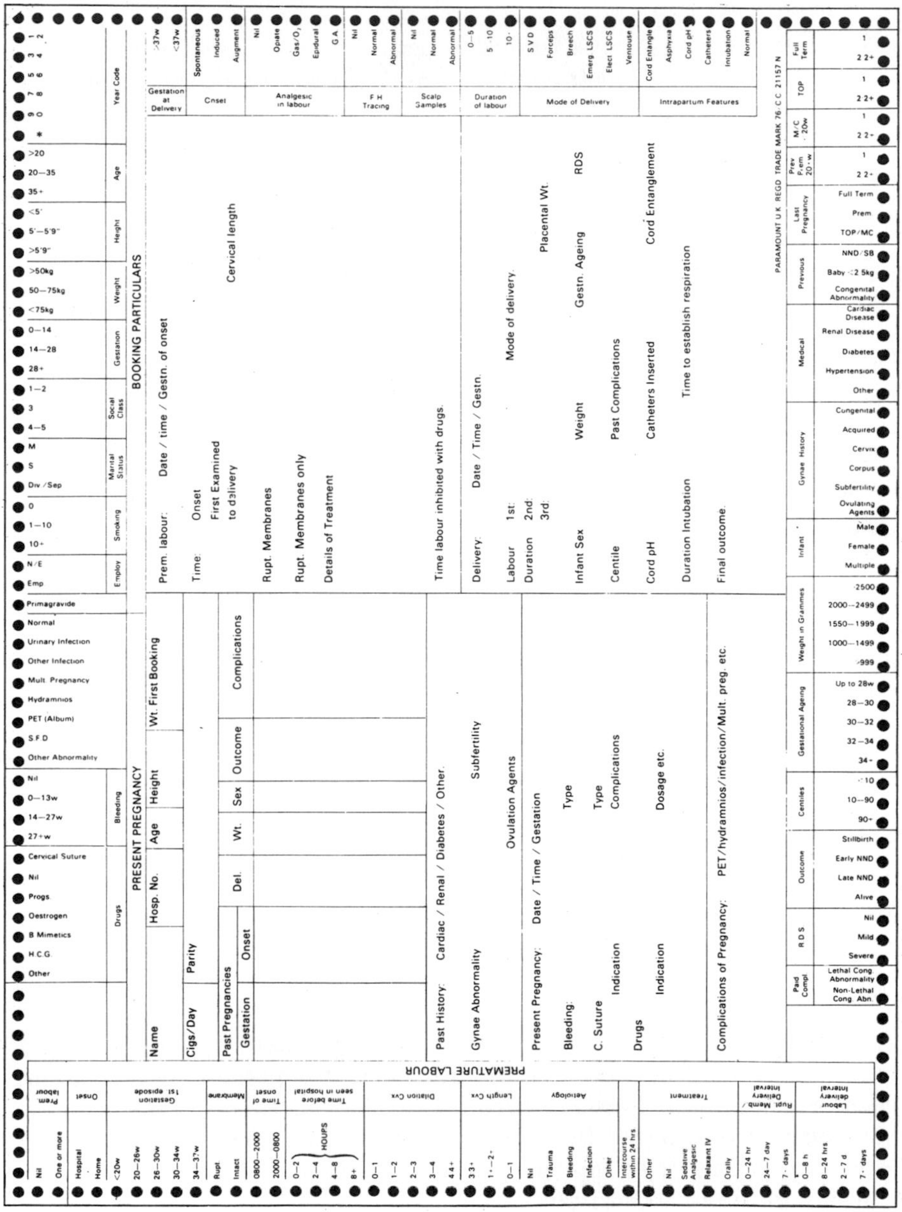

Fig. 15.2. The edge-punched card (printed).

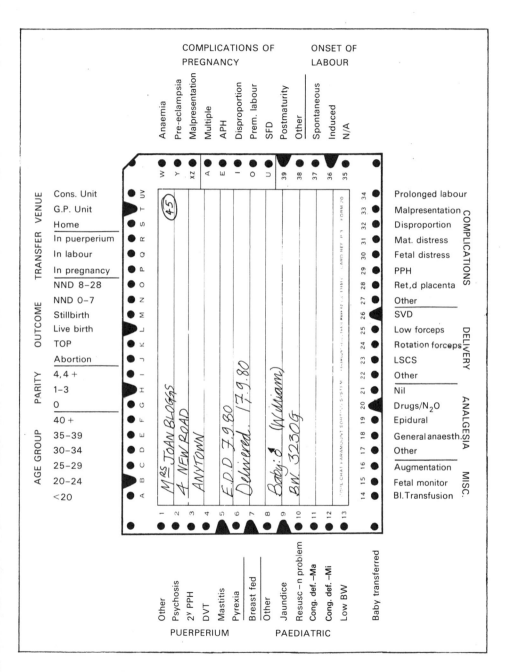

Fig. 15.3. The edge-punched card (template method).

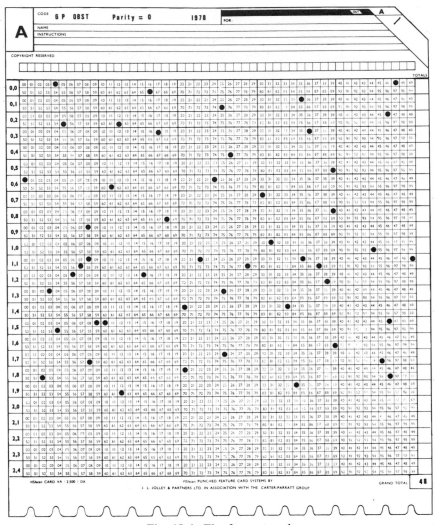

Fig. 15.4. The feature card.

used as computer input documents. This system was the basis of the RCOG standardized Maternity Hospital Medical Report System (RCOG 1949), and is also appropriate for general practitioner maternity units delivering several hundred patients each year (Bull 1980).

Computers

Computers with their massive storage capacity and facility for rapid sorting and analysis of complicated data sets are particularly appropriate for obstetric audit. A mainframe system operating in batch mode was described

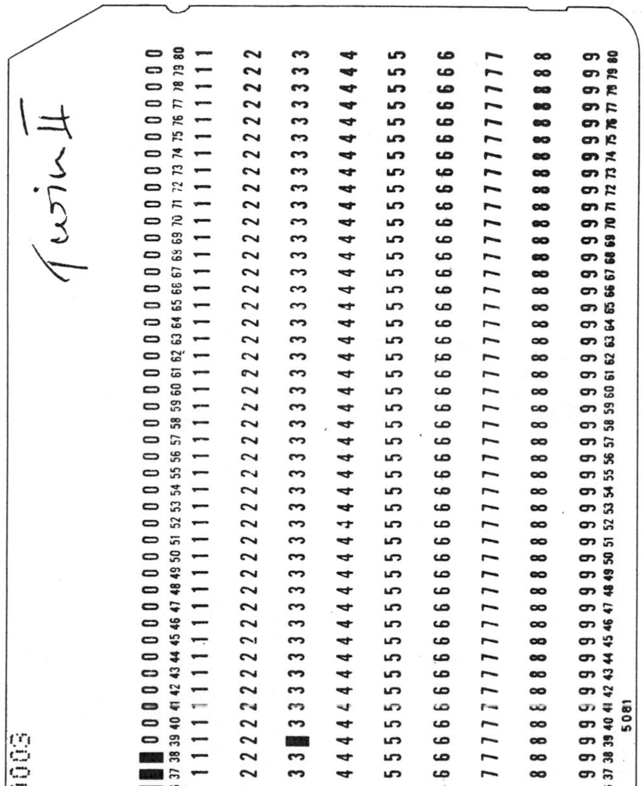

Fig. 15.5. The Hollerith card.

G.P. OBSTETRIC SURVEY

1–6 National GP Code $\boxed{6|2|2|9|7|4}$ 7–10 Serial No. $\boxed{0|4|3|5}$

Surname ...... *NOAKES* ......   Forenames ...... *SUSAN* ...... E.D.D. *3/4/81* ......

11–12 Age $\boxed{1\,9}$ 13–14 Gravida $\boxed{0\,1}$ 15–16 Para $\boxed{0\,0}$ 17–18 Stature $\boxed{6\,1}$
(inches)

Husband's Occupation ...... *BUS DRIVER* ...... Employment Status
.... 1 Self-employed – with employees
2 Self-employed – without employees
3 Manager
19. Social Class $\boxed{3}$ 4 Foreman
⑤ Other employee

Civil States: Risk Group:
20. At booking   21. At Confinement 22. Primigravida   23. Multigravida   24. Blood Group
1 Single   1 Single   ① Low   1 Low   ① 0+ 6 B –
② Married   ② Married   2 Intermediate   2 Intermediate   2 0– 7 AB+
3 Widowed   3 Widowed   3 High   3 High   3 A+ 8 AB–
4 Other   4 Other   4 N/K   4 N/K   4 A– 9 N/K
5 N/K   5 N/K   5 B+

25. Place of Booking
    0 Not booked
    1 Home
    ② GP unit
    3 Hospital – GP care
    4 Hospital – Consultant care
    5 Other ....

26. Transfer of Booking
    0 Not transferred
    ① Transferred in pregnancy
    2 Transferred in labour
    3 Transferred, in puerperium

27* Place of Delivery
    0 N/A (Abortions)
    1 Home
    2 GP unit
    3 Hospital – GP care
    ④ Hospital – Consultant care
    5 Other ....

28* Complications of Pregnancy (select principal c.)
    0 None or N/A
    ① Toxaemia
    2 APH
    3 Anaemia
    4 Multiple pregnancy
    5 Malpresentation
    6 ? disproportion
    7 Premature labour
    8 Postmaturity
    9 Other ....

29 Onset of Labour
    0 No labour (elective CS)
    1 Spontaneous
    2 Induction – stretch and sweep
    3 Induction – ARM
    4 Induction – Oxytocin
    ⑤ Induction – 3 + 4
    6 Induction – Other
    9 N/K

Complications of Labour:
30* Stage 1
    ⓪ N/A or none
    1 Ruptured membranes – not in labour
    2 Prolonged first stage
    3 Malpresentation – breech
    4 Malpresentation – other
    5 Intrapartum haemorrhage
    6 Hypertension
    7 Disproportion
    8 Fetal distress
    9 Other ....

31* Stage II
    0 N/A or none
    ① Delay – OA
    2 Delay – OP
    3 Malpresentation – breach
    4 Malpresentation – brow
    5 Malpresentation – face
    6 Malpresentation – other (including
    7 Maternal distress   twins)
    8 Fetal distress
    9 Other ....

32* Stage III
    0 N/A or none
    1 Retained placenta
    ② PPH (over 500 ml)
    3 1 + 2
    4 Third degree laceration
    5 Other ....

33–34 Duration of labour $\boxed{0\,7}$ hours

35.   N Mode of Delivery
    1 Vertex spontaneous
    ② Low forceps
    3 Rotation and forceps
    4 Breech
    5 Ventouse
    6 LSCS
    7 Other ....
    8 Abortion
    9 N/K

Fig. 15.6. A data coding sheet.
(Reverse not shown)

in the early 1970s (South and Rhodes 1971) and many large district maternity hospitals must now have the advantage of such facilities, although as yet not on a standardized basis. More recent developments in the field relate to the use of relatively inexpensive microcomputers with online applications for both service functions such as antenatal care (Lilford and Chard 1982) and audit (Maresh *et al.* 1983). Even now programmes are being developed in individual general practices (Kelly 1982) for the use of home computers to undertake obstetric and other forms of audit.

INDICES FOR OBSTETRIC AUDIT

How then shall we examine the quality of care that general practitioners provide in obstetrics? Maternal characteristics (structure) and styles of care (process) are traditionally examined in terms of outcome. As the result of major surveys (the triennial confidential enquiries into maternal deaths and the Perinatal Mortality Surveys of 1958 and 1970) guidelines have been laid down concerning selection of patients for general practitioner care. Broadly, these are:

A 'normal' medical and obstetric history
Nulliparae — age between 17 and 29 years at booking
             — stature more than 152 cm.
Multiparae — age less than 35 years at booking
             — parity less than 4

One application of audit, therefore, may be to determine if these criteria are being adhered to or indeed whether they are in need of modification. Some conventional process and outcome variables will now be discussed.

Perinatal mortality rate (PNMR)
Traditionally the perinatal mortality rate calculated thus

$$\frac{(\text{Stillbirths} + \text{early NNDs}) \times 1000}{\text{Total births}}$$

has been regarded as the standard yardstick of obstetric care. However, while there may be some justification for its use in large cohorts of patients, for small numbers it is a very insensitive instrument. The average practitioner in the United Kingdom has some 2200 patients on his NHS list amongst whom, at current fertility rates, and assuming a normal practice age distribution, no more than 30 women may be expected to give birth each year. In some districts, perinatal mortality is already below ten per 1000 births so each general practitioner will on average expect only one perinatal death in his practice every 3 years. Even for larger numbers (for example general practitioner maternity units delivering 500–1000 women per annum) the validity of crude perinatal mortality rates is questionable if used as an index of quality of care. For example, perinatal mortality rates relating to women actually *delivered* in general practitioner units will give no reliable indication of appropriate selection for general practitioner care because patients developing problems in pregnancy or labour (which may result in perinatal death) will usually be transferred to specialist care before delivery occurs. Thus, figures for perinatal losses for general practitioners admissions will be artificially low and it is only by examining the mortality rates for all *original* bookings that success in selection can be measured. Even so, perinatal mortality rates may still be far from reliable indicators of quality of care (Chalmers 1979). In developed countries the three principal causes of perinatal mortality now are lethal congenital abnormalities, extreme immaturity and intrauterine hypoxia. Congenital abnormalities and immaturity together account for over 70 per cent of fetal wastage and, while some of these cases may be detectable by screening routines in pregnancy, few could have confidently been predicted at booking. The principal *avoidable* cause of perinatal death therefore remains intrauterine hypoxia which includes pre-eclampsia, placental abruption, intrauterine growth retardation (IUGR), cord problems and so on. These conditions are potentially detectable during pregnancy and labour and all require modification of management routines to avoid disaster. Thus, until cause-specific death rates are generally available, audit of fetal losses due to reasons *other* than congenital defect or preterm delivery may give a more accurate indication of quality of obstetric care than crude perinatal mortality rates. The calculation now is as follows:

$$\text{Adjusted PMNR} = \frac{(\text{SB} + \text{NND} - \text{PTD} - \text{LCD}) \times 1000}{\text{Total births}}$$

where
   SB   = number of stillbirths
   NND = number of first week neonatal deaths
   PTD = number of pre-term deliveries before 37 weeks
   LCD = number of fetuses with lethal congenital defects.

Nulliparae *vs.* multiparae

In the examination of other process and outcome variables it is almost always wise to distinguish between nulliparous and parous women. The reason is that the course of pregnancy and labour (Chapter 23) in the former often follows a rather different pattern from the latter. For example, nulliparae are more prone to pre-eclampsia, delay in the first stage of labour, and cephalopelvic disproportion; multiparae on the other hand, more frequently experience malpresentation, postpartum hemorrhage and so on. Since parity is a prime selection factor for general practitioner care (see

Chapter 9) it is of particular importance to validate this criterion independently by means of cross-tabulation with other outcome variables.

Transfer of care

Transfer of care either antenatally or in labour because of complications has already been mentioned as a process variable and is often worthy of special scrutiny. A high transfer rate across the board might imply either poor selection of patients initially or lack of practical skills amongst general practitioner obstetricians. Low transfer rates antenatally with high rates in labour might suggest less than optimal antenatal care. On the other hand, low rates generally could be held to suggest good case selection and above average competence of practitioners and midwives. Results may be shown in the form demonstrated in Fig. 15.7 and (when patients are divided into nulliparae and multiparae) in Fig. 15.8. The diverse outcome pattern when compared with the original selections is very apparent.

It is insufficient simply to tabulate transfer rates, however: reasons must also be examined and alternative selection or management policies considered. For example, in one general practitioner maternity unit the third most common reason (after pre-eclampsia and antepartum hemorrhage) for transfer to specialist care before labour was uncomplicated postmaturity. The introduction of a protocol (Chapter 22) to permit general practitioners to use prostaglandin pessaries for induction of their patients in suitable cases resulted in a very significant reduction in the transfer rate over the next 2 or 3 years. Similarly, the introduction of active management techniques during labour can be expected to reduce the number of nulliparae transferred in the first stage of labour and will thus enable a higher proportion of women to remain in the care of the community obstetric team.

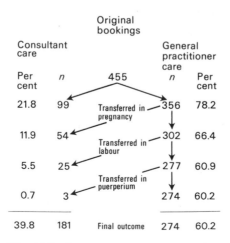

Fig. 15.7. Transfer of care—all parities.

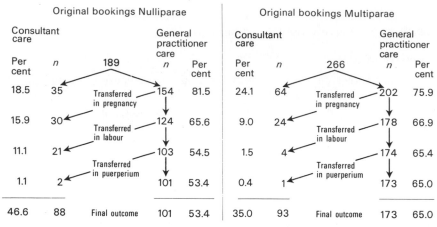

Fig. 15.8. Transfer of care—nulliparae *vs.* multiparae.

LABOUR OUTCOMES

At the end of the day, whatever the system of obstetric care the patient has received, it will be her experiences during labour that measure the success of selection and management procedures. A number of the more apposite outcome variables will therefore be briefly discussed.

Duration of labour

It has been stated elsewhere (O'Driscoll and Meagher 1980), that more than any other measurable factor, duration of labour determines the impact of parturition not only on mothers and on babies but also on the medical staff who care for them. Labour of short duration tends to equate with successful outcome and the mother's recollection of it is usually favourable since she has not become exhausted nor suffered loss of morale. Long labours suggest inefficient uterine action or obstruction (Chapter 22) and may require unpleasant interventions. Whatever the case, duration is clearly a significant outcome variable; the problem in its measurement is, when does labour start? O'Driscoll states his criteria for the diagnosis of labour, but for the purpose of meaningful audit a more specific point of origin is required. Hendricks, Brenner and Kraus (1970) recommended the time of admission to the delivery room, but experience demonstrates how fallible a notion this is. A more scientific starting point (based on the work of the same authors) might however, be the onset of the active phase of labour. Again this can be clinically difficult to identify, but when cervicographic records are used in labour, retrograde extrapolation of the plot back to the 3 cm line will give a reasonably reliable indication of time of origin. On the other hand, the time of birth is usually noted with accuracy.

Mode of delivery

The mode of delivery of the baby, whether spontaneous, instrumental (forceps or ventouse, with or without rotation) or operative (caesarean) is almost always correctly recorded. Spontaneous delivery implies normality so low instrumental and operative delivery rates suggest successful outcomes in terms of selection and management of patients. In most general practitioner obstetric units the spontaneous delivery rate should approach 90 per cent and should be considerably higher than that for parent or neighbouring specialist units which needs must accept women in all risk categories.

The accoucheur

The status as well as the name of the person actually delivering the baby should be recorded. Again straightforward births are generally attended (in the United Kingdom at any rate) by midwives either trained or in training, whereas the more complicated the delivery, the more senior the specialist involved. Tabulation of transfer of care against either accoucheur or mode of delivery will thus give some index of justification for alteration of plans during pregnancy or labour.

What however, is the role of the general practitioner obstetrician? If a delivery is easy it will be undertaken by a midwife; if too difficult, almost certainly by a specialist. The general practitioner's contribution should perhaps be monitored by his presence during labour and especially at the delivery. A high attendance rate, particularly if complemented by low intervention and transfer rates, implies sound selection of patients and good management procedures, and (perhaps even more important) a strong personal commitment to the care of his patients.

Specific intervention rates

Instrumental and operative delivery have already been discussed, but other procedures in pregnancy or labour (Table 15.2) can be used as process and outcome indices if presented as percentage rates for various cohorts of women. These figures can then be untilized in a comparative manner (see below) for different systems of care or management protocols. Other events, such as the incidence of postpartum hemorrhage or retained placenta or the use of blood transfusion can be used in a similar manner.

The neonate

The condition of the neonate is, of course, next to maternal mortality and morbidity, the most important outcome indicator of maternity care. Perinatal mortality has been already discussed but there are other prime variables. Birth weight, especially coupled with gestational age, is a good

Table 15.2 *Some specific interventions in pregnancy and labour*

Pregnancy	Labour
Sonar examination	Induction
Radiology	Acceleration
Amniocentesis	Continuous monitoring
Haematological examinations	Fetal blood sampling
Oestriol estimations	Regional analgesia
Cardiotocography	Drugs in labour
	Episiotomy
	Instrumental or operative delivery
	Blood transfusion

indicator of fetal health and maturity. Apgar scores at 1 and 5 minutes after delivery respectively monitor intrapartum fetal hypoxia and can give important prognostic pointers for immediate management and future development. Transfer of care to neonatal intensive care units or special care baby units imply problems beyond the scope of the general practitioner obstetrician and the follow-up of all of these should be an important aspect of any audit system.

COMPARATIVE STUDIES

The basis of selective community obstetric care (as opposed to specialist care for all) is a system embodying continuity of care for low-risk women provided by small numbers of primary care team professionals. With continually improving standards in obstetrics measured by objective outcome variables such as those described above, it is essential to ensure that such alternative systems of care as may seem to be aesthetically preferable do not fall short on performance. Audit of differing styles of care is therefore of vital importance but the problem is one of ensuring comparability. Clearly there is little value in presenting results from, for example, a general practitioner maternity unit delivering only normal multiparae against those from a consultant unit handling women in all risk categories. Like must be compared with like, and even so outcomes from matched cohorts may be biased, for example, by transfer of care before or during labour. Though there are numerous reports in the literature concerning the working of individual general practitioner maternity units, few have attempted any serious comparisons either with each other or with competing systems.

Roseveare and Bull (1982) tried to compare two markedly differing styles of community care but, although results in terms of outcome seemed to be very similar, firm statistical validation could not be achieved owing to differences in age groups, social class and ethnic origins in the cohorts examined.

Taylor and his colleagues (1980) mounted a better designed study to compare outcomes between low-risk woman in general practitioner maternity units in West Berkshire with matched groups in consultant care in both Rochdale and the Isle of Wight, units where there was no community care alternative. In spite of relatively high perinatal mortality rates in all three situations, the authors concluded: 'Booking into a general practitioner maternity unit can be as safe for low risk women as booking into a consultant unit'. This study was also open to the criticism that, since the groups studied were so widely dispersed geographically, ethnic and socioeconomic comparability could not have been assured and biases could thus have occurred.

Black (1982) examined birthweight-specific perinatal mortality rates in neighbouring district hospitals which apparently had high and low respective proportions of women delivered in general practitioner care. In both units the rates for mature babies were satisfyingly low (2.54/1000 births) but the suggestion that the rate for the hospital with seemingly low general practitioner participation rate (12 per cent) could have been reduced by dilution with low-risk cases in consultant care failed to take into account the fact that the catchment area for the general practitioner unit in that hospital was very much smaller than that of the consultant unit and general practitioners were actually responsible for delivery of over 30 per cent of possible cases.

The three studies above are quoted, not with any perjorative motives in mind, but simply to illustrate the pitfalls of what might seem at the outset to be straightforward exercises in comparative audit. Perhaps the most significant study in this respect in the United Kingdom to date has been that published by Klein and his colleagues (1983). They compared carefully matched cohorts of low-risk women booked in either consultant (shared) care or general practitioner (community) care in the same hospital and analysed them by a number of outcome variables. In spite of the fact that interventions in labour such as induction, acceleration, drugs, regional analgesia, forceps delivery and intubation of the neonate occurred significantly less often in community care than in the shared care group, there was no significant difference in perinatal mortality rates and Apgar scores were actually higher in the community care group. The conclusions were that not only were short-term outcomes for low-risk mothers and their babies better when delivered in community care, but when similar women were delivered in consultant care there seemed to be a tendency for high-risk techniques to spill over into their management, perhaps not always to their advantage. This latter view supports the conclusion of a much larger survey (Fryer and Ashford 1972) over a decade ago and gives substance to the idea that the general practitioner obstetrician and community midwife still have a valuable role in contemporary maternity care.

OBSTETRIC AUDIT—THE FUTURE

Examination of maternity care at national level on a continuing basis would not only enable comparisons to be made between different systems of care but would have demographic uses and important implications for health care planning. Such a system is already in operation in Scotland (Cole 1980) but in England and Wales agreement on a format has not yet been reached. For some years the Office of Populations and Censuses (OPCS) has published maternity statistics as part of the hospital inpatient enquiry (HIPE), but these figures are based only on a 10 per cent sample of admissions and become available often several years in arrears. A development of HIPE was maternity hospital activity analysis (Mat.HAA) but this again was not very successful partly because it was profligate of computer services but also because it examined statistics in terms of hospital admissions rather than maternities (births), thus introducing errors.

Clearly more comprehensive and up-to-date information is required. In 1976 the Child Health Computing Committee was set up by the Department of Health and Social Security to advise on paediatric data collection. Their deliberations resulted in a comprehensive neonatal discharge system (NDS) (Dunn 1980), but its use is voluntary at local area level and it does not seem to have been widely adopted. Brown, Elbourne and Mutch (1981) proposed a standard minimum perinatal data set (MDS) for national use the criteria for which were that the items incorporated should be unequivocally definable, be readily available for all maternities and should provide useful information. Their final list of some 40 items includes identification and social data and current pregnancy, labour, delivery and neonatal details for every birth.

Both the NDS and MDS proposals tend to concentrate on data for the investigation of perinatal outcomes rather than the more esoteric problems of pregnancy and labour management. In 1977, the Northern Region Health Authority convened a steering committee to develop for national use a satisfactory system for maternity statistics to embrace all registerable births including home confinements. This exercise has resulted in the Standard Maternity Information System (SMIS) (Thomson and Barron 1980) and pilot studies are presently in operation in three areas. Mutch and Elbourne (1983) have compared these last three systems and a fourth (the Korner Maternity Information System commissioned by the Steering Committee on Health Services Information) and have suggested basic tabulation packages that could be used for both obstetric and perinatal audit. While all four systems have much in common, SMIS seems the most appropriate for use in both perinatal and obstetric audit by either specialist or general practitioner obstetricians.

REFERENCES

Black, N. (1982). Do general practitioner deliveries constitute a perinatal mortality risk? *Br. Med. J.* **1**, 488–90.

Brown, I., Elbourne, D., and Mutch, L. (1981). Standard national perinatal data: a suggested minimum data set. *Commun. Med.* **3**, 298–306.

Bull, M. J. V. (1980). Ten years experience in a general practice obstetric unit. *J. Roy. Coll. Gen. Practit.* **30**, 208–15.

Chalmers, I. (1979). The search for indices. *Lancet* **2**, 1063–5.

Cole, S. (1980). Scottish maternity and neonatal records. In *Perinatal audit and surveillance* (eds. I. Chalmers and G. McIlwaine) RCOG, London, p. 39.

Donabedian, A. (1966). Evaluating the quality of medical care. *Millbank Mem. Fund Q. (Suppl.)* **44**, 166–206.

Dunn, P. M. (1980). A standard neonatal discharge record. In *Perinatal audit and surveillance.* (eds. I. Chalmers and G. McIlwaine) RCOG, London, p. 93.

Fryer, J. G. and Ashford, J. R. (1972). Trends in perinatal and neonatal mortality in Engalnd and Wales. *Br. J. Prev. Soc. Med.* **26**, 1–9.

Harden, K. A., Harden, R. McG., and Reekie, D. (1974). New approach to information handling in general practice. *Br. Med. J.* **2**, 164–6.

Hendricks, C. H., Brenner, W. E., and Kraus, G. (1970). Normal cervical dilatation patterns in late pregnancy and labour. *Am. J. Obst. Gynecol.* **106**, 1065–82.

Kelly, S. (1982). Letting the patient talk to the computer. *Computer Update* **1**, 111–14.

Klein, M. *et al.* (1983). A comparison of low risk women booked for delivery in two systems of care: shared care (consultant) and integrated general practice unit. *Br. J. Obst. Gynaecol.* **90**, 118–28.

Lilford, R. J. and Chard, T. (1982). Computers in antenatal care. *Br. J. Hosp. Med.* **28**, 420–6.

Maresh, M. *et al.* (1983). Selection of an obstetric database for a microcomputer and its use for on-line production of birth notification forms, discharge summaries and peri-natal audit. *Br. J. Obst. Gynaecol.* **90**, 227–31.

Mourin, K. (1976). Auditing and evaluation in general practice. *J. Roy. Coll. Gen. Practit.* **26**, 726–33.

Mutch, L. and Elbourne, D. (1983). Standard national perinatal data: a suggested common core of tabulations. *Commun. Med.* **5**, 251–9.

O'Driscoll, K. and Meagher, D. (1980). *Active management in labour. Clinics in obstetrics and gynaecology: supplement 1.* W. B. Saunders, Eastbourne.

Roseveare, M. P. and Bull, M. J. V. (1982). General practitioner obstetrics—two styles of care. *Br. Med. J.* **1**, 958–60.

Royal College of Obstetricians and Gynaecologists. (1949). Maternity medical report. *J. Obst. Gyn. Brit. Emp.* **55**, 478–94.

South, J. and Rhodes, P. (1971). Computer service for obstetric records. *Br. Med. J.* **4**, 32–35.

Taylor, G. W. *et al.* (1980). How safe is general practitioner obstetrics? *Lancet* **2**, 1287–9.

Thomson, A. M. and Barron, S. L. (1980). A standard maternity information system. In *Perinatal audit and surveillance.* (eds. I. Chalmers and G. McIlwaine) RCOG, London, p. 79.

16 Different settings for intrapartum care: the integrated general practitioner unit

M. J. V. Bull

INTRODUCTION

A striking feature of maternity care in the United Kingdom during the last three decades has been the increasing reliance on delivery of mothers within specialist obstetric units. Reasons for this trend may have been both the identification of risk factors by successive maternal and perinatal mortality surveys and the increasing availability of beds in district general hospitals due to a falling birth rate coupled with shorter postnatal hospitalization. Development of increasingly sophisticated techniques for the management of labour has also played its part but, by the 1980s, a degree of reaction had set in and both doctors and mothers began to question the necessity for high-risk technology for low-risk women. Unfortunately, even the most careful selection of mothers for low-risk status cannot guarantee the absence of complications at delivery (Cox *et al.* 1970; Curzen and Mountrose 1976) and avoidable mortality or morbidity could result unless facilities for emergency delivery and neonatal resuscitation are readily available at the chosen place of confinement. Nevertheless, the disadvantages of universal delivery of women in specialist departments (for example, impersonal attitudes, unnecessary interventions and lack of continuity of care) have recently been highlighted (Boyd and Sellers 1982) and alternative systems of care are now increasingly being sought.

The concept of the combined or integrated maternity unit, wherein general practitioner obstetricians and community midwives attend low-risk cases in district hospitals alongside specialist staff, is not new (Barnard *et al.* 1970; O'Sullivan, 1961; Oldershaw and Brudenell, 1968)
The advantages are manifest:

1. For the women—continuity of care by her family doctor and community midwife through pregnancy, parturition and puerperium with, in the absence of complication, a relaxed style of management and a flexible regime.
2. For the general practitioner obstetrician and community midwife—the

opportunity to play their respective roles safe in the knowledge that specialist expertise and equipment is readily to hand should an emergency arise.

3. For the specialist—easing of the burden in crowded hospital antenatal clinics and relief of pressure on the specialized facilities of the consultant unit delivery suite (Brudenell 1983).

The structure of the obstetric care team in the integrated general practitioner maternity unit is displayed in Fig. 16.1. Continuous lines indicate the normal channels of consultation whereas broken lines show the routes for emergency access.

Setting up an integrated general practitioner maternity unit may not however be easy. The problems fall broadly under two heads. The first is geographical: most specialist obstetric departments (which necessarily form the parent unit) are situated in district hospitals in the larger conurbations; clearly only doctors and patients in the immediate vicinity will be able to take advantage of them. However, since approximately three-quarters of the population of the United Kingdom reside in urban districts, there would seem to be considerable scope for the expansion of general practitioner obstetric care in a field that has erstwhile been the province of the rural practitioner in more isolated circumstances. The second problem is interpersonal and concerns relationships between general practitioners and specialists, community midwives, and hospital staff. Unless there is a tight system of

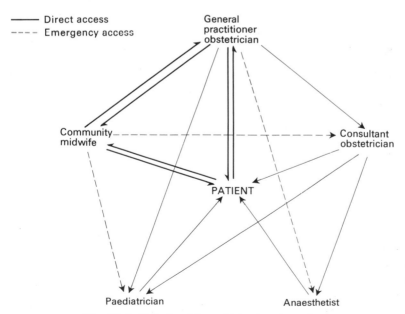

Fig. 16.1. Relationships within the obstetric care team.

management and a close arrangement for liaison and consultation, friction due to suspicion and mistrust may well arise. It may be useful therefore to describe the organization of an integrated general practitioner unit that has functioned successfully in a large district obstetric hospital for over 13 years (Bull 1980).

MANAGEMENT

Overall organization is the responsibility of a management committee consisting of:

> six general practitioners appointed by the District Local Medical
>   Committee
> two consultant obstetricians
> one consultant pediatrician
> one hospital administrator
> one divisional nursing officer (midwifery)
> one nursing officer (community midwives)
> one in-post community midwife
> one secretary

This committee meets on a regular basis and is concerned with drawing up an operational policy for the unit (see Appendix A, p. 247), guidelines for general practitioner obstetricians (see Appendix B, p. 248), provision of reports and statistics and dealing with *ad hoc* problems. Administration is simplified if one practitioner (preferably a clinical assistant working with the specialist unit) is nominated to supervise day-to-day functioning of the unit and a senior community midwife is appointed to receive and scrutinize bookings.

CRITERIA FOR GENERAL PRACTITIONER OBSTETRICIANS

General practitioners wishing to deliver their patients in the unit must reside within a realistic distance (not more than 15 km) of the unit and must be on the special obstetric list of the Family Practitioner Committee or have approved obstetric experience. They must also hold (for medicolegal reasons) an honorary contract from the District Medical Officer to practice within the hospital. For the future, in line with national recommendations, it may be necessary to require participant general practitioners to admit and attend a minimum number of women each year to maintain their competence and skills.

SELECTION OF PATIENTS

The criteria for the booking of low-risk women for delivery in the unit are substantially those recommended by Cranbrook (1959). Women should fulfill the following conditions:

(i) An unexceptional medical and obstetric history.
(ii) If primigravid, be between the ages of 18 and 29 at booking; over 152 cm. in stature.
(iii) If multigravid, under the age of 35 at booking; not more than three previous deliveries.

Women in these categories are accepted without question. However, because of the special nature of the integrated unit, with specialist advice and assistance so readily to hand, booking criteria need not be too rigidly enforced. Where an identifiable risk factor is potential (for example, a woman over 35 years with a normal obstetric history, or greater than para 4, or with a history of, say, a single postpartum haemorrhage or retained placenta) rather than actual (for example diabetes, hypertension, scar on the uterus, previous difficult operative delivery) a woman may still be accepted provided the opinion and consent of a consultant obstetrician has been obtained. For this reason the general practitioner obstetrician working in an integrated unit can book a greater number of women in his personal care than would apply if he were working in isolation.

RECORDS

A further feature that enhances the team approach to maternity care is that general practitioner booked women use the same obstetric case notes as do those booked for consultant care. Indeed the case note was specifically designed to cater for the needs of both categories of mother. The women carry these notes personally so that the updated record is always available whether to the community midwife visiting the home, to the general practitioner at the health centre, to the consultant in his clinic if the patient is referred, to the radiologist if sonar examination is required, and so on (see Chapter 13). When the woman is delivered and (after her return home) is finally discharged by the community midwife, the records are returned to the hospital for coding for statistical purposes and ultimate archiving. Records are seldom if ever lost and the fact that they are in the mother's own possession increases her understanding of her condition and confidence in her attendants.

LABOUR

When a mother goes into labour, she is admitted without formality into the hospital delivery suite in the care of her community midwife. The midwife is then responsible for the management of the labour but she will inform the general practitioner so that he can maintain a watching brief on progress. In the event of problems the doctor may intervene personally (Chapters 21, 22, 23 and 24), request advice or assistance from consultant unit staff or, if need be, arrange transfer of care. Even in the last eventuality both general practitioner and community midwife can remain involved and so maintain that continuity of care that is the lynchpin of community obstetrics. Problems resolved and the woman delivered, mother and baby then return to the designated general practitioner unit postnatal beds.

AUDIT

In a situation where generalists are working alongside specialists, it is of paramount importance that the former examine and publish their results on a regular basis for general appraisal. When women are selected by absence of risk factor for general practitioner unit booking and when transfer of care or assistance is so readily available if complications arise, the final figures in terms of outcome indices such as perinatal mortality, mode of delivery and neonatal morbidity (see Chapter 15) should be very good indeed. Statistics should be collected monthly and collated annually into a formal report. A quarterly audit meeting attended by general practitioner obstetricians, community midwives and members of the specialist department should be held to discuss results and examine problems especially when a perinatal death, unexpectedly difficult delivery or neonatal illness has occurred. Such meetings have considerable educational content and do much to maintain and improve relationships between community and hospital staff.

CONTINUING EDUCATION

In obstetrics, as in any branch of medicine, continuing education is of paramount importance and can take various forms. The value of audit meetings has been mentioned, and, in the context of the integrated maternity unit, it is not difficult to arrange relevant lectures by specialists on a regular basis. However, the most effective form of learning probably takes place in the delivery room itself when problems in labour have been encountered and consultant advice or assistance has been invoked. On these occasions the general practitioner obstetrician should make every attempt to remain involved in the care of his patient, and, by means of consultation or by undertaking operative interventions under supervision, he will be enabled to enhance practical knowledge and maintain manipulative skills. This is a peculiar advantage of the integrated maternity unit not normally encountered when deliveries take place elsewhere. There is a risk, however, that full advantage may not be taken and, if transfer of care is too readily available, personal commitment may wane and confidence thereafter diminish.

It will be clear from the foregoing account that, in the circumstances of this particular integrated general practitioner unit, both doctors and community midwives have a very considerable degree of autonomy in the management of their patients in labour which is the logical extension of their roles in antenatal care. Provided the guidelines are adhered to no mandatory supervision by consultants is necessary and yet, because of the excellent relationships that have been fostered over the years, advice or assistance is immediately forthcoming in time of need.

In conclusion, experience has shown that such is the flexibility and acceptability of this particular form of obstetric care that domiciliary confinement is rarely requested. Perhaps the integrated unit could be said to encompass the best of both worlds: continuity of care, relaxed and flexible management during labour and the puerperium, yet offering the maximum of safety to both mother and child.

APPENDIX A: GENERAL PRACTITIONER MATERNITY UNIT, JOHN RADCLIFFE HOSPITAL, OXFORD

Operational policy

1. The unit will consist of delivery suite facilities and 12 lying-in beds accommodated in the John Radcliffe Hospital.
2. The administration of the unit, appointment of staff and granting of honorary contracts is the responsibility of the Oxford District Health Authority. A Management Committee will be formed as a link in the administration of the unit and to advise the Maternity Liaison Committee and the Oxford District Health Authority as required.
3. Access to the beds will be restricted to general practitioners on the special obstetric list of the Oxfordshire Family Practitioner Committee who hold an honorary contract with the District Health Authority. Patients will only be admitted to the unit under the care of a general practitioner obstetrician and will remain the clinical responsibility of that general practitioner unless or until formal transfer of responsibility to a consultant (or a member of his staff) becomes necessary.
4. Each general practitioner will be responsible to the District Health Authority for the continuing clinical care of his patient and for ensuring that during his absence a deputy holding a similar honorary contract will assume responsibility.
5. The District Health Authority may consider the grant of sessional contracts to three general practitioner assistants for at least one session per week working with a consultant. These general practitioner medical assistants will act as administrative links with the nursing, medical and general administrative personnel of the hospital.
6. General practitioners granted honorary contracts will have access to pathological and radiological facilities in the hospital and will be entitled to use library and restaurant services whilst working therein.
7. Statistics and reports concerning the unit will be rendered annually to the Maternity Liaison Committee and will form part of the annual statistics for the Maternity Department of the John Radcliffe Hospital.

APPENDIX B: GENERAL PRACTITIONER MATERNITY UNIT,
JOHN RADCLIFFE HOSPITAL, OXFORD

Memorandum for Guidance of General Practitioner Obstetricians

1. Eligibility to use the unit is restricted to general practitioners included in the Special Obstetric List of the Oxfordshire Family Practitioner Committee and residing within a practicable distance of the hospital. They must hold an honorary contract with the District Health Authority to practise on hospital premises and must be a member of a medical defence organization.
2. Responsibilities

    (i) Each general practitioner obstetrician will have complete clinical responsibility for his patients (both mother and child) but is advised to be conversant with and abide by patient management policies currently in operation in the hospital.
    (ii) He must ensure that during his absence a deputy duly qualified as defined in para 1 above, is nominated. He shall not make use of junior hospital medical staff for this purpose.
    (iii) He shall retain the right and obligation to call for help from hospital consultant staff in case of difficulty. This responsibility shall not devolve upon the midwife attending his patient except in cases of extreme urgency. Responsibility for any patient requiring continuing specialist care must be transferred to a consultant.
    (iv) He shall be responsible for ensuring the fitness of both mothers and babies for discharge from the unit and, in the case of early discharge, should confirm with the community midwife that home conditions are suitable.
    (v) He should ensure that the obstetric case notes concerning his patients are fully completed prior to their discharge from the hospital.

3. Booking of patients
   A patient will be considered suitable for booking in the general practitioner maternity unit

    (i) if her physical, mental and obstetric histories are satisfactory;
    (ii) if she is a primigravida between the ages of 18 and 29 years at booking and over 152 cm in stature, or she is pregnant for the second, third of fourth time and is under the age of 35 years.
    (iii) if she has no rhesus or other antibodies.

Patients who do not conform to these criteria shall only be booked with the approval of a consultant.
Bookings should be made on the triplicate form approved by the Maternity Liaison Committee and should include full information regarding the patient especially in connection with ABO and Rh blood group, past medical and obstetric history (if any) and domiciliary conditions. Applications should be forwarded to the Maternity Liaison Sister at the General Practitioner Maternity Unit, John Radcliffe Hospital.

4. Facilities

Approved general practitioner obstetricians shall have full access to pathology, radiology, library and restaurant facilities while working in the hospital.

5. Obstetric meetings

General practitioner obstetricians are encouraged to attend monthly meetings with consultant and midwifery staff (approved under Section 63 of the NHS Act) which are convened with the intention of providing continuing education in obstetrics, gynaecology and paediatrics.

REFERENCES

Barnard, M. J. *et al.*, (1970). A combined maternity unit. *J. Roy. Coll. Gen. Practit.* **19**, 211–14.

Boyd, C. and Sellers, L. (1982). In *The British way of birth*. Pan Books Ltd., London.

Brudenell, J. M. (1983). Future of general practitioner obstetrics: discussion paper. *J. Roy. Soc. Med.* **76**, 197–99.

Bull, M. J. V. (1980). Ten years' experience in a general practice obstetric unit. *J. Roy. Coll. Gen. Practit.* **30**, 208–15.

Cox, C. A. *et al.* (1976). Critical appraisal of domiciliary obstetric and neonatal practice. *Br. Med. J.* **1**, 84–6.

Cranbrook, The Earl of (1959). *Report of the Maternity Services Committee*, Ministry of Health. HMSO, London.

Curzen, P. and Mountrose, U. M. (1976). The general practitioner's role in the management of labour. *Br. Med. J.* **2**, 1433–4.

Oldershaw, K. L. and Brudenell, J. M. (1968). The use by general practitioners of obstetric beds in a consultant unit: report of first 500 cases. *Br. Med. J.* **1**, 139–42.

O'Sullivan, J. V. (1961). General practitioner maternity beds in a large general hospital. *Br. Med. J.* **2**, 1349–50.

17 Different settings for intrapartum care: the alongside unit

G. N. Marsh

DEFINITION

By 'alongside' is meant a general practitioner unit which is either underneath —connected by lift or stairs—or along the corridor from, the consultant unit. Not included are units which are so separate that ambulances are required to convey women from one place to the other. 'Flying squad' facilities, either paediatric or obstetric, may occasionally be used in the alongside unit for sudden unexpected emergencies where transfer could increase the morbidity, for example, torrential haemorrhage, shocked baby. Similarly paediatricians attending at marginally abnormal deliveries, such as forceps, or erratic fetal heart in the second stage, can be a normal arrangement.

The joint report of the RCOG and the RCGP (1982) describes three alternatives for general practitioners—the 'isolated' unit, the 'alongside' unit and the 'integrated' unit. Of the latter two the RCOG preferred the integrated unit. In these units it would be patently easier to ordain, and adhere to consultant protocols. 'Control' would be easy to enforce on all labours. The RCGP representatives saw advantages in the alongside unit since the general practitioner would be working 'in his own right' and would be able to establish his own systems and standards. He would, of course, also be responsible for them. It is the purpose of this chapter to describe the benefits and drawbacks of the alongside unit for the women and their general practitioners.

FUNCTION

Alongside units are customarily open to all general practitioners within a reasonable distance who wish to be responsible for deliveries. For the most part they will be on the obstetric list for the area since those not on the list have patently no interest in deliveries and the financial differential is certainly a deterrent. Case selection for the alongside unit can be slightly less rigorous and exclusive than for an isolated unit or home delivery since major technology including instant emergency caesarean section is only 'next door'. The number of general practitioner bookings can therefore increase.

ALTERNATIVE BOOKING SYSTEMS

1. Open access is provided and the general practitioner books what he feels he can cope with. In practice, since consultants have to respond to and be responsible for the results of emergencies, this system is uncommon. In it consultants are totally unprotected from the 'lunatic fringe' of general practitioner who book inadvisedly. Nevertheless in some areas such a system does operate and a general practitioner obstetric committee monitors the women in the unit.

2. A very common system is for the consultant to see every woman at booking, or at 36 weeks, or sometimes on both occasions. Thus the consultant spends a large amount of time seeing normal women, but effectively ordains which of them will be booked in the general practitioner unit. Much responsibility is taken from the general practitioner.

3. A third, and very effective system which minimizes consultant effort, introduces cooperation, and leaves the general practitioner with responsibility, is for the notes of women booking for the general practitioner unit to be reviewed by a consultant (Fig. 17.1). Where there is doubt about the suitability the notes are then referred to a booking committee. This committee consists of equal numbers of consultant obstetricians and general practitioners the latter possibly nominated by the local general practitioner 'cogwheel' committee. There are also representatives of district midwives and senior hospital nursing staff from both consultant and general practitioner units. General practitioners in the area are informed of the contraindications to booking for the general practitioner unit, hence the number of cases referred is fairly small. Table 17.1 lists absolute contraindications

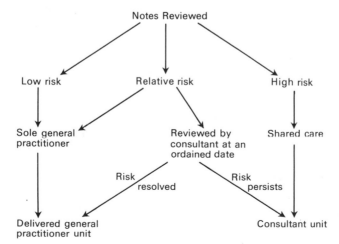

Fig. 17.1. Booking system for alongside unit using notes review.

Table 17.1   *Absolute contraindications to booking in general practitioner alongside unit*

1. Previous caesarean section
2. Infertility especially over 30
3. Previous multiple abortions with no live children
4. Postpartum haemorrhage and/or retained placenta
5. Intrauterine growth retardation and low birth weight at term in previous pregnancy
6. Certain maternal diseases—especially diabetes and essential hypertension
7. Twins (if detected by time of booking)
8. Pelvic abnormality

to booking in an alongside unit and Table 17.2 some relative contraindications. It is women in Table 17.2 that are discussed and the committee then assesses other factors such as the general practitioner's experience, availability, and enthusiasm which are often known to the consultants and even more perhaps to the general practitioner unit midwifery staff.

A refinement of this booking system is also illustrated in Fig. 17.1. This accepts the concept that a relative 'risk' in early pregnancy may have resolved by the end of it. An example would be a multigravid woman less than 150 cm who at 36–38 weeks' gestation has a moderate-size baby with the vertex deeply engaged and has already had 3600 g spontaneous delivery last time. In such a woman the initial delivery arrangements can be left open and finalized by the consultant, with appropriate suggestions from the general practitioner, at a later attendance at the consultant clinic.

Nevertheless the majority of women booked by general practitioners will not be referred to the booking committee, they will be their entire responsibility, and the latter will concentrate their minds dramatically.

OBLIGATIONS OF THE GENERAL PRACTITIONER

In an 'alongside' unit the general practitioner has the following obligations:

(i)   24-hour availability either of himself, or an equally qualified deputy.

Table 17.2   *Relative contraindications to booking in an alongside general practitioner unit*

1. Primigravidae less than 152 cm
2. Multigravidae less than 150 cm
3. Fifth baby or more
4. Primigravidae over 30
5. Multigravidae over 40
6. Primigravidae under 18
7. Previous baby needed difficult forceps delivery

(ii) To be within 10 minutes of the labour suite.

(iii) Aim to be present in labour and ideally at delivery.

(iv) A minimum number of deliveries—say 10 per year.

(v)   To attend refresher courses.

Hence the use of a deputizing service whose doctors are not known, whose qualifications may not be satisfactory and whose availability may be problematic would preclude intranatal care. However, some deputizing services specifically provide obstetrically qualified doctors in order to facilitate user doctors participating in care of their women in labour. Nevertheless this is second rate compared with personal general practitioner care, or partner deputizing.

OPPORTUNITY FOR AUDIT

By using the standard hospital record, audit of the general practitioner unit can be undertaken and possibly done in parallel with the consultant unit. Audit can be unit or practice-orientated. Factors such as perinatal mortality rate, length of labour, frequency of episiotomy and forceps delivery and analysis of transferred cases can all prove interesting and increase the database of general practitioners doing obstetrics.

VISITS TO PRACTICE BY GENERAL PRACTITIONER UNIT STAFF

Where the staff of an alongside general practitioner unit are in post for some time they can make visits to the general practitioners' antenatal clinics in the area and see the style and type of care offered. They can also get to know the receptionists and telephone staff of the practice thus facilitating instant access to doctors.

THE 'PHILOSOPHY' OF THE ALONGSIDE UNIT

What follows in this section is not precluded in an integrated unit, but may be more difficult to achieve in that setting.

In the alongside unit general practitioners can have a sense of pride in their 'own' place, a sense of identity, a sense of responsibility to their 'own' unit. Invitation to specialist staff to come and help with problems can be easily arranged, but is by invitation rather than automatic. They can develop a personal knowledge of the senior nursing staff in the unit, who hopefully will be fairly permanent. They will prefer to work with relatively few people. Because the women have been rigorously selected and are all potentially normal cases, the majority of whom are delivered totally normally, the atmosphere can be a relaxed 'hotel-like' one and schedules and routines can be less rigid. On the whole drugs will be avoided and 'people' (such as father, midwife, mother, general practitioner) used in their place. 'Technology' (for example, continuous fetal monitoring) is not available, carrying with it the well-documented disadvantages for the normal case (see Chapter 23). There is evidence that abnormal protocols are used more frequently on normal cases in an integrated unit. There is always the comforting thought that should matters go awry the necessary technology is virtually instantly available 'upstairs' or 'along the corridor'. From first stage to discharge the whole family should be involved and there should be maximal children's visiting. Discharge dates can be arranged on an individual basis. Because the unit is alongside, and not integrated, the women will not be exposed to abnormal obstetrics, sick babies, mothers recovering from caesarean section or other mechanized labours. They will not be associated with women with unhappy experiences to relate.

Because of the somewhat different philosophy pertaining in the alongside unit many ideas can spin sideways via communal midwives to the consultant unit and the latter can change as a result. Thus an alongside unit can have benefits that are not possible in an integrated unit.

DISADVANTAGES OF THE ALONGSIDE UNIT

Midwives rotating from the alongside general practitioner unit to the specialist one can become confused by the somewhat different approach to normal labour. Some of them feel lost without the safety that technology appears to provide, and also in having to work in a unit where the doctor is usually not present, but contacted by telephone. Occasionally there can be worrying delays and hitches in transfer arrangements.

Because of their isolation in their own unit general practitioners do not necessarily learn of the new techniques and technology available, and 'what can be done'. Epidurals, ventouse etc. are usually not available in the alongside unit and occasionally would be applicable for a normal woman; they would be more available in an integrated unit. Changes in obstetric protocols are often decided by the consultants without reference to their general practitioner colleagues and tend to be passed to the general practitioner unit via the midwives. This causes offence and problems with compliance. Midwives become caught in any crossfire.

CONCLUSION

Where consultant and general practitioner attitudes differ, and aims do not necessarily coincide, it seems that the alongside unit is an ideal setting in which general practitioner can work. Still necessary, however, are cooperation and collaboration around women who develop problems. Many alongside units currently provide happy settings in which the women are safely and normally delivered.

REFERENCE

Royal College of General Practitioners and Royal College of Obstetricians and Gynaecologists. (1982). Obstetrics and gynaecology for general practitioners. Report on Training. Joint Working Party. *J. Roy. Coll. Gen. Practit.* **32**, 116–22.

18 Different settings for intrapartum care: the isolated unit

A. H. Melhuish

INTRODUCTION

In 1960 the general practitioner maternity unit provided a significant part of maternity care in Britain. Some 25 per cent of all mothers delivered their babies in such units, while a further 50 per cent of deliveries took place under the supervision of the general practitioner obstetrician at home. In 1980, just 20 years later, the whole pattern of maternity care has altered. Only about 1 per cent of deliveries take place at home; hospital deliveries have become the rule. General practitioner units, which had nearly all been isolated, in fact if not in situation, have become polarized into those units close to or within the consultant unit, and into isolated units. In 1980, deliveries in isolated units in England and Wales had come down to 4.4 per cent of all deliveries and the proportion continues to fall. If present trends continue, the isolated unit may well become extinct during the decade 1980–90.

Medicine must progress and it may be argued that the isolated general practitioner maternity unit has outlived its usefulness. Most practising general practitioners will remember the extinction of another isolated unit, the tuberculosis sanatorium. This occurred, however, through the virtual elimination of a disease process and was paralleled in other European countries with similar socioeconomic cultures. The closure of the general practitioner maternity unit, however, reflects the decision of a society advised and guided by politicians and hospital consultants that mothers should have no choice as to where they have their baby; indeed that society has the right to dictate where babies should be born. It is not surprising that such an authoritarian decision has been questioned strongly during the last 10 years, notably by Sheila Kitzinger and John Davis in their book *The place of birth* (1978); nor that modern maternity care was singled out by Ivan Illich in his lecture to the College of General Practitioners in Dublin in April 1982 as a prime modern example of the takeover by the authorities of the patient's individual freedom (Illich 1982).

It is perhaps pertinent to ask how many modern general practitioners are on the side of the authorities, and how many on the side of the mother. The answer may be disquietening. As general practitioners do we allow our patients the right to choose; or is the evidence that consultant unit deliveries are best for our patients—in physical, social and psychological terms—so clearcut that such deliveries for all must be accepted uncritically. Is there still a place for the general practitioner obstetrician and the isolated unit, or is the concept extinct like the tuberculosis sanatorium? The answer is obviously complex and is influenced by financial and social factors and policies, by scientific advances and by the attitudes of both doctor and the mother. This chapter looks at the present situation regarding the isolated general practitioner unit and the literature about it; it suggests some guidelines for the running of such units; and finally it tries to answer the question: is there still a place for the isolated unit?

THE FACTS

The use made of the isolated general practitioner unit will depend on the number of women becoming pregnant each year, the facilities available for their care (hospital and general practitioner unit beds, together with the general practitioners prepared to provide maternity care) and the attitudes to the place of delivery of the mother and the general practitioner. Table 18.1 shows the steady decline (expressed as a percentage) in the number of deliveries in isolated general practitioner units between 1975 and 1980.

Table 18.1 *Series FM1 (1–7) Birth Statistics England and Wales, OPCS*

	1975	1976	1977	1978	1979	1980
NHS:A Isolated general practitioner units	7.0	8.0	6.8	6.0	5.1	4.4
NHS:B Hospital and integrated general practitioner units	88.0	88.0	89.9	91.2	92.3	93.1
Other hospitals (private etc.)	2.0	1.0	1.3	1.2	1.1	1.2
At home	3.0	3.0	1.9	1.6	1.4	1.2
Elsewhere	0.0	0.0	0.1	0.1	0.1	0.1

Some consolation for those concerned about the number of general practitioner unit deliveries lies in the fact that the number of deliveries in England and Wales actually increased between 1975 (603 445), and 1980 (656 234)—a reversal of the downward trend between 1960 and 1975. So at least the actual number of general practitioner unit deliveries has not decreased quite so dramatically.

The number of mothers delivered in isolated general practitioner units is also influenced by the number of general practitioners committed to provide full maternity care. Recent trends in the number of general practitioners involved in providing care in general practitioners units makes depressing reading. Lloyd (1975) looked at various measures of general practitioner involvement in obstetrics and found that, for instance, between 1963 and 1971 more general practitioner unit beds became available to general practitioners, but less general practitioners were prepared to train for, or provide, full maternity care. Equally depressing is the number of deliveries fully supervised by those general practitioners who do provide care and who need as many deliveries as possible to maintain their experience and standards. The RCGP report (1981) refers to the fact that in 1979 15.4 per cent of all maternity claim forms included delivery. This meant that approximately 100 000 deliveries were supervised by the general practitioner in that year, and with only one in three general practitioners taking full responsibility for delivery, some 8000 general practitioners individually looked after ten to twelve deliveries each year, a bare minimum for safe obstetrics.

The most up-to-date details of isolated general practitioner units have been compiled by Dr A. J. M. Cavenagh (personal communication). Using questionnaires he found that in July 1983 there were 131 isolated general practitioner units in England and Wales with 2268 general practitioners on their staff (21 per unit). There was an average of twelve beds per unit with thirteen deliveries for each bed per year, and with eight midwives working full time in each unit. The typical unit was found to be 25 km (16 miles) from the nearest district general hospital. 20 per cent of the units had operating theatres, 68 per cent had general anaesthesia available, 61 per cent had an incubator and 91 per cent had the availability of a flying squad.

THE PRESENT SITUATION

Theoretical considerations
It is difficult, if not impossible, to measure the value of the isolated general practitioner unit. One possible guide is the safety of the unit in terms of maternal and fetal mortality. This measure is impractical for high-risk patients are usually transferred from the general practitioner unit to the consultant unit before or during labour. The cost of the unit is another possible measure, but again assessment of cost is complex and reports vary. There is, therefore, a tendency to assess the value of the unit in terms either of the number of deliveries at the unit or the bed occupancy. The number of deliveries will depend upon the decision of the mother as to where to have her baby after consultation with the general practitioner. The mother's decision will also affect the bed occupancy but this is in addition influenced by the policy of the consultant unit in discharging patients either to the general practitioner unit or home.

The place of birth will be influenced by: the medical situation, the emotional situation, and the geographical situation.

The medical situation

(i)   pre-existing medical and obstetric problems;

(ii)   problems arising during the antenatal period or early labour;

(iii)   availability of appropriate beds (influenced by economic considerations and medical priorities).

Isolated general practitioner units represent an obvious economy for hard-pressed regional or district authorities. They are thus threatened by the economies now taking place.

The emotional situation

The mother's feelings   Her preference for scientific hospital delivery or for the more personal care which the general practitioner can provide in the relaxed atmosphere of the general practitioner unit. In general it seems that the increasing preference of younger mothers for hospital deliveries has been balanced by the reaction of many older mothers against impersonal care in consultant units.

The doctor's feelings   Many general practitioners obtain great satisfaction in taking on the full responsibility of delivering their patients in an isolated general practitioner unit. But the price can be high. Time and skills are needed and the younger general practitioner in particular may be unwilling to commit himself to provide these. His recent in-hospital training may have succeeded in convincing him that the general practitioner is not the right person to be in charge of a delivery. And general practitioner obstetrics, particularly in isolated units, is extremely time-consuming. Time spent by a doctor with a patient can be time spent away from his family, often at unsocial hours. The younger general practitioner, in common with most other young professionals, often sees the priorities of care in a different light from his older colleague, and wants and needs more time with his family.

The geographical situation

Improved transport and communication have played their part in the increased use of the central consultant unit. However, the distance from the patient's home to the hospital can produce a number of problems. At a medical level, the obstetric risks may be increased by a long journey—particularly if there is a history of precipitate deliveries—while the support of visiting during the puerperium is influenced by the distance that family and friends must travel to the hospital. In country areas public transport is usually inadequate; not all families have cars, and it is often those without who are most at risk for depression in the puerperium. The isolated general practitioner unit: close to the doctor, mother and family is the ideal solution.

Because so many factors apply and because the British remain committed to free choice about where to have the baby, conflict will always be present as to the most appropriate place of birth. One thing is certain however; for most mothers there is no right or wrong place, only more or less appropriate sites for delivery. Compulsion to consultant unit deliveries with the phasing out of the remaining isolated general practitioner units would seem insensitive, impractical and risky. A number of mothers will decline to go to consultant units in towns or cities; if there is no alternative they will deliver at home. There is a clear warning in the statistics from the technologically advanced state of California where 15 per cent of deliveries take place at home.

General practitioners need no reminding of the danger of relying too much on hard scientific data in such an emotional matter as having a baby. A live mother and baby are not the most important outcome of pregnancy; a happy mother and baby are. This point is clearly expressed by Marsh (1977) as follows: 'Future perinatal, neonatal and maternal mortality and morbidity statistics will increasingly be viewed not in absolute terms, but will be set against the amount of deviation from the normal process'.

Practical considerations

The isolated general practitioner unit has two main functions:

1. The provision of facilities for full antenatal care, delivery, and postnatal care of carefully selected mothers—who still represent some 60 per cent of all deliveries.

2. Provision of shared antenatal care and 'lying-in' of mothers who for medical reasons must have the baby in a consultant unit.

Some particular benefits of the isolated unit are:

(i)   It provides the ideal focus for maternity care in the isolated area. The midwives working full time in the unit can take calls and answer queries for their district colleagues with their statutory duty to provide community midwifery care.

(ii)   The provision of antenatal care at the isolated unit allows the mother to get to know the doctor and midwife in the environment in which she will have her baby.

(iii) Delivery without unnecessary intervention and with a mobile relaxed patient stands a high chance of a natural outcome.

(iv) The availability of general practitioner unit beds allows the rapid discharge of patients from the consultant unit after delivery.

(v)   Anxiety in the postnatal period will be reduced by the small nature of the unit and by the ease of visiting. Breast-feeding etc. will be helped by the time available for teaching from the midwives who are spared time-consuming visiting in the district by the admission of their patients to the central general practitioner unit.

(vi) The facility for the consultant obstetrician to do regular clinics at the unit improves the care of the mother and the skills of the general practitioner.

GUIDANCE FROM RECENT LITERATURE

Official guidelines

The last 5 years have seen three important discussion documents. In 'Obstetrics and gynaecology for the GP' (RCGP 1981), the working party of the RCGP discussed general arguments for and against full general practitioner care and quoted a number of facts about this. The second document published in 1982 (RCGP and RCOG 1982) produced more practical suggestions—particularly that one or two partners in each practice should have special obstetric experience and carry out all the obstetric care.

The GMSC report, published in 1981, reaffirmed the view that maternity care is an integral part of general practice while recognizing that not all doctors wish to provide it, now or in the future. It suggested that doctors wishing to give obstetric care should be split into two groups—skilled obstetricians, and those providing just antenatal and postnatal care.

Published papers

Safety of general practitioner unit deliveries

Many recent papers have demonstrated the safety of general practitioner unit care and reports exist from as far afield as Gwynedd, Stockton-on-Tees, Colchester, Oxford and Derbyshire. They all highlight the provision of care by an organized and dedicated team of doctors. On the other hand Curzen and Mountrose (1976), and Fedrick and Butler (1978) provide arguments against home delivery and in favour of consultant unit delivery.

A more specific look at the safety of general practitioner unit deliveries was undertaken by Taylor *et al.* (1980). The outcome of the pregnancies of low-risk mothers with access to general practitioners units was compared with the outcome in similar mothers in areas where there were no general practitioner units who were thus delivered in a consultant unit. The authors concluded that low-risk women could be delivered as safely in a general practitioner unit as in a consultant unit, and that the cost was almost certainly less.

Economics

Tew (1977) and Steele and Gray (1981) have looked at the cost involved in deliveries in consultant units and in general practitioner units. Such costs are hard to estimate but both papers concluded that the general practitioner unit was much cheaper.

General papers

The arguments of home or isolated general practitioner unit delivery against hospital delivery are well summarized by Barry (1980) and by Bull (1981).

Information particularly related to isolated general practitioner units

The two most important papers on this have come from a group of obstetricians and general practitioners at Southampton (Elstein *et al.* 1975) and from Shapland (1979). The former recommended that peripheral units should (*a*) be more than a quarter hour's car drive from the big unit: (*b*) be run by a small number of highly qualified general practitioners: (*c*) should receive regular consultant visits; and (*d*) that a flying squad should be available.

Shapland studied four isolated units and concluded that excellent results could be achieved at such units.

PRACTICAL PROCEDURES

Booking policy

In general, this must be flexible for the policy must depend on the skills of the general practitioner obstetrician in charge, the distance from the nearest consultant unit and the amenities available at the isolated unit. In practice, booking policies for isolated units must be more rigid and better enforced than for those units close to the consultant unit. Primiparae represent the main bone of contention; most general practitioner obstetricians feel that they should be delivered in a consultant unit unless the general practitioner who has undertaken to be present at the delivery has some higher qualifications in obstetrics.

Intrapartum care

Equipment must be up to date and well maintained. A 'sonicaide' should be available for each mother in labour. Carefully kept partograms on each patient are vital. When possible, the membranes should be ruptured early in labour.

General practitioner obstetrician in charge

There seems little doubt that the most effective care can be provided by a small number of committed and well-qualified general practitioner obstetricians. How such general practitioners can be identified and encouraged remains uncertain.

Audit

Audit can be carried out in conjunction with the consultant unit or by regular meetings of the doctors using the general practitioner unit. The subject is well covered by Marsh (1977), and also in Chapter 15.

Cooperation from the hospital

Ideally the consultant obstetrician will attend the general practitioner unit every 2–4 weeks to vet bookings and to check any worrying aspect of antenatal care. Anaesthetists and paediatricians are two very useful extras for any isolated general practitioner delivery.

Availability of flying squad

The decreased number of home deliveries has led to less call for the flying squad and many hospitals are now unsatisfactorily equipped to provide such care. It is obviously of concern that in July 1983, 9 per cent of isolated general practitioner units had no access to a flying squad. General practitioner obstetricians should be fully aware of their local flying squad facilities.

CONCLUSION

There is no doubt that there is a place for the isolated general practitioner unit. Many mothers live well away from consultant units. If these mothers are considered suitable for general practitioner unit delivery such a delivery will usually be a happy and safe occasion for the mother, and a source of satisfaction for the general practitioner obstetrician. If they are not suitable, delivery at a consultant unit followed by the earliest possible transfer back to the general practitioner unit will produce a happy mother and family.

Unfortunately there are two major threats to the isolated general practitioner unit. First is the threat of closure due to financial constraints. The general practitioner in charge of the isolated unit may find himself spending more time in committees fighting for his unit than in the delivery room looking after his patient. The second lies in the lack of enthusiasm of the younger general practitioner for obstetrics, and it must be hoped that those general practitioners involved in training can perhaps influence their trainees to a more positive attitude to maternity care (see Chapter 30).

REFERENCES

Barry, C. N. (1980). Home versus hospital confinement. *J. Roy. Coll. Gen. Practit.* **30**, 103–7.
Bull, M. J. V. (1981). Ten years' experience in a general practice obstetric unit. *J. Roy. Coll. Gen. Practit.* **31**, 357–67.

Curzon, P. and Mountrose, U. M. (1975). The general practitioner's role in the management of labour. *Br. Med. J.* **2**, 1433.

Elstein, M. *et al.* (1975). The general practitioner obstetrician—the evolution of his role in the next decade. *J. Coll. Gen. Practit.* **25**, 373–6 (Wessex Faculty region report).

Fedrick, J. and Butler, N. R. (1978). Intended place of delivery and perinatal outcome. *Br. Med. J.* **1**, 763–5.

General Medical Services Committee Maternity Services Subcommittee (1981). General practitioner obstetrics—a policy for the '80s. *Br. Med. J.* **282**, 1171–2.

Illich, I. (1982). Lecture to the Royal College of General Practitioner in Dublin, April. *J. Roy. Coll. Gen. Practit.* **32**, 463–70.

Kitzinger, S. and Davis, J. A. (1978). *The place of Birth*. Oxford University Press, Oxford.

Lloyd, G. (1975). The general practitioner and changes in obstetric practice. *Br. Med. J.* **1**, 79–82.

Marsh, G. N. (1977). Obstetric audit in general practice. *Br. Med. J.* **2**, 1004–6.

Royal College of General Practitioners (1981). Obstetrics and gynaecology for general practice. Working Party report. *J. Roy. Coll. Gen. Practit.* **31**, 72–9.

Royal College of General Practitioners and Royal College of Obstetricians and Gynaecologists (1982). Obstetrics and gynaecology for general practitioners. Report on Training. Joint Working Party. *J. Roy. Coll. Gen. Practit.* **32**, 116–22.

Shapland, D. E. (1979). Extended role for general practitioners in obstetrics? A medical audit. *Br. Med. J.* **1**, 1199–1200.

Steele, R. and Gray, A. M. (1981). The economics of specialist and general practitioner maternity units. *J. Roy. Coll. Gen. Practit.* **31**, 586–92.

Taylor, G. W. *et al.* (1980). How safe is general practitioner obstetrics? *Lancet* **2**, 1287–9.

Tew, M. (1977). Obstetric hospitals and general practitioner maternity units—the statistical record. *J. Roy. Coll. Gen. Practit.* **27**, 689–94.

19 Different settings for intrapartum care: home

B. A. Sides

Planned home confinements are no longer recommended by most authoritative medical opinion. (Peel report 1970; Barron and Thompson 1977). The falling birth rate, increased consultant and general practitioner hospital beds (Short 1980) and facilities, combined with an effective educational programme that 'hospital is best', have resulted in a massive reduction in home deliveries. Over the last 20 years they have fallen from over 50 per cent to less than 1 per cent of all births. In one urban study of 1746 pregnancies the change is demonstrated as follows (Sides 1981):

	1966 (per cent)	1981 (per cent)
Home confinement bookings	51.4	0.7
Consultant unit bookings	48.6	65.7
General practitioner unit bookings	nil	33.6

The accompanying reduction in the perinatal mortality rate from 35 to less than twelve per thousand might support the conclusion that fewer home confinements have been a contributory factor although there are obviously many other factors (Barron and Thompson 1977, and Chapter 14).

HOME BIRTH GROUPS

Home births fall into two groups:

Group A consists of those who deliver at home unexpectedly, in other words, not as planned by the mother/midwife/doctor team. The usual causes are:

(i)   precipitate and/or premature labour of mothers booked for hospital confinement who are unable to get to the hospital;
(ii) concealment of pregnancy until it is too late to transfer;
(iii) intentional rejection of conventional medical 'wisdom' and medical care;

This whole group contains many high-risk women.

Group B consists of women who deliver as planned at home. These are a very carefully selected group. Many misleading and exaggerated conclusions have been drawn by considering the results and statistics of both groups as a single entity. As the perinatal mortality rate (PNMR) is about twenty times greater in group A than it is in group B (Burnett *et al.* 1980), it is important to define clearly to which group perinatal statistics are attributed (Ellam 1984).

Efforts should be made to continue to reduce the numbers in group A by continuing patient education.

Women in group B are now usually those who consider that they have made a well-informed decision to have a normal delivery in the natural setting of their own home. They wish to experience a most significant family event in the family situation. The request is almost always initiated by them. Several procedures are necessary to help the woman and her partner to finalize their decision or, if necessary, dissuade them from it. A reasonable procedure is as follows:

1. The prospective parents must be aware of the increased risks involved. These are difficult to quantify but it is probable that the PNMR is increased by less than one per thousand.

If the couple still express a strong desire to continue the next step is the medical selection.

2. Selection is vitally important and aims to exclude as many risks as possible at the time of booking. The reasons for exclusion are usually quite specific. A typical list would be (Stirrat 1983):

   (i)   primigravidae under 18 or over 30;
  (ii)   multigravidae over 35;
 (iii)   unsatisfactory home conditions (more likely in social classes iv and v);
 (iv)   significant medical conditions such as diabetes, rheumatic heart disease, thyrotoxicosis etc.;
  (v)   previous third stage abnormalities or other bad obstetrical history, including previous preterm delivery or low birth weight infant;
 (vi)   previous uterine or gynaecological operations such as caesarean section, myomectomy, cone biopsy, colporrhaphy;
 (vii)   those who have had more than four previous pregnancies;
(viii)   those with rhesus or other forms of isoimmunization.
 (ix)   those with elevated serum alphafetoprotein (with or without neural tube defect)

Following these exclusions the next step is the arrangement of appropriate medical and midwifery services.

3. It is important that the general practitioner and community midwife should both be willing, confident and competent to provide total care for a home delivery. This is becoming less available. Many general practitioners no longer do provide intrapartum care and there are fewer midwives who have

any experience of, or confidence in, the home setting. The doctor must have had adequate training including a 6 month residential obstetrical hospital appointment. He must be accessible and available at all times, and in his absence be covered by an equally competent colleague. Only the highest standard of antenatal care is acceptable. He must have easy access to consultant obstetrical, radiological, pathological, and anaesthetic facilities. He should have had experience in neonatal resuscitation. The confidence of the doctor/midwife team should be reflected in the mother. Her attendance at relaxation and parent craft classes in the later weeks of her pregnancy can be very beneficial.

As far as possible 'non-interference obstetrics' should be the rule. Practical procedures will be minimal and limited to the administration of systemic and inhalation analgesics, local anaesthetics, episiotomy and perineal repair if necessary.

4. The final step is the necessity for the woman to realise that there will be at least a one in five chance (Bull 1980; Sides 1981) that she will have to be transferred to hospital at some time before the completion of labour. Of women booked for hospital 16–23 per cent will be transferred before the onset of labour. The reasons will include malpresentation, problems regarding maturity, toxaemia of pregnancy, social problems, antepartum haemorrhage, anaemia, suspected fetal abnormality, hydramnios, premature rupture of the membranes without onset of labour, the late detection of multiple pregnancy, fibroids, and developing medical conditions. Between 6 and 8 per cent of booked women will require transfer after the onset of labour. The reasons will include premature labour, delay in the first or second stage, antepartum haemorrhage, malpresentation, prolapsed cord, undiagnosed multiple pregnancy, fetal distress, retained placenta, and postpartum haemorrhage.

CONDITIONS GIVING RISE TO CONCERN

There are three particular conditions (Moore 1979) which give rise to most concern in home confinements and which may occur unpredictably after the onset of labour. They are as follows.

Cord prolapse

Even if the known predisposing causes of this condition are excluded there remains an incidence of about one in 2000 in the supposedly normal case. When this occurs in hospital the baby has a good chance of survival following urgent caesarean section. If it occurs at home the baby will probably die.

Postpartum haemorrhage (PPH) retained placenta

The tragedy of maternal death from a postpartum haemorrhage can only be minimized if home confinements take place in areas with an efficient obstetrical flying squad. It is usually safer for the flying squad to resuscitate the mother if she is shocked, and to remove the placenta in the home under a general anaesthetic, than it would be to remove her to hospital first.

Fetal distress and birth asphyxia

About 6 per cent (Moore 1979) of babies require some assistance at or immediately after birth. Delay in getting the baby to a special care unit could be fatal. It is essential that the doctor be present at the delivery to help with resuscitation if necessary.

It is in these three situations that the increased risks of home confinements lie.

CONCLUSIONS

The problems facing those requesting home confinements are therefore considerable, however, they need not be insurmountable. The question of justification of any increased risk, no matter how small, is a difficult one. Before condemning it as totally unacceptable the rights of the woman regarding freedom of choice must be considered. The advantages, to some mothers, of having a normal delivery in their own home, with continuity of care from familiar attendants, are sufficient in their opinion, to outweigh the slight increase in risk. The satisfaction and peace of mind in fulfilling her desire to have what is probably a most significant natural event in a family life, in a natural family situation, on her terms and with a minimum of interference, is such that the trend away from home confinements may yet be reversed by women's demands. However this can only be justified if the woman's decision is made with a full knowledge of all the facts and so long as there are competent general practitioner obstetricians and community midwives willing to accept the responsibility.

REFERENCES

Baron, S. L. and Thompson, A. M. (1977). Home and hospital confinement in Newcastle-upon-Tyne 1960–1969. *Br. J. Obstet. Gynaecol.* **84**, 401–11.

Bull, M. J. V. (1980). Ten years experience in a general practitioner obstetric unit. *J. Roy. Coll. Gen. Practit.* **30**, 208–21.

Burnett, C. A., Jone, J. A., Rooks, J., Chen, C. H., Tyler, C. W. and Miller, C. A. (1980). Home delivery and neonatal mortality in North Carolina. *JAMA* **244(24)**, 2741–5.

Ellam, G. A. (1984). Department of Community Medicine, West Berkshire Health Authority. Delivery outcome and its relationship to intended place of confinement—a review. (Publication pending).

Moore, W. M. O. (1979). Preparation for home confinement. *Update* **15 July**, 147–53.

Short, R. (1980). Social Services Committee. Perinatal and neonatal mortality. *Second report from the Social Services Committee*. HMSO, London.

Sides, B. A. (1981). Problems and trends of home confinements. A 15-year survey (1966–80) of obstetrical practice in an urban area. *Practitioner* **225**, 1231–4.

Stirrat, G. M. (1983). The general practitioner's role in obstetrics. *Update* **1.1**, 26–37.

20 Physiological labour and natural birth

Jean Towler

Childbirth in itself is a natural phenomenon and the large majority of women need no interference whatsoever—only close observation, moral support and protection against human meddling. A healthy woman who delivers spontaneously performs a job that cannot be improved upon.

(Kloosterman 1972)

Physiological labour, which implies a natural process without the imposition of birth technology, should be the experience of the 80 per cent or so of mothers who fall into the low risk category. As a consultant Paediatrician has put it: 'If only we could regain our confidence in normality and leave women in the care of midwives and husbands then there would be ample time to put the remaining twenty per cent under the obstetrical microscope' (Dunn 1976). Over the last 20 years there has been unprecedented interference in the birth process by the unselective use of technology on a scale sufficient to arouse the comment that 'childbirth is not now something women do but something done unto them by doctors' (Tweedie 1975). Obstetric and neonatal technology may be beneficial in high-risk and complicated cases but its indiscriminate routine application has resulted in an increasing number of women rebelling against interventionist policies and demanding a more natural, humane and sensitive approach to childbirth. 'In the subtle system of nature, technology and in particular the super-technology of the modern world, acts like a foreign body, and *there are now numerous signs of rejection*' (Schumacher 1975).

The attainment of the very high standard of *physical* care at present delivered to pregnant women has been at the expense of other aspects of care and in consequence psychological and emotional needs and choices of individual women have been largely neglected or ignored. There has been a tendency to regard the woman solely as a pregnant *body* with precious little consideration given to the other components of mind and spirit (personality) which together with her body make her a person in her own right, whole and worthy of respect. Healthy low risk women have been treated as obstetric *patients* (implying illness) and have had the medical will imposed on them in terms of technological interference simply because it has become the 'norm' to view pregnancy as a pathological state. The psychosomatic effects of this concept are deep disturbance to the mind and emotions of the mother during her pregnancy which can also affect her performance in labour, and clear relationships have been shown to exist between anxiety and fear during the antenatal period and labour complications. When disturbed by the often total and unreasonable disregard of her subjective desire for non-intervention, the woman ceases to be an integrated harmonious whole and the resulting psychological damage may make her tense, sad, and despondent. 'Body functions are dependent on ease of mind, and ease of mind is more effective than technology in promoting normal parturition and lactation' (Holt 1977). Because a relaxed mother is likely to have an easier labour it is essential that couples should be physically, mentally, psychologically, and emotionally prepared for labour, birth, and parenthood. Ideally they should be able to interact on a personal level with their midwife and general practitioner so that fears and anxieties can be discussed and allayed, and plans made for the labour and birth with contingency plans in the event of complication. The relationship with the midwife is particularly important as she will have the female attributes of empathy, sensitivity, and compassion and will recognize emotional as well as physical needs. The midwife together with the general practitioner can provide continuity of care during pregnancy and birth which are invaluable to the promotion of confidence and relaxation in the mother. Unfortunately male characteristics, demonstrated by the enthronement of intellect, logic, reasoning, science, and technology have dominated obstetrics with male obstetricians tending to be more interested in the mechanics of birth and the safe 'production of the goods' than in the parturient woman herself. From the birthing woman's point of view it is vitally important that the female characteristics of instinct, intuition and emotion at least *balance* if not override the male aspects of human nature.

PREPARATION

The mother must be adequately instructed in the actual physiological processes of labour and delivery and she must be taught how to relax and how to cope with the unfamiliar physical sensation of uterine contractions. She must be taught how to mentally accept that she must work *with* her contractions and not *against* them. She may learn to relax through modified psychoprophylaxis, yoga or other exercise techniques. The mothers are aiming towards the sense of achievement and self-fulfilment which comes from physiological conscious birthing. The method itself is not important as long as the mother learns to relax deeply and to surrender herself to the experience rather than attempt to resist it. The practice of yoga or other exercise techniques will stretch and tone the muscles and the mother will be able to practise poses and postures which may be useful to her while labouring and giving birth. Many mothers now enjoy the discipline and gentle exercise of 'keep fit' classes in pregnancy which lead to an increase in self-awareness and enhance physical and mental health and the sense of wellbeing.

Initiation of labour

During pregnancy the uterus is never entirely relaxed, but as with all smooth muscle, it undergoes rhythmical movements. As the pregnancy advances and the muscle bulk of the uterus increases so the contractions increase in their amplitude and are subjectively interpreted as 'tightenings'. Labour is an extension of this physiological activity and while the precise mechanism which brings about this increased activity in the uterine muscle is not completely understood it appears to be due to mechanical, hormonal, and chemical factors working in concert. However, 'the "final common event" in the action of all myometrial smooth muscle stimulants involves the release of calcium into the cytoplasm of cells where it reacts with myofibril contractile proteins to cause contraction' (Hillier 1977).

Signs of impending labour

The onset of labour is frequently rather insidious. The mother may experience one or all of a variety of symptoms to which there is no particular pattern. She may be aware of dull low backache which gradually increases in intensity or she may have abdominal discomfort similar to 'period pain'. Others may become aware of more regular 'tightenings' accompanied by mild discomfort due to brief low amplitude contractions. Alternatively the first sign of activity may be a 'show' indicating displacement of the operculum from the cervical os.

THE FIRST STAGE OF LABOUR

Physical and emotional support

There will be heightened emotional satisfaction if the mother has a supportive companion with her throughout the labour. This will indicate to her that she is valued, and serves to enhance her self-esteem and help raise her tolerance for what otherwise might be perceived as intolerable pain. On the other hand the absence of a companion may pose a threat to her self-image so lowering her morale. The companion, who should encourage her, may be her husband, partner, or woman friend while the midwife should be her constant professional associate, preceptor and friend, sensitive to her feelings and respectful of her aspirations. In addition to the psychological benefit from human companionship several studies suggest that the presence of a supportive companion reduces catecholamine levels, significantly shortens the labour and enhances maternal behaviour in the immediate postdelivery period (Klaus and Kennell 1982). The companion can coach the mother to relax, help her into comfortable postures and provide physical contact by handholding, back massage or by abdominal stroking. Conversation is often superfluous if the couple communicate with their eyes, or by touch and gesture. The partner should remain to support his wife during vaginal and other examinations. 'A significant low incidence of problems of labour and birth has been reported for the group of infant–mother pairs who had a supportive companion' (Klaus and Kennell 1982).

Practical aspects

Predelivery shaving of pubic and perineal hair is not necessary in a low-risk mother, although some consultants still require this procedure to be performed on their high-risk patients in case they require an operative delivery. A survey (Romney 1981) revealed that leaving the pubic and perineal hair intact did not affect the incidence of infection but removal of the hair caused multiple small abrasions and discomfort and itching during regrowth.

The administration of enemata in labour is now a contentious issue and their effectiveness has been questioned. Many mothers certainly seem to dread this procedure and so unless a full bowel is obviously obstructing the course of labour, the enema is often omitted. It is also excluded where the labour is well advanced. However there seem to be certain good reasons for giving a generous soap and water enema early in the first stage. Firstly, the lower bowel will be emptied so more space will be made available in the pelvis for descent of the baby's head. An empty bowel overcomes the problem of extrusion of faeces immediately before or during the birth and so, in addition to the aesthetic considerations, the area is cleaner for delivery. A large enema may also, by reflex action, stimulate uterine contractions and thus enhance the progress of labour. If the mother has strong objections to being subjected to the rigours of an enema then glycerine suppositories or a small disposable phosphate enema are alternatives which will at least ensure that the lower bowel is emptied, with the minimum of discomfort to the mother.

The volume of urine voided will be measured, recorded and then tested, particularly for ketones. However 'the presence of ketones in labour is common . . . and its significance remains an enigma' (Foulkes and Dumoulin 1983). These authors point out that there is no good evidence that even moderate ketosis is deleterious to the fetus. While a trace of ketones may be acceptable their study of a large number of women suggests that uterine performance may be impaired in the presence of ketosis. However prophylactic intravenous infusion of dextrose during labour does not seem to be the answer and 'is not without significant hazard to both mother and fetus' as it may create the risk of hyponatraemia (Foulkes and Dumoulin 1983).

During labour gastric motility is reduced and the digestive processes are almost at a standstill so any nutriment taken should be in a form which requires little or no digestion. It is not unreasonable to allow a healthy woman in early physiological labour to have something light and easily assimilated such as natural yoghurt or very thin bread and butter spread with honey, or eaten with dates. As labour progresses nourishment may be given such as cold or warmed milk, sweetened tea or one of the many refreshing herbal teas. Raspberry leaf tea, which claims to make labour easier, is at present enjoying a revival. The mother may also like to suck glucose or 'barley sugar' sweets.

Environment

The environment should be one in which the physiological process can take place without disturbance. The birth room should ideally be attached to a small ward made 'homely' by pictures, curtains and television. The atmosphere in the ward and birth room should provide the psychologically optimum conditions for the mother to relax and become responsive to her instincts. The birth room may be carpeted, papered and simply furnished with the minimum amount of surgical equipment stored on shelves behind a curtain. There may be floral and net curtains, comfortable chairs, a small table and a bed with counterpane. There should be a large wedge, cushions, bean bags, birthing chair, table lamp, fan, mattress, and mirror. A cassette player is useful to provide soothing music and the room should be kept warm. Couples may wish to play Scrabble or card games in early labour. The subdued lighting and the quiet and homely atmosphere should serve to minimize mental and sensory stimuli and prevent fear and tension. Removal of spectacles and closure of the eyes during contractions also seem to aid relaxation. Anxiety will cause release of catetholamines which can disturb the physiological pattern of contractions. 'Epinephrine (adrenaline) has a direct effect on uterine muscle, decreasing uterine contractions and thereby increasing the length of labour' (Zuspan 1962); 'Fear and tension influence the inner biological rhythms' (Dick-Read 1968). A warm bath induces a feeling of wellbeing and relaxation and in fact some mothers benefit from spending long periods of time in the bath during the first stage of labour. A few mothers find such soaking so helpful that they spend almost the entire labour in the bath. The husband and midwife can chat or listen to music with the mother and the fetal heart checks can be made with the aid of a Bosch electronic stethoscope or a Sonicaid although the abdomen has to be dried and oiled when the latter is used.

The consultant obstetrician Michel Odent who has pioneered a natural birth unit at Pithiviers in France believes that environment is an important aid to regression or a sinking below culturally acquired 'norms' and expectations (Odent 1983). He believes that such regression alters the mother's state of consciousness and produces a positive feeling of wellbeing which protects her against the effects of pain possibly by the release of endorphins. The environment is designed to spare the intellect and senses and the mother is encouraged to separate herself from the everyday world and discover and respond to what is instinctive inside herself as if listening to an older and more primitive part of the brain. The decor in his non-conventional birth rooms is plain with walls painted a warm brown, orange curtains and a single light bulb covered by a raffia shade. There is a low platform covered with brightly coloured cushions on which the mother gives birth in a supported-squat position. There is also a wooden birthing chair and a record player.

It is interesting that Percivall Willughby wrote thus in the sixteenth century 'And, for the labouring woman's chamber, let it be made dark, having a glimmering light or candle light. Let her walk gently in her chamber, or come to her knees' (Willughby 1596).

Ambulation and pain relief

'Adoption of the recumbent posture in labour is an obstetric fashion: it has no scientific basis' (Engleman 1882). When the labour is physiological the mother, not confined to bed by drips or attachment to machines can stand or walk about with gravitational pressure aiding both descent of the baby's head and certical dilation. Lying down may adversely affect the progress of labour so the mother should not be confined to bed and unless she specifically wishes to lie down to rest for short periods it is advantageous for her to walk, stand, sit, or kneel during the first *and* second stages. She may lean or bend forwards during contractions or be supported by her husband in the *en face* position. She may prefer to sit astride a chair leaning over the chair back or find a comfortable position supported by bean bags and pillows. An alternative posture is for her to kneel with her arms and chest supported by a bed, a chair, or her husband's thighs. Ambulation facilitates the progress of labour and when the mother is standing contractions are of greater amplitude but are nevertheless not as painful. 'The records of intra-uterine contractions have a greater intensity when the mother is in the vertical position than when she is in the supine position. Their efficiency for dilating the uterine cervix is also greater in the vertical position. These beneficial effects of the vertical position are most significant before cervical dilation has reached 7 or 8 centimetres' (Mendez-Bauer 1975). These conclusions were reached after mothers in labour were asked to stand for half an hour and then lie down for half an hour alternately. The contractions were found to be weaker when the mothers were lying down and doubly effective in dilating the cervix when they were standing up although less painful. These findings were endorsed by a Latin American collaborative study which concluded that 'in normal spontaneous labours the vertical position facilitates the progress of labour, shortens its duration and reduces maternal discomfort and pain' (Caldeyro-Barcia 1979). If the mother is able to relax she seems less aware of pain and it is thought that together with emotional contentment this may help to trigger the release of endogenous endorphins. Discomfort and pain during contractions may be relieved by bending forwards, back massage, heat from a warm water bottle or radiant heat lamp, or by controlled breathing/concentration, self-hypnosis, or downward stroking of the uterus and these aids may obviate the need for analgesic drugs. Medication will be available at the mother's request or if deemed necessary in the clinical judgement of the doctor or midwife. The degree of pain experienced in labour certainly seems to be related to the *state of mind* of the mother and to the amount of affection and emotional support she is given and so mothers who are ambulant, calm, and relaxed seem to feel considerably less pain than those who are tense, frightened, or not interacting on an emotional level with their 'significant other'. 'Pain perception varies with individuals depending on the state of the brain when it receives the message, and this is affected by cultural expectations about the outcome of pain' (MacFarlane 1977). Although pethidine has been used consistently over the last 30 years as an antispasmodic drug in labour it is known to cross the placenta and in a trial on its effectiveness only 50–60 per cent of mothers regarded the analgesic effect as satisfactory (Grant *et al.* 1970). As pain is not inevitable in a normal labour pethidine or other pharmacological means of pain relief need not be used routinely and the wishes of the mother regarding medication should be considered. 'If the baby is born with any of the drugs in his bloodstream, he is then dependent on his own liver to complete the process of detoxification. The neonate's liver is one of the last systems to mature so a drug like pethidine . . . may persist in the baby for several days' (Inch 1982).

Babies born after injudicious administration of pethidine to the mothers are drowsy and behave as if drugged whereas babies born to mothers who have not had analgesic drugs are awake, alert, and perceptive. Workers studying mother–infant interaction concluded that 'Meperidine (pethidine) produces outstanding neonatal differences in the ability to process information' (Brackbill *et al.* 1974).

Self-hypnosis has proved to be valuable in childbirth as the mother learns to think of a uterine contraction as a warm positive experience rather than as something to be endured. If pain does intrude she minimizes it by concentrating on counting backwards from 100 aloud during the contraction.

While epidural analgesia may lower the blood pressure and reduce pain perception in certain *high-risk* cases, mothers in the *low-risk* group, who have been adequately prepared for labour and who are in an environment which dispels apprehension and promotes positive thinking, should not require epidural anaesthesia. The mother with an epidural *in situ* has to lie inert in bed and while it may be in her interest to have a relatively pain-free labour this procedure is certainly not without risk to her and her baby

(Aleksandrovicz 1974; Nugent 1935). Moreover, a recent survey on 1000 women revealed that they preferred the pain of childbirth to the numbness of an epidural anaesthetic. They were generally less satisfied than those who had been allowed to give birth naturally and their labours were significantly longer (Morgan *et al.* 1982 a and b) 'Immediately after delivery infants with greater exposure to bupivacaine in utero were more likely to be cyanotic and unresponsive to their surroundings. Visual skills and alertness decreased significantly with increases in the cord blood concentration of bupivacaine, particularly on the first day of life, but also throughout the next six weeks'. (Rosenblatt 1981).

Inhalational analgesia

The premixed gases nitrous oxide and oxygen may be inhaled by the mother to produce a satisfactory level of analgesia without any disadvantage to the fetus. Entonox is not unpleasant, does not produce nausea, and the 50 per cent oxygen content is psychologically attractive to the mother and physiologically beneficial to her baby. This somewhat underrated inhalational analgesia can be used in the first and second stages of labour and the fact that it is self-administered is important to the mother who wishes to be fully conscious when giving birth. Concentration on the machine, and on the mental and respiratory efforts which are required for effective pain relief, serve to divert the mother's attention away from the contracting uterus.

Assessment of progress

The midwife will make a written record of the history and progress of the labour which will include the strength and character of the contractions. An orderly rhythmical pattern of intermittent contractions is essential for progress. In early labour the contractions should be regular, infrequent, of short duration and low amplitude but as labour progresses they increase in strength, frequency and duration until they are expulsive and last a full minute or more with a minimum relaxation period of 1 or 2 minutes. A 'normal' contraction rises gently to a peak and then declines gradually and is followed by a period of relaxation. During normal uterine action a contraction may be felt by the examiner some seconds *before* the mother experiences discomfort and for a few seconds *after* the discomfort has ceased. When the uterine action is uncoordinated and disorderly the uterus may feel tense *between* contractions and the mother may experience pain before an appreciable contraction can be felt by the examiner. The midwife can use her tactile sense to assess the amplitude of contractions. She should be able to feel the muscle fibres start to contract gently in the region of the cornua, spread to the fundus where the contraction is at its maximum intensity and then feel the wave of contraction travel down the uterus with diminishing intensity. The body of the uterus has many more bundles of muscle fibres than the lower segment and so the force of the contraction is much stronger in the upper uterine segment than in the lower segment. This 'fundal dominance' overcomes the weak contraction of the muscle fibres in the lower segment and as the upper segment thickens and shortens due to retraction so the lower segment thins and stretches, and the cervix is steadily pulled open.

The effect of intermittent contractions which slowly gather momentum is to cause *descent* and rotation of the presenting part and to dilate the cervix. It may be necessary to perform a vaginal examination at the onset of labour to determine or confirm the presentation, and also during the labour to ascertain the dilation of the cervix and the position and station of the head in the pelvis. It is usual for the mother to lie or sit in bed for a vaginal examination but a satisfactory alternative posture is for the mother to stand with one leg supported on a low stool. Gloves will be worn for this sterile procedure, although the use of masks for such procedures and for normal deliveries has now largely been abandoned.

Maternal and fetal wellbeing

The midwife will make a record of the maternal and fetal conditions throughout the labour. After ausculation of the fetal heart rate she must also check and record the mother's pulse rate. She will expect a slightly faster beat than usual due to the increased physical activity but will advise the general practitioner if the pulse rate is persistently above 100 beats/minute.

The mother's blood pressure will be estimated at the onset of labour but if she is normotensive and up and about it will not be necessary to make regular recordings. If, however, the mother consistently lies in bed thus creating the potential for supine hypotensive syndrome then it is a wise precaution to measure the blood pressure at frequent intervals. Auscultation of the fetal heart should be made as often as every half hour in the first stage and between every contraction in the second stage. The normal rate of between 130–150 beats/minute may alter during a contraction. It may accelerate before the peak of the contraction, decelerate at the height and then pick up to its normal rate and rhythm as the contraction dies away. The midwife will listen for one full minute counting the beats and listening for any variation in the rate. She may use a Pinard's stethoscope, Sonicaid or an electronic stethoscope. As a 'human monitor' the midwife must be extremely vigilant and careful in her fetal heart counts yet at the same time be as unobtrusive as possible. If the fetus is distressed due to oxygen deprivation this will manifest itself by tachycardia, bradycardia or a failure by the heart to 'pick up' and resume its normal rate and rhythm after a contraction, and the midwife will notify the general practitioner and/or consultant obstetric staff depending on the degree of distress and the point in labour. Continuous fetal heart monitoring using a cardiotocograph machine confines the woman to bed and its indiscriminate use on low as well as high-risk mothers is one of the most contentious aspects of modern labour ward care as it can be argued that this could potentiate fetal distress (see Chapter 23).

The conclusion drawn from a recent paper entitled 'Second thoughts on routine monitoring in labour' (Parsons *et al.* 1983) is that 'the continuously monitored patient is at greater risk of caesarean section whether she is obstetrically of low or high risk'. Four studies mentioned in this document failed to show any benefit in terms of perinatal outcome from continuous fetal heart monitoring even in high risk cases with an exception in the case of premature labour. Moreover, damage can be caused to the fetal scalp by the application of spiral electrodes. Complications in 2 per cent of babies were recorded in a recent study on 192 mothers with *low-risk* labours (De Souza, Black and MacFarlane 1982). Other studies have reported abrasions, abscess formation, haemorrhage, sepsis, and osteomyelitis (Corderio and Hon 1971). Michel Odent asserts that 'Obstetricians may be right to monitor intensively the labours of women lying on their backs because this position is dangerous'. Continuous monitoring has been shown to treble the risk of cacsarcan section 'because fluctuations in fetal heart rate are little understood, and so unnecessary action is taken. It has not been shown to save babies' lives, nor to increase their Apgar scores' (Gordon 1982).

Calculations on the efficiency of electronic fetal heart monitors seriously question the usefulness of a monitor in detecting abnormalities in practice. When monitors are used, tragedies occasionally occur when staff disregard an ominous tracing, assuming that the machine is not working properly. An operational research scientist writing in the *Lancet* calculated that this situation is the expected result of the rate of false alarms. He claims that 'even if a machine detects 95 per cent of all abnormalities, and has a low probability of raising the alarm when there is no abnormality, the fact that there are so many more normal than abnormal labours means that 67 per cent of all alarms will be false. The staff reaction, of course, depends on the rate of false alarms: they will always take action if there are no false alarms, never take action if there are only false alarms, and sometimes take action if there are sometimes false alarms. Thus the probability of detecting an abnormality in practice depends both on the machine's raising the alarm (95 per cent chance) and on staff reacting (maybe as low as 35 per cent chance), so the overall detection rate in practice would be only 31 per cent. Of course staff reacting more readily would mean reacting to a high proportion of false alarms, and would explain the high caesarean rate associated with electronic fetal monitoring' (Royston 1982).

THE SECOND STAGE OF LABOUR AND THE BIRTH OF THE BABY

When we are born we cry that we are come to this great stage of fools' (Shakespeare, *King Lear*, **IV, 6**). 'It would seem that a woman being given permission to be a birthing human animal, in touch with her instincts, takes birth in her stride' (Combe 1981).

When the contractions are expulsive and the cervix is fully dilated the parturient woman should be encouraged to adopt any position she finds conducive to greatest ease and comfort. Such postures are likely to be physiologically advantageous as the mother is then pushing with gravity rather than against it. The mother may frequently change position and may like to stand *between* contractions and kneel, squat or crouch *during* contractions. The midwife should ensure that the bladder is empty and should count and record the fetal heart and maternal pulse rate between each contraction. Organized directed breath holding and pushing sessions should not take place but the mother should be asked to bear down naturally when *she* feels an irresistible urge to push. The mother herself should control the force, length, and number of 'bearing down' efforts per contraction. It has been shown that spontaneous expulsive efforts, which are short and made with an open glottis, decrease the incidence of fetal hypoxia, (Caldeyro-Barcia *et al* 1979). Lung expansion and maternal oxygenation are improved when the mother is in a vertical position. A squatting or sitting position also prevents compression of the inferior vena cava, aorta, and iliac arteries. These vessels are compressed between the pregnant uterus and the spine when the mother is in the lithotomy position; the resulting circulatory disturbances may reduce the maternal perfusion of the placenta causing fetal hypoxia, hypercapnia and acidosis (Humphrey *et al.* 1974). Provided that the mother is in a vertical position for delivery, and her pushing is physiological, analysis of blood gases showed 'better' levels than when the pushing is forced and prolonged (Caldeyro-Barcia *et al.* 1979).

For the actual birth any upright posture will position the body in an ideal configuration for gravity-assisted descent and expulsion of the fetus. The mother may wish to deliver on a birthing chair which has the front cut away to facilitate the baby's exit, or she may wish to be propped up in bed or on a mattress on the floor supported by a wedge and cushions. On the other hand she may wish to squat between her sitting husband's legs resting her arms and elbows on his thighs, or she may be supported from behind in a semi-squatting position. Once the pelvic floor has been displaced so that more and more of the head comes into view the mother should be asked to pant during contractions and then gently *breathe* the head out *between* contractions. In this way the head will be crowned slowly and it is likely that the perineum will remain intact. The birth can take place with the mother kneeling on all fours either with her trunk horizontal and supported, or inclined downwards as in the knee—chest postition. If the mother has remained relaxed and in control so that the baby's head has emerged slowly, it is quite likely that a perineal tear will be avoided.

For giving birth the mother may like to change from her own nightdress into a large pyjama jacket or tunic. This will keep her shoulders warm and will allow for her naked baby to be lifted directly on to her warm abdominal skin to be caressed, admired and put to the breast. The baby can lie, covered with a warm towel, inside the jacket.

To prevent perineal tearing the midwife may massage the perineum with olive oil, or 'hot compresses placed over the labia and perineum, are soothing and stimulate circulation' (Hoare and Weig 1982). The midwife may wish to flex the head up to the point of crowning and then extend it away from the perineum using the biparietal hold.

In addition to the advantages already mentioned the squatting position allows for expansion of the pelvis to its maximum dimensions. 'The pelvic capacity depends on the mother's position at delivery. For maximum outlet dilation the squatting position is best. Perhaps the old fashioned birth stool is due for reassessment' (Russell 1973). In this century the second stage of labour has had time limits put upon its duration, and its length has been so 'doctor contracted' that midwives have become conditioned to thinking in terms of *delay* if the baby is not delivered within 1 hour. However, provided the mother is not distressed, has physical and emotional support, and the fetal heart rate is satisfactory and within normal limits, the second stage should be allowed to continue without time-imposed stress affecting the mother. It has been shown that when the mother is in the sitting position for birth not only are the blood gases better but that 'no differences were found in pH, Po_2, Pco_2 or base deficit in fetal blood at birth between the group of labours in which the second stage lasted 16–60 minutes and in that in which it lasted 60–120 minutes' (Caldeyro-Barcia *et al.* 1979).

There is no evidence to substantiate the oft repeated statement that the clean straight cut of an episiotomy is 'better' than a jagged tear (see Chapter 24). There is no justification for routine episiotomy, even in primigravidae. It has been found that women who had episiotomies for normal deliveries had more pain at the end of 7 days than those who had tears. Episiotomy is a deterrent to breast-feeding as mothers find it painful to sit in suitable positions, and they are also more likely to suffer from dyspareunia (Kitzinger, and Walters 1981). Episiotomy should certainly be discussed with the mother, as a 'routine (unnecessary and objected to) episiotomy is a serious assault (and battery) against a patient. It is no different in law from a knife wound delivered in a fight. Likewise the giving of drugs, say pethidine, against a person's will is an assault' (Finch 1982). Should an episiotomy be judged necessary, and agreed to by the mother, a midwife is licensed to infiltrate the perineum with local anaesthetic, make the incision and repair the perineum afterwards. On the other hand if the family practitioner is present at the delivery he may like to perform and/or repair the episiotomy himself.

Delivery of the placenta and membranes

The third stage of labour which can take up to 1 hour is concerned with the separation and expulsion of the placenta and membranes and the control of bleeding from the placental site. The bladder should be kept empty as if full it can cause uterine inertia which may interfere with placental separation and control of bleeding. If the placenta has not become detatched with the last expulsive birth contraction the uterus may go into a resting phase for 5 or 10 minutes prior to resuming contraction and retraction.

If the baby suckles in the first few minutes after birth this will stimulate the release of natural oxytocin which will aid contraction, separation and control of bleeding. Separation is a physiological process and if the mother is vertical, rather than horizontal, the placenta often swiftly follows the birth of the baby stripping the membranes off the uterine wall as it falls by gravity. The uterine muscle then controls bleeding by a natural haemostatic mechanism. If the mother is upright theoretically the risk of postpartum haemorrhage is reduced as a result of improved venous return. If the mother is in bed signs of separation of the placenta may be awaited. The fundus will rise and become hard, narrow, and mobile. When the placenta separates there is inevitably a trickle of blood from the placental site and as the placenta descends the cord will be seen to lengthen at the vulva. The mother may experience backache and have a desire to bear down. The placenta and membranes may then be expelled by maternal effort, or gentle fundal pressure may be applied providing the fundus is firm and signs of separation have been observed. The fundus should remain firm and well contracted with a blood loss of 200 ml or less, but if the uterus should relax and cause bleeding Syntometrine should be given intramuscularly. There is as yet limited but increasing evidence from practice which suggests that mothers delivering in the sitting or squatting position have a small, if not smaller, blood loss than those mothers given Syntometrine prior to controlled cord traction.

It is current obstetric fashion to give Syntometrine routinely, either with the birth of the anterior shoulder, or immediately following delivery of the baby in order to produce a sufficiently powerful contraction to accelerate placental separation and to aid the 'living ligature' action. Such active management is usually followed by delivery of the placenta by controlled cord traction. This pharmacological 'active' management of the third stage of labour was the obstetrician's response to potential post-partum haemorrhage but, 'as so often with developments in obstetrics *all mothers* came to be treated in the same manner, *irrespective of the degree of risk*' (Moore, Chard and Richards 1977).

The conclusions drawn from a study by Howard *et al.* (1964) were that the *routine* use of oxytocic drugs benefited only 7 per cent of women, and their findings of hypertension in the groups of women given oxytocin concurred with the findings of Hacker and Briggs. 'The giving of drugs which interfere with the physiological process of separation and haemostasis has increased the need for general anaesthetic and manual removal of the placenta, which may become trapped due to contraction of the cervix in response to oxytocin' (Dewhurst and Dutton 1957). So should such 'prophylactic' oxytocic drugs be used indiscriminately or should the third stage be physiological and Syntometrine reserved for certain selected cases, or when the need arises? Hacker and Briggs compared three small groups one of which received intravenous ergometrine, one intramuscular Syntometrine, and the other no drug at all. They found a postpartum blood loss of less than 200 ml *in each of the mothers*. However, although all the mothers had been normotensive, the mothers in the ergometrine group and 60 per cent in the Syntometrine group had moderate to severe *increases in blood pressure* whilst there were no such increases in the control group (Inch 1982).

Controlled cord traction precipitates the need to cut the umbilical cord, whereas delaying the infant's detachment from the placenta, by later cord clamping could, Leboyer asserts, confer certain benefits on the baby, particularly in relation to the transition from placental to pulmonary respiration.

The whole process described in the preceding paragraphs has been summarized in the right-hand column of Table 20.1. The alternative and frequently employed 'active' system is described in the left-hand column.

PROFESSIONAL RESPONSIBILITY

The midwife, who is licensed to conduct normal labour and delivery on her own responsibility, will be the principal professional participant and caregiver to mothers during physiological labour. It is usual for the midwife to inform the general practitioner that labour has started and to keep him informed of its progress although he accepts that the primary responsibility for continuous care belongs to the midwife. The doctor may wish to visit the mother during the course of the labour to support the midwife in her decision-making, and to encourage not only the mother but also the relatives who are supporting her. Acknowledging the importance of *continuity of care* and having established a rapport with the mother, the midwife may remain on duty until the delivery is completed. 'A good and friendly relationship between the mother and the midwife is vital to the subsequent and long term relationship between the mother and her child . . . in no other branch of medicine is the attitude of the attendant to her patient so productive of positive results as in midwifery' (Central Midwives Board 1952).

Table 20.1 *'Unnatural' and 'natural' labour*

'Unnatural' Labour/birth	'Natural' Labour/birth
INTRODUCTION or ACCELERATION (pharmacological)	SPONTANEOUS ONSET (no interference)
Conventional 'clinical' labour ward	Quiet room Subdued lighting Soft music Minimal mental and sensory stimulation

Artificial rupture of membranes
Intravenous infusion (syntocinon and/or
             levulose/dextrose)
          → Potential for uterine
               hyperactivity
	Relaxation
	  freedom to move
	  choice of position
	Ambulant. Walking,
	leaning, kneeling during
	contractions.

Mother confined to *bed* (wet)	Contractions less painful but more effective

Tension/anxiety–adrenaline
          Potential for supine
          hypotensive syndrome
	Use of Pinard's stethoscope
	or Sonicaid/
	intermittent human
	  monitoring.

Fetal scalp electrode/continuous Cardiotocograph monitoring	

Painful sharp syntocinon contractions	Natural endorphins
	  released due to
	      relaxation/trust
	      emotion/affection

Increase in anxiety, tension and perception of pain	
Need for analgesia pethidine or *epidural* Delivery in 'stranded beetle' position	Warm bath Use of bean bag

Semi-recumbent. Loss of gravity
      Loss of pelvic mobility
      Breath holding for pushing
	Natural posture for delivery
	Kneeling
	Standing
	Squatting
	Sitting–birth chair

Time limited second stage	Upright posture positions Mother's body in an optimal configuration for gravity assisted descent and delivery–so naturally shortened second stage. Head 'breathed out' *between* contractions.
Episiotomy Forceps	

Third stage. Active management
  Syntometrine–CCT
  Noise, harsh lights	

Baby to resuscitaire	*Baby* Immediate skin to skin contact

May have/acquired 'Hangover'
        drowsiness
        impaired sucking reflex
        jaundice
	To breast
	Release of oxytocin
	Physiological third stage
	
	Alert
	Aware
	Perceptive

The midwife will consult with the general practitioner during the labour should she detect any minor deviation from the normal but she can, in the event of an emergency, call the consultant obstetric or paediatric team or the flying squad as well as the doctor. The doctor may wish to enjoy the fruits of his preconceptual counselling and antenatal care by sharing with the family and midwife in the moment and celebration of birth.

There is a good deal of hard research which shows that how a mother feels in labour has an enormous influence on how she delivers. If her emotions are positive and she is relaxed and uninhibited there is a high chance of a trouble-free birth but if her emotions are negative and she is constrained and apprehensive the risk of having a difficult birth rises (Verny 1981).

If a baby is born into an atmosphere of peace, tranquillity and joy it is likely that this will confer important emotional advantages to the baby. The conclusion must be drawn that the quality of the birthing experience *does* matter and that this may influence the quality of parenting and the quality of life.

'Spontaneous labour in a healthy woman is an event marked by a number of processes which are so complex and so perfectly attuned to each other that any interference, will too often change true physiological aspects of human reproduction into pathology. Many Western doctors hold the belief that we can improve everything; even natural childbirth in a healthy woman' (Dunn quoting Kloosterman 1980).

REFERENCES

Alexsandrowicz, M. (1974). The effects of pain-relieving drugs administered in labour on the behaviour of the newborn. *Merrill-Palmer Q.* **20**.

Brackbill, Y. Kane, B. S., Manniello, R. L., and Abramson, D. (1974). Obstetric premedication and infant outcome. *Am. J. Obstet. Gynaec.* **118**.

Caldeyro-Barcia, R. *et al.* (1979). Physiological and psychological bases for the modern and humanised management of normal labour. Presented at *Symposium on recent progress in perinatal medicine, Tokyo*.

Central Midwives Board. (1952). Annual report.

Chan, W. H., Paul, R. H., and Toews, J. (1973). Intra partum fetal monitoring, maternal and fetal morbidity and perinatal mortality. *Obstet. Gynaec.* **41**, Quoted in De Souza *et al.* (1982).

Combe, E. (1981). Liberation of childbirth. *J. Early Childh.* March.

Corderio, L. and Hon, E. H. (1971). Scalpabscess: a rare complication of fetal monitoring. *J. Paediat.* **78**. Quoted in De Souza *et al.* (1982).

De Souza, S., Black, P., MacFarlane, T., and Richards, B. (1982). Fetal scalp damage and neonatal jaundice; a risk of routine fetal scalpelectrode monitoring. *J. Obstet. Gynaec.* January.

Dewhurst, J. C. and Dutton, W. D. (1957). Recurrent abnormalities of the third stage of labour. *Lancet* 9 October, 764–76.

Dick-Read, G. (1968). *Childbirth without fear*. Pan, London.

Dunn, P. (1976). Obstetric delivery today: for better or for worse. *Lancet* 10 April.

Dunn, P. (1980). Quoting G. J. Kloosterman, from *Proceedings of the 7th European Congress of Perinatal Medicine, Spain*
Engleman, G. J. (1882). *Labour amongst primitive peoples.* J. H. Chambers, St Louis.
Finch, J. (1982). Legal route to life. *Nursing Mirror* 27 October.
Foulkes, J. and Dumoulin, J. G. (1983). *Br. J. Hosp. Med.* **29**, 562–4.
Gordon, Y. (1982). *International Conference on Active Birth.* Wembley, London, October 1982.
Grant, A. M., Holt, E. M., and Noble A. D., (1970). A comparison between pethidine and phenazocine for relief of pain in labour. *J. Obstet, Gynaec. of Br. Commonw.* **77**.
Hacker, M. F. and Briggs, J. (1979). Blood pressure changes when uterine stimulants are used after normal delivery. *Br. J. Obstet. Gynaec.* **86**.
Haddad, F. (1982). Alternative positions for labour. *Midwife, Health Visitor and Community Nurse,* July.
Hillier, K. (1977). Uterine contractility. *Br. J. Hosp. Med.* March.
Hoare, S. and Weig, M. (1982). *How to avoid episiotomy.* Birth Centre document, London.
Holt, J., MacLennan, A. H., and Carrie, L. E. S., (1977). Lumbar puncture analgesic in labour; relation to fetal malposition and instrumental delivery. *Br. Med. J.* **1** Quoted in *Place of birth*, by Kitzinger and Davis, Oxford University Press.
Howard, W. F., McFedden, P. R. and Keettel, W. C., (1964). Oxytocic drugs in fourth stage of labor. *J. Am. Med. Assoc.* **189 (6)**.
Humphrey, M. D. Chang, A., Wood, E. C., Morgan, S. and Hounslow, D. (1974). A decrease in fetal pH during the second stage of labour when conducted in the dorsal position. *J. Obstet. Gynaecol. Br Commonw.* **81**.
Inch, S. (1982). *Birthrights.* Hutchinson, London.
Kitzinger, S. and Walters, R. (1981). *Episiotomy.* National Childbirth Trust, London.
Klaus, M. and Kennell, J. (1982). *Parent–infant bonding.* C. V. Mosby, St. Louis.
Kloosterman, G. J. (1972). Obstetrics in the Netherlands. Survival or a challenge. *Paper presented at meeting on problems in obstetrics.* Pitman, Tunbridge Wells.
Leboyer, F. (1975). *Birth without violence.* Knopf, New York.
MacFarlane, A. (1977). *Psychology of childbirth.* Fontana, London.
Mendez-Bauer, C. *et al.* (1975). Effect of standing position on spontaneous uterine contracting and other aspects of labour. *J. Perinat. Med.* **3**.
Moore, W. M. O., Chard, T. and Richards, M. (1977). *Benefits and hazards of the new obstetrics.* Heineman, London.
Morgan, B., Bulpitt, C., Clistan, P., and Lewis, P. (1982a). Analgesia and satisfaction in childbirth. *Lancet* 9 October.
Morgan, B. *et al.* (1982b). Effectiveness of pain relief in labour. *Br. Med. J.* 11 September.
Nugent, F. B. (1935). *Am. J. Obstet. Gynaecol.* **30**.
Okada, D. M., Chow, A. W., and Bruce, V. T. (1977). Neonatal scalp abscess and neonatal monitoring. *Am. J. Obstet. Gynaec.* **129**. Quoted in De Souza (1982).
Parsons, *et al.* (1983). Second thoughts on fetal monitoring In *Progress in obstetrics and gynaecology.* (ed. J. Studd), Vol 1. Churchill Livingstone, Edinburgh.
Paul, R. H. and Hon, E. H. (1973). Experience with a spiral electrode. *Obstet. Gynaec.* **41**. Quoted in De Souza (1982).
Romney, M. (1981). Pre-delivery shaving; an unjustified assault. *J. Obstet. Gynaecol.* **1**.

Rosenblatt, D. B., Belsey, E. M., Lieberman, B. A., Redshaw, M., Caldwell, J., Notarianni, L., Smith, R. L., and Beard, R. W. (1981). The influence of maternal analgesia on neonatal behaviour: II. Epidural Bupivacaine.

Royston, G. H. D. (1982). Fetal heart monitoring: a systems view. *Lancet* **10 April**, 861.

Russell, J. G. B. (1973). *Radiology in obstetrics and antenatal paediatrics*. Butterworths, London.

Schumacher, E. (1975). *Small is beautiful*. Abacus, London.

Tweedie, J. (1975). Polished delivery. *Guardian*, 13 October.

Willughby, P. (1596). *Observations in midwifery*. Edited from original MS by Henry Blenkinsop. Published 1863 by Shakespeare Press, Warwick.

Winkel, C. A., Snyder, D. G., and Sehlaerth, J. B. (1976). Scalp abscess: a comlication of the spiral electrode. *Am. J. Obstet. Gynaec.* **126**. Quoted in De Souza 1982).

Verny, J. (1981). *Secret life of the unborn child*. Sphere Books, London.

Zuspan, F. P. (1962. Myometrial and cardiovascular responses to alterations in plasma epinephrine and norepinephrine. *Am. J. Obstet. Gynaecol.* **84**.

FURTHER READING

Inch, S. (1982) *Birthrights*. Hutchinson, London.

Kitzingers and Davis, J. (1978). *The place of birth*. Oxford University Press.

Klaus, M. and Kennell, J. (1982). *Parent–Infant bonding* C.V. Mosby. St. Louis.

Macfarlane, A. (1977). *The psychology of childbirth*. Fontana and Open Books Publishing Ltd., Glasgow.

Odent, M. (1984). *Birth reborn*. Souvenir Press Ltd., London.

Post, Laurens van der (1978). *Jung and the story of our time*. Hogarth Press and Penguin, Hammondsworth.

21 Intervention in labour: drugs in normal labour

K. B. Lim and D. F. Hawkins

The choice and careful use of drugs in labour not only affect the outcome of labour, but also the safety of both mother and baby.

SEDATION IN LABOUR

The cultural background, emotional state and ingrained attitudes of the patient towards childbirth and the antenatal education she has received strongly influence her reaction to the confinement. Preconceived ideas of the observer also affect the apparent requirements of the patient.

In theory a sedative allays anxiety but may produce drowsiness; a hypnotic induces sleep resembling natural sleep; a tranquillizer relieves anxiety without affecting clarity of consciousness. In practice, the drugs used in labour have all three effects.

Opposition to the use of sedatives during labour developed because of the suspicion that they might cause fetal asphyxia and damage the newborn brain (Schreiber 1938; Schreiber and Gates 1938). Further resistance to the use of these drugs developed when other studies suggested that they adversely affect the infant's short and long-term behaviour (Conway and Brackbill 1970; Friedman *et al.* 1978; Stechler 1964). The concepts of Dick-Read (1944) and Lamaze (1970) of the practice of muscle relaxation and breathing exercises during labour strengthened some women's resolve to refuse sedatives.

Other studies support the view that sedatives are beneficial, reducing maternal anxiety and fear. Maternal anxiety early in labour, combined with high plasma adrenaline concentration, is associated with altered fetal heart rate patterns indicative of asphyxia (Lederman *et al.* 1981). Maternal anxiety has been found to be associated with prolonged labour (Beck *et al* 1980). When pain and anxiety are relieved with drugs, sympathetic nervous tone is reduced. This reduces circulatory levels of catecholamines and may improve uterine action.

Oral sedatives can only be of value in very early labour. Once labour is established they are not absorbed adequately and only parenteral sedatives are helpful.

Barbiturates

Barbiturates act as central nervous system depressants, with a range of effect from mild sedation up to general anaesthesia. The most commonly used preparations, in increasing order of the duration of action that is claimed are quinalbarbitone, pentobarbitone, cyclobarbitone, amylobarbitone and butobarbitone. In clinical practice there is little objective difference between their effects or their duration of action. Once absorbed they pass readily to the fetus and levels in the fetus are comparable to those in the mother. They pass the placenta freely and large doses may cause neonatal respiratory depression, or even a newborn sedative withdrawal syndrome. Babies born to mothers having had both pethidine and quinalbarbitone throughout labour had more depressed Apgar scores than babies whose mothers had pethidine alone or no medication (Shnider and Moya 1964). Lower Apgar scores and delays in establishing respiration in the newborn have been shown to occur with the administration of vinbarbitone to mothers in labour compared with babies whose mothers had received pethidine alone or with a phenothiazine (Batt 1968). Poor suckling rates, suckling pressures and milk intake were found in babies born to mothers who were given 200 mg of quinalbarbitone intravenously between 10 to 180 minutes before delivery (Kron, Stein and Goddard 1966). The quality and quantity of sucking behaviour in the newborn was reduced in the first 4 days.

Attentive behaviour has been found to be reduced in 2–4 day old newborn where the mother had received barbiturates within 90 minutes before delivery (Stechler 1964). The newborn also showed electroencephalographic changes in about 30 per cent of the medicated group that paralleled their general behavioural depression (Borgstedt and Rosen 1968). Myers and Myers (1979) thought that barbiturates have some protective effect on the hypoxic fetus by reducing stress and maternal sympathetic nervous system activity, thus improving uterine blood flow, tending to prevent lactic acidosis.

A small dose of barbiturate given to a woman when there is doubt if she has started to labour will do no harm, but there are more desirable alternatives, and in general barbiturates should not be used as routine sedatives in established labour.

Benzodiazepines

Chlordiazepoxide

Early in the first stage of labour 25–50 mg of chlordiazepoxide may be given orally, though whether or not it is absorbed effectively is doubtful. As much as 50–100 mg of chlordiazepoxide parenterally has no effect on either spontaneous tone or oxytocin-induced contractions of the uterus (Mark and

Hamel 1968; Stucki and Gross 1962). Mark and Hamel (1968) found chlor-diazepoxide to be of little value as a tranquillizer in labour. Chlordiazepoxide readily crosses the placenta, but any effect on the infant is usually mild (Decanq, Bosco and Townsend 1965; Mark and Hamel 1968). With very large doses maternal drowsiness, ataxia and hypotension may occur, and fetal side effects are probably similar to those of diazepam.

Diazepam

The newborn, especially if preterm, has a limited capacity to metabolize diazepam and its active metabolite desmethyldiazepam. Diazepam readily crosses the placenta, and concentrations in the fetal blood may be higher than in the mother owing to the greater degree of protein binding in fetal serum (Cree, Meyer and Hailey 1973; Mandelli *et al.* 1975). The drug may accumulate in fetal tissues, particularly in the nervous system. Neonatal hypotonia, hypothermia, respiratory depression and poor feeding can occur when doses of 30 mg or more of diazepam are given to the mother in the 15 hours before delivery (Cree, Meyer and Hailey 1973). In infants at risk, feeding difficulties and hypothermia can be caused by smaller doses of diazepam. The elimination of bilirubin may be impaired by diazepam because both the drug and the pigment are conjugated with glucuronic acid before excretion (Erkkola and Kanto 1972).

The effectiveness of oral diazepam as a sedative in labour is doubtful. Diazepam 10–20 mg given parenterally does not have any consistent effect on the course of uterine action (Bepko, Lowe and Waxman 1965; Nisbet, Boulas and Kantor 1967). Elder and Crossley (1969) found diazepam with pethidine no more effective than injections of a placebo with pethidine. The dose requirements of pethidine were unaltered when diazepam and pethidine were given together to mothers in labour (Davies and Rosen 1977).

It seems inadvisable to use diazepam routinely in labour when other sedatives and tranquillizers are available, though the drug may be required as an anticonvulsant with hypertensive mothers.

Nitrazepam

There have been no reports of any special hazards to the newborn with the use of nitrazepam as a hypnotic in labour, though its effects differ little from those of diazepam. It is suitable in very early labour if sleep is required. It can be given in doses between 2.5–10 mg orally and this acts in 30–60 minutes to produce sleep, lasting for 6–8 hours. It is best avoided in patients with chronic obstructive lung disease.

Chloral hydrate and related drugs

Chloral hydrate, dichloralphenazone and triclofos are metabolized into tri-chlorethanol after absorption from the gastrointestinal tract. Trichlorethanol is the compound responsible for the mild sedative and hypnotic action. For use in labour, these drugs are generally safe alternatives to the barbiturates.

Chloral hydrate, 500 mg to 1 g, has been used as a hypnotic, but its unpleasant taste makes it unpopular with patients. It is best avoided in patients with dyspepsia as it may cause gastric irritation. Occasionally, skin rashes may occur and rarely, excitement or delirium are encountered.

Dichloralphenazone is more palatable. A single dose of 0.5–2 g with milk can be used when anxiety is a problem at the onset of labour.

Triclofos, 0.5–1 g tablets, or in syrup, is a suitable hypnotic; gastro-intestinal disturbances are less common and it is not irritant to skin and mucous membranes.

Phenothiazines and related drugs

Phenothiazines have been extensively prescribed for their sedative and anxiolytic properties. They can also be used for their antiemetic actions.

Variable results have been obtained with respect to the action on uterine activity. Initial reports suggested that these drugs in the usual therapeutic doses did not affect uterine contractions (Caldeyro-Barcia 1958). Occasionally promethazine, 25–100 mg parenterally, caused a temporary reduction of contractions (Pannullo and Cerone 1960). A decrease, lasting 1–2 hours in both amplitude and frequency of contractions after promazine, 50 mg intramuscularly, was demonstrated by Zourlas (1964). Matthews (1963) found no effect on the overall duration of labour. Most reports were that prochlorperazine and perphenazine had no effect on uterine contractions.

Most clinicians would agree that promazine has a calming and perhaps a pethidine-sparing action. Promazine 50 mg with pethidine 50 mg was thought to be superior to 100 mg pethidine alone by MacVicar and Murray (1960). The effectiveness of promazine was disputed by McQuitty (1967). The apparent analgesic action may be due to an anxiolytic effect, rather than true analgesia.

There is no known risk to the newborn when a 25–50 mg intramuscular injection of promazine or promethazine is given in labour.

Chlorpromazine is now rarely used routinely in labour.

Conclusion

There is no harm in giving a small dose of an oral sedative to a woman in early labour, particularly if the patient is anxious. We prefer to use dichloralphenazone or triclofos. If a sedative is needed in established labour the best choices are either promazine, 50 mg intramuscularly or promethazine, 25 mg intramuscularly.

FLUIDS IN LABOUR

Oral fluids in labour should be restricted to sips of water to prevent thirst. In established labour absorption of fluid by the oral route is usually inadequate to prevent dehydration occurring. Should general anaesthesia be required, aspiration of gastric contents is highly dangerous and remains a significant cause of maternal death.

Records of urinary output or the occurrence of ketosis can indicate the risk of dehydration, but any woman who has been in established labour for 8 hours needs intravenous fluids. Five per cent dextrose at a rate of a litre each 6–8 hours is appropriate; labours are not usually permitted to proceed to more than 20 hours, when electrolyte replacement might be indicated. There is no excuse for inadequate supervision of intravenous infusions and fluid overload now drip counters are available.

VOMITING IN LABOUR

Vomiting in labour is common even if no drugs are used, but as many as 50 per cent of women develop nausea and vomiting when narcotic analgesics are given in labour. Vomiting may also indicate full dilatation of the cervix. When vomiting is recurrent during labour, possible medical or surgical causes should be considered. While the patient retains her cough reflex the risk of aspiration of gastric contents is small.

Remedies

Antiemetics

Phenothiazine derivatives are helpful in the prevention and treatment of nausea and vomiting in labour. For this purpose, promethazine 25–50 mg, promazine 50 mg, perphenazine 5 mg or prochlorperazine 12.5 mg intramuscularly are recommended. No more than two doses should be given in labour before reassessment by the physician. Other useful antiemetics are trifluoperazine 1 mg or cyclizine 50 mg. Drowsiness, dry mouth, skin rashes, hypotension and oculogyric crises may occasionally occur.

Antacids

There has been debate about the practice of repeated administration of antacids in labour. This has arisen because of some reports of 'acid aspiration' occurring in mothers in whom apparently adequate antacids had been given before its occurrence. Magnesium trisilicate, 10–15 ml orally, every 2 hours, is generally suitable for the patient in labour. Some clinicians prefer the use of a non-particulate antacid such as 0.3 mol/l sodium citrate if general anaesthesia can be anticipated (Lahiri, Thomas and Hodgson 1973).

It must be emphasized that regular use of antacids in labour is only one of the measures taken to reduce the risk of aspiration of gastric contents. When general anaesthesia is required, other vital measures include rapid induction and careful application of cricoid pressure.

PAIN IN LABOUR

Patterns of behaviour during the pains of established labour vary widely between different individuals. The need for pain relief by each patient should be assessed on a personal basis. Dick-Read (1944) and O'Driscoll (1975) have stressed that good personal care given continuously throughout labour reduces emotional stress and significantly reduces the need for analgesic drugs. There is no good evidence that relaxation exercises or psychoprophylaxis alone modify the requirement for analgesia. In a later edition of his book, Dick-Read (1954) states that when women in labour appear to have any discomfort from which they desire to escape, their attention should be drawn to the available means of pain relief.

Parenteral drugs used for pain relief in labour should provide effective analgesia and avoid risks to mother and baby. All analgesics cross the placenta and the main restriction to the administration of powerful narcotic analgesics is the possibility of causing neonatal respiratory depression. The fetus and the newborn have an impaired ability to metabolize these drugs.

An analgesic drug is best offered at the earliest indication of pain because of the time delay before the onset of action; when effectiveness begins to diminish a further dose should be given.

Pethidine

This is commonly prescribed for pain relief in labour. It is a cortical analgesic and an antispasmodic. In active labour, the analgesic effect usually begins about 15 minutes after intramuscular injection, has its maximum effect for 1–2 hours and takes about 1 hour to wear off.

For the first stage of labour 100–150 mg should be given intramuscularly every 3–4 hours as required. When there is severe maternal distress, the dose may have to be repeated 2 hourly, or resort made to epidural analgesia. Intramuscular injection of pethidine 150 mg gave useful but incomplete relief of pain to 50–60 per cent of mothers (Grant, Holt and Noble 1970) and 50–100 mg of pethidine was helpful only to 40 per cent of women in labour (Moore, Carson and Hunter 1970). The reasons for this may be due to failure to anticipate the need for analgesia and for repeated doses. There is no sound basis to withhold the drug because the cervix is not dilated to a given extent or is nearly fully dilated. A few surveys have indicated that if the drug is given in early or late labour, it facilitates progress (Barnes 1956; Sica-Blanco, Rosada and Remedio 1967).

If an intramuscular injection of pethidine is given to the mother within 3 hours before delivery, it may cause respiratory depression in the newborn (Shnider and Moya 1964). It has been claimed that sucking, feeding and bonding between mother and infant may be adversely affected even in infants born with high Apgar scores (Brackbill, *et al.* 1974; Weiner, Hogg and Rosen 1977) though most British obstetricians consider these claims have little substance. It is desirable that a narcotic antagonist is available in the delivery room, though there is some doubt as to whether or not its use of value if respiratory maintenance is adequate. Naloxone is the agent of choice. After ventilatory resuscitation, neonatal injection of naloxone 0.04 mg may be administered into the umbilical vein. There is no point in giving the drug intramuscularly to an asphyxiated baby with poor perfusion of the muscles. The use of preparations combining a morphine antagonist with pethidine in the hope that neonatal respiratory depression will be prevented has largely been abandoned, as some of the antagonists available impaired the analgesic action of pethidine.

Self-controlled intermittent intravenous injection of pethidine provides better analgesia than intramuscular injections. The procedure may pre-dispose to neonatal respiratory depression as considerably larger doses of pethidine may be administered.

As maternal nausea and vomiting are common, pethidine is often used in conjunction with either promazine or promethazine. Pethidine should not be given to mothers taking monoamine oxidase inhibitors, or who have obstructive airway disease.

Pentazocine

This can be used as an alternative to pethidine. Its analgesic effectiveness is intermediate between those of pethidine and codeine. In labour, 30–60 mg intramuscularly may be given every 3–4 hours. Pentazocine, 40 mg, is claimed to be effective as 100 mg pethidine. It has minimal effect on neonatal respiration and should respiratory depression occur, it may be reversed with naloxone. Pentazocine causes less nausea and vomiting (Moore and Ball 1974), but it causes vertigo in some patients and sometimes hallucinations.

Morphine

The need for morphine has been greatly reduced in modern obstetrics, and the use of morphine in labour should be restricted to highly selected cases with good preparations for infant resuscitation. The ability of morphine to penetrate the infant's brain makes it more likely to depress neonatal respira-tion (Way, Costley and Way 1965). Maternal nausea, vomiting, constipation and euphoria are more common than with pethidine.

Diamorphine

This is not recommended for routine use in labour. Total doses of 10 mg or more decrease amplitude and frequency of uterine contractions. It is the most addictive drug of the series. In very anxious patients 5 mg intra-muscularly may be given in the first stage of labour.

Meptazinol

A number of recent studies have suggested that safe and effective analgesia in labour can be obtained with meptazinol in doses between 100–150 mg intramuscularly. Pain relief is rapid in onset and lasts between 45–90 minutes. Meptazinol causes very little dysphoria and has no serious side-effects. It seems to have less depressant effect on the newborn than pethidine (Nicholas and Robson 1982). The Committee for Safety of Medicines are still requesting special reporting of side-effects of this drug.

Inhalation agents

In the later phases of the first stage and in the second stage of labour, nitrous oxide, methoxyflurane and trichloroethylene are equally effective for pain relief. In British obstetrics, the use of trichloroethylene has diminished.

Equal volumes of nitrous oxide and oxygen is premixed and dispensed from the 'Entonox' apparatus. The cylinders containing premixed oxygen and nitrous oxide should be stored in a room above 10°C (50°F) for at least 2 hours before use or there is a chance of the gases separating and when the cylinder is almost empty lower proportions of oxygen are supplied. The amount of the mixture inhaled is controlled by the patient. Entonox is approved for use by midwives throughout the United Kingdom. The 'Lucy Baldwin' machine can give a higher concentration of nitrous oxide, but no more than 70 per cent nitrous oxide should be administered. The gas mixture takes about 20 seconds to relieve pain. The mother should be encouraged to start breathing from the mask of the apparatus as soon as a contraction is felt; the effect is at a maximum after 45–60 seconds. A mouthpiece can be used when a patient dislikes the use of an anaesthetic mask. Nitrous oxide with oxygen is safe for both mother and fetus. Occasionally nausea, vomiting or confusion may occur.

The optimal concentration of methoxyflurane for use in labour is 0.35 per cent in air. This mixture is delivered by the Cardiff inhaler. The apparatus should be stored in a temperature similar to that of the delivery room, as an abnormally high concentration of methoxyflurane vapour may be delivered when the apparatus is moved from a hot to a cold environment. Opinions differ as to whether methoxyflurane is more likely to cause drowsiness, confusion and loss of co-operation than nitrous oxide. Methoxyflurane is probably more suited for short but painful labours where delivery is imminent.

There may be complete failure to relieve pain in about 30 per cent of patients with either of the inhalation techniques. Parenteral or epidural analgesia is indicated in these patients.

Local anaesthetics

Lignocaine

Lignocaine in concentrations between 0.5 and 2 per cent is mainly used for pudendal nerve blocks and local anaesthesia. Analgesia develops within 1–2 minutes and lasts for about 45 minutes with the plain solution; total dose for local infiltration should not exceed 20 ml of the 1 per cent solution (200 mg).

Analgesia may be prolonged to 1½–2 hours by addition of a vasoconstrictor such as adrenaline, in a concentration not exceeding 1 in 200:000. With adrenaline, up to 25 ml of 2 per cent lignocaine (500 mg) can be given for local infiltration but such quantities are rarely needed. The main toxic effects relate to overdose or inadvertent intravenous infusion and result in excitation of the central nervous system and depression of the cardiovascular system.

DRUGS USED FOR THE MANAGEMENT OF THE THIRD STAGE OF LABOUR AND POSTPARTUM HAEMORRHAGE

The introduction of the use of oxytocic drugs before the onset of the third stage of labour greatly reduced the incidence of postpartum haemorrhage (Dumoulin 1981; Kimbell 1959; Martin and Dumoulin 1953). Ergometrine, oxytocin or a combination of both by intramuscular or intravenous injection, have been used routinely for this purpose. The following mean times between administration of an oxytocic and the onset of contraction in the puerperal uterus were found by Embrey (1961): intravenous ergometrine, 41 seconds; intramuscular ergometrine, 7 minutes; intramuscular oxytocin, 2 minutes 32 seconds; intramuscular oxytocin and ergometrine, 2 minutes 37 seconds.

Ergometrine

An intramuscular injection of 0.5 mg of ergometrine maleate can be given with the crowning of the fetal head for the prophylaxis of postpartum haemorrhage. There is no significant increase in the need for manual removal of the placenta if the placenta is delivered promptly with controlled cord traction (Gate and Noel 1967; Mathie and Snodgrass 1967). It has some pressor activity, due to peripheral vasoconstriction and ergometrine is best avoided in patients with hypertension in labour. This is not so much because these patients are particularly prone to a hypertensive response, as because such an effect could be more dangerous if the patient is already hypertensive. Rare cases of postpartum eclampsia have been associated with the use of ergometrine.

When additional doses of ergometrine are used for the management of postpartum haemorrhage associated with uterine atony, the drug should be injected intravenously in a dose of 0.25 mg. Nausea and vomiting sometimes result.

Oxytocin

With the crowning of the fetal head at vaginal delivery, 10 units of oxytocin may be given intramuscularly. When the baby is delivered, the placenta is delivered by controlled cord traction.

An infusion of oxytocin, 20–50 units in one litre of 5 per cent dextrose solution should be initiated in the presence of postpartum haemorrhage associated with uterine atony. The infusion is commenced at 25 u/minute (25 drops/min of 20 u/1) and increased by adding more oxytocin, 20 u/1 at a time to the infusion fluid, until the uterus contracts and maintained at this rate for an hour.

Oxytocin has an antidiuretic action and water intoxication has been reported when very large volumes of fluid have been administered concurrently. Transient hypotensive episodes with tachycardia may rarely occur when intravenous injection of a concentrated solution of 5 units of oxytocin is made too rapidly.

Oxytocin with ergometrine

Oxytocin 5 units with ergometrine maleate 0.5 mg in 1 ml used intramuscularly, is widely used in British obstetrics in the management of the third stage of labour. The combined preparation is given intramuscularly with the crowning of the fetal head, and provides the more rapid action of oxytocin together with the sustained effect of ergometrine on the uterus.

Prevention of postpartum eclampsia

A rise in blood pressure can occur following delivery in an otherwise normal pregnancy. If the blood pressure is above 140/85 mmHg, immediately after delivery or 1 hour later, sedation with a prophylactic anticonvulsant should be initiated. For this purpose, phenobarbitone sodium 200 mg or diazepam 10 mg may be given intramuscularly. The blood pressure should be monitored hourly for 24 hours. Hypotensive agents such as hydralazine, in doses of 5–10 mg intramuscularly can be used when systolic blood pressure is elevated, over 150 mmHg, or diastolic blood pressure is over 100 mmHg.

REFERENCES

Batt, B. L. (1968). Are large doses of intravenous barbiturates justified for use as premedication in labor? *Am. J. Obstet; Gynecol.* **102**; 591.

Barnes, J. (1956). Quoted by Hingson, R. A. and Hellman, L. M. In *Anaesthesia for obstetrics*, p. 15. Lippincott, Philadelphia.

Beck, N. C., Siegel, L. J., Davidson, N. P., *et al.* (1980). The prediction of pregnancy outcome: maternal preparation, anxiety and attitudinal sets. *J. Psychosom. Res.* **24**, 343.

Bepko, F., Lowe, E. and Waxman, B. (1965). Relief of the emotional factor in labour with parenterally administered diazepam. *Obstet. Gynecol.* **26**, 852.

Borgstedt, A. D. and Rosen, M. G. (1968). Medication during labour correlated with behaviour and EEG of the newborn. *Am. J. Dis. Child.* **115**, 21.

Brackbill, Y., Kane, J., Manniello, R. S., and Abramson, D. (1974). Obstetric meperidine usage and assessment of neonatal status. *Anesthesiology* **40**, 116.

Caldeyro-Barcia, R. (1958). Uterine contractility in obstetrics. In *Second International Congress of gynaecology and obstetrics in Montreal*, 1958, vol. 1, p. 65. Beauchemin, Montreal.

Conway, E. and Brackbill, Y. (1970). Delivery medication and infant outcome: an empirical study. *Mon. Soc. Res. Child. Devel.* **35**, 24.

Cree, J. E., Meyer, J., and Hailey, D. M. (1973). Diazepam in labour. Its metabolism and effect on clinical condition and thermogenesis of the newborn. *Br. Med. J.* **4**, 251.

Davies, J. M. and Rosen, M. (1977). Intramuscular diazepam in labour. A double-blind trial in multiparae. *Br. J. Anaesth.* **49**, 601.

Decanq, H. E., Bosco, J. R., and Townsend, E. H. (1965). Chlordiazepoxide in labour. *J. Pediatr.* **67**, 836.

Dick-Read, G. (1944). *Childbirth without fear. 2nd edition*, p. 192. Harper and Brothers, New York.

Dick-Read, G. (1954). *Childbirth without fear. 3rd edition*, p. 110. Heinemann Medical, London.

Dumoulin, J. G. (1981). A reappraisal of the use of ergometrine. *J. Obstet. Gynaecol.* **1**, 178.

Elder, M. G. and Crossley, J. (1969). A double-blind trial of diazepam in labour. *J. Obstet. Gynaecol. Br. Commonw.* **76**, 264.

Embrey, M. P. (1961). Simultaneous intramuscular injection of oxytocin and ergometrine: a tocographic study. *Br. Med. J.* **1**, 1737.

Erkkola, R. and Kanto, J. (1972). Diazepam and breast feeding. *Lancet* **1**, 1235.

Friedman, S. L., Brackbill, Y., Caron, A. J., and Caron, R. F. (1978). Obstetric medication and visual processing in 4 and 5 month-old infant. *Merril-Palmer Q.* **24**, 111.

Gate, J. M. and Noel, J. D. O. (1967). Syntocinon and ergometrine in the prevention of postpartum haemorrhage. *J. Obstet. Gynaecol. Br. Commonw.* **74**, 49.

Grant, A. M., Holt, E. M., and Noble, A. D. (1970). A comparison between pethidine and phenazocine (Narphen) for relief of pain in labour. *J. Obstet. Gynaecol. Br. Commonw.* **77**, 824.

Kimbell, N. (1959). Discussion on the uses and abuses of ergometrine. *Proc. Roy. Soc. Med.* **52**, 569.

Kron, R. E., Stein, M., and Goddard, K. E. (1966). Newborn sucking behaviour affected by obstetric sedation. *Pediatrics* **37**, 1012.

Lahiri, S. K., Thomas, T. A., and Hodgson, R. M. H. (1973). Single-dose antacid therapy for the prevention of Mendelson's syndrome. *Br. J. Anaesth.* **45**, 1143.

Lamaze, F. (1970). *Painless childbirth: psychoprophylactic method.* Reginery, Chicago.

Lederman, E., Lederman, R. P., Work, B. A. Jr., and McCann, D. S. (1981). Maternal psychological and physiologic correlates of fetal-newborn health status. *Am. J. Obstet. Gynecol.* **139**, 956.

MacVicar, J. and Murray, M. H. (1960). Clinical evaluation of promazine as an adjuvant to pre-delivery sedation. *Br. Med. J.* **1**, 595.

Mandelli, M., Morselli, P. L., Nordio, S., Pardi, G., Principi, N., Sejeni, F., and Tognoni, G. (1975). Placental transfer of diazepam and its disposition in the newborn. *Clin. Pharmacol. Therap.* **17**, 564.

Mark, P. M. and Hamel, J. (1968). Librium for patients in labour. *Obstet. Gynecol.* **32**, 188.

Martin, J. D. and Dumoulin, J. G. (1953). Use of intravenous ergometrine to prevent postpartum haemorrhage. *Br. Med. J.* **1**, 643.

Mathie, I. W. and Snodgrass, C. A. (1967). The effect of prophylactic oxytocic drugs on blood loss after delivery. *J. Obstet. Gynaecol. Br. Commonw.* **74**, 653.

Matthews, A. E. (1963). Double-blind trials of promazine in labour. *Br. Med. J.* **2**, 423.

McQuitty, F. M. (1967). Relief of pain in labour. *J. Obstet. Gynaecol. Br. Commonw.* **74**, 925.

Moore, J. and Ball, H. G. (1974). A sequential study of intravenous analgesic treatment during labour. *Br. J. Anaesth.* **46**, 365.

Moore, J., Carson, R. M., and Hunter, R. J. (1970). A comparison of the effects of pentazocine and pethidine administered during labour. *J. Obstet. Gynaecol. Br. Commonw.* **77**, 830.

Myers, R. E. and Myers, S. E. (1979). Use of sedative, analgesic and anesthetic drugs during labour and delivery: bane or boon? *Am. J. Obstet. Gynecol.* **133**, 83.

Nicholas, A. D. G. and Robson, P. J. R. (1982). Double-blind comparison of meptazinol and pethidine in labour. *Br. J. Obstet. Gynaecol.* **89**, 318.

Nisbet, R., Boulas, S. H., and Kantor, H. I. (1967). Diazepam (Valium) during labour. *Obstet. Gynecol.* **29**, 726.

O'Driscoll, K. (1975). An obstetrician's view of pain. *Br. J. Anaesth.* **47**, 1053.

Pannullo, J. N. and Cerrone, D. M. (1960). Promethazine in obstetrics. *J. Med. Soc. NJ.* **57**, 65.

Schreiber, F. (1938). Apnea of the newborn and associated cerebral injury. *J. Am. Med. Assoc.* **111**, 1263.

Schreiber, F. and Gates, N. (1938). Cerebral injury in the newborn due to anoxia at birth. *Michigan Med.* **22**, 145.

Shnider, S. M. and Moya, F. (1964). Effects of meperidine on the newborn infant. *Am. J. Obstet. Gynecol.* **89**, 1009.

Sica-Blanco, Y., Rozada, H., and Remedio, M. R. (1967). Effect of meperidine on uterine contractility during pregnancy and pre-labour. *Am. J. Obstet. Gynecol.* **97**, 1096.

Stechler, G. (1964). Newborn attention as affected by medication during labour. *Science* **144**, 315.

Stucki, D. and Gross, J. (1962). Étude clinique du 'Librium' au cours de l'accouchement. *Praxis* **51**, 624.

Way, W. L., Costley, E. C., and Way, E. L. (1965). Respiratory sensitivity of the newborn infant to meperidine and morphine. *Clin. Pharmacol. Therapeut.* **6**, 454.

Weiner, P. C., Hogg, M. I. J., and Rosen, M. (1977). Effects of naloxone on pethidine-induced neonatal depression. *Br. Med. J.* **2**, 228.

Zourlas, P. A. (1964). *In vitro* and *in vivo* effects of sparine (promazine hydrochloride) on human uterine contractility. *Am. J. Obstet. Gynecol.* **88**, 770.

22 Intervention in labour: acceleration, induction, and other 'active' procedures

M. J. V. Bull

Once the point of fetal viability in pregnancy is attained, labour is acknowledged to the point of highest risk of either mortality or morbidity for mother and child; it thus demands the highest standards of care from both doctor and midwife. As far as the general practitioner obstetrician is concerned, efficient primary selection and secondary referral should ensure that only women without identifiable risk factors are booked for delivery outside a specialist obstetric department. Even so, a small number of low-risk women will develop life-threatening conditions in labour (both fetal and maternal) that could not have been foreseen yet need medical intervention (Curzen and Mountrose 1976). The degree to which the general practitioner obstetrician can respond to emergency situations will depend on three main factors: his or her personal skills and experience, the scale of equipment and facilities to hand, and the availability of specialist assistance. Clearly the doctor who delivers his patients in either the integrated or alongside maternity unit is more favourably placed than the colleague working in an isolated unit or in the home (Chapters 16, 17, 18, 19). While alternatives other than direct intervention are available in the latter situations, the ultimate option of the obstetric flying squad inevitably takes time to organize and the transfer of women in labour from home (or isolated maternity units) to hospital has long been known to increase the hazards (Hobbs and Acheson 1962).

A generation ago, medical students and midwives were taught to adopt an attitude of 'watchful expectancy' to women in labour. Unfortunately, this did not always culminate in an expeditious outcome and eventually hasty and even heroic operative procedures ensued, sometimes to the detriment of either mother or neonate. A better understanding of the physiological pattern of normal labour has, however, enabled a prospective approach to be made by which many problems can be anticipated or averted before critical situations arise. This approach, now widely accepted internationally and termed 'active management of labour', was pioneered by Kieran O'Driscoll at the National Maternity Hospital, Dublin. His work (O'Driscoll and Meagher 1980) should be mandatory reading for all obstetricians whether specialist or generalist and the following precepts are unashamedly based on his teaching.

NORMAL LABOUR

Understanding of the mechanical and physiological pattern of normal labour is of paramount importance (Chapter 20). The time scale in terms of dilatation of the cervix and descent of the presenting part was first quantified by Friedman (1967). In normal labour (Fig. 22.1) the first stage can be divided into a latent and an active phase; the former may be variable in duration but the latter (which usually commences at about 3 cm dilatation of the cervix) progresses at a regular and relatively rapid rate in the absence of delaying factors. In the nullipara this rate should be not less than 1 cm/hour, and in the multipara, it may be considerably faster.

The second stage of labour can also be divided into two phases: the first is that of descent of the presenting part through the vagina and rotation to the occipito-anterior position; the second is dilatation of the introitus and expulsion of the baby to the exterior.

NULLIPARAE AND MULTIPARAE

Next in importance is the realization that patterns of labour in nulliparae and multiparae are very different. Indeed, so great is the disparity, O'Driscoll avers that the two categories might well belong to different biological species! In the nullipara inefficient uterine action is by far the

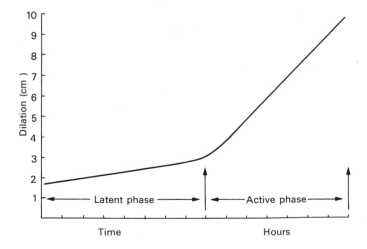

Fig. 22.1. The Friedman curve.

most common complication and the reason why long and difficult labour occurs so often. In the multipara on the other hand, the uterus is an efficient organ and delay is much more commonly due to obstruction through malpresentation or disproportion. A further fundamental truth in clinical practice is that the uterus of the nullipara is virtually immune to spontaneous rupture even when oxytocin is used. Finally, the nullipara and her child are more likely to sustain trauma due to the apparent need for instrumental delivery. Thus the archetypal woman to whom the basic principles of active management of labour apply is the nullipara with a singleton pregnancy at term and with a cephalic presentation.

DIAGNOSIS OF LABOUR

Diagnosis of labour is a crucial issue since in practical terms it means a decision to commit a woman to delivery and wrong diagnosis leads to inappropriate treatment. Painful uterine contractions alone do not warrant a confident diagnosis but must be supported by one or more of the following features:

  (i)   a 'show' (implying cervical effacement);
  (ii) spontaneous rupture of the membranes;
  (iii) perceived dilatation of the cervix

The two main mistakes are to institute treatment on the basis of painful uterine contractions alone or to withold treatment due to inaccurate diagnosis.

DURATION OF LABOUR

Duration is a prime indicator in the problems of management in labour. This factor, more than any other, determines the impact of the labour on both mother and fetus and, in particular, on the mother's subsequent recollection of her experiences (O'Driscoll and Meagher 1980). Duration of labour is sometimes equated with the number of hours spent in the delivery unit (Hendricks, Brenner, and Kraus 1970) and the ability to restrict duration, without increasing the use of operative delivery, represents a major advance in the management of labour. This approach has further advantages in reduction in maternal dehydration and ketosis and the demand for analgesia. If labour is of short duration a woman is better able to maintain her morale and, because she is not exhausted, to deliver herself.

RECORDING LABOUR

A further advance relevant to management of labour has been the development of a graphic record of progress, the partogram (Philpott 1972), which

forms the basis for any system of active management. Based on the concept
of the Friedman curve (see above, and Fig. 22.1), its plots cervical dilatation
and descent of the presenting part against time as well as recording other
factors such as the quality of the contractions, fetal heart rate, state of the
liquor, maternal pulse and blood pressure, and so on, so that the whole picture of the progress of the labour can be seen at a glance. On this chart,
Philpott superimposed 'alert' and 'action' lines to provide criteria for progress and as a cue for intervention in the event of delay. Developments such
as nomograms of cervical dilatation (Studd 1973) and a partographic stencil
(Bull 1982) to simplify this approach have since been suggested.

Once labour is diagnosed, the patient is assessed at regular intervals, say
3-hourly. When the active phase commences, labour should thenceforth
proceed at a regular rate of not less than 1 cm/hour of cervical dilatation
and, dependent upon the slope of the line representing dilatation, the duration of the first stage should be predictable with reasonable accuracy. If
progress is delayed however, the plot will fall to the right of the 'alert' line
(Fig. 22.2). In this event, dehydration and ketosis if present should be corrected and analgesia administered if necessary. If however, the plot crosses
the 'action' line, labour is frankly delayed and acceleration with oxytocin is
indicated (see below).

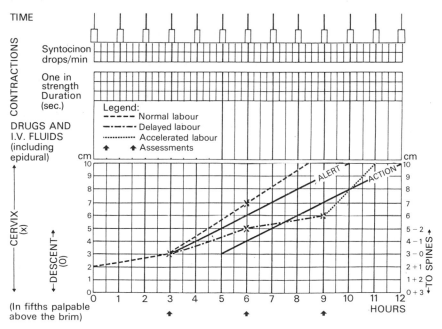

Fig. 22.2. The partogram; patterns of cervical dilatation.

MANAGEMENT OF LABOUR: THE FIRST STAGE

Artificial rupture of membranes

A good case can be made for artificial rupture of the membranes in every patient once labour has entered the 'active' phase (3 cm dilatation, see above). Firstly, the quality of the contractions will be stimulated and dilatation will proceed more efficiently because the presenting part is better applied to the cervix and the need for acceleration of labour with oxytocin may thus be diminished. Secondly, the quality of the liquor released gives a good indication of placental function and therefore of fetal wellbeing. Copious clear liquor indicates good placental function, but meconium staining or very scanty liquor suggests placental (and therefore fetal) embarrassment. Fresh meconium staining is an indication for a specialist opinion and, if it is heavy, transfer of care is advisable.

Acceleration of labour

In any nullipara, a plot of cervical dilatation falling to the right of the 'action' line on the partogram is an indication for acceleration with intravenous oxytocin. Routines may vary but an eminently satisfactory technique is as follows: an intravenous infusion of 4 per cent dextrose in half molar saline is set up. To the first ½ litre 1 unit of oxytocin is added. The drip rate is adjusted to 15 drops/minute and subsequently increased at 15-minute intervals to 30, 45 and 60 drops/minute. Supervision is greatly simplified by the use of an electronic drip monitor. If the quality of contractions in terms of duration, strength and frequency is not sufficiently improved, the first ½ litre is replaced by a second containing 4 units of oxytocin and a regime of 20, 30, 40, 50, 60 drops/minute is continued. Once reassessment has indicated that progress is continuing at a satisfactory rate it may well be prudent to reduce the infusion rate by one half. In some cases, even higher concentrations of oxytocin may have to be employed, but before proceeding a general practitioner obstetrician would be wise to consult his specialist colleagues.

In the multipara, delay in the first stage must be approached with more caution. Problems here are more often associated with malpresentation or obstruction and, since the multiparous uterus is *not* immune to rupture, oxytocin should be used only after both have been excluded. Specialist advice is advisable and even so oxytocin should be used at only half the rate suggested above, that is, ½ a unit in the first ½ litre, 2 units in the second ½ litre.

Problems of accelerated labour

While the precepts of active management such as diagnosis of labour, artificial rupture of membranes, and partographic recording may be applied in whatever situation a labour is conducted, it should be categorically stated that acceleration with oxytocin should never be employed unless specialist back-up is readily to hand. First, acceleration often increases the need for analgesia and while drugs such as pethidine may provide sufficient relief in a proportion of cases, in others, especially those associated with an occipito-posterior position, regional analgesia may be required which will require the services of a specialist anaesthesiologist (see Chapter 16, Fig. 16.1). Second, acceleration of labour with oxytocin may cause embarrassment to a fetus with diminished but as yet undiagnosed placental function. Clearly then this technique must only be used in situations where there are facilities for continuous electronic fetal monitoring (see Chapter 23) and there is recourse to emergency delivery by caesarean section. Third, in any patient where intravenous fluid infusion is used during labour, the water intoxication syndrome must be guarded against. In practice this is most unlikely to occur where the total infusion volume is less than 1500 ml. Finally, patients in whom oxytocin has been used in labour are more prone to postpartum haemorrhage (Brinsden and Clark 1978). To prevent this, the result of subsequent uterine relaxation, 0.5 mg ergometrine should be given intramuscularly after delivery of the baby and the oxytocin infusion left running at its final rate for a further hour.

ACTIVE MANAGEMENT: THE SECOND STAGE

The aim of the obstetrician is to achieve delivery of the infant naturally by means of uterine contractions and maternal expulsive effort. Operative interference (except in the event of acute fetal distress) should be resisted as it is a potential cause of both fetal and maternal morbidity. Again, an understanding of the natural process is important (see above, p. 301).

In the management of the second stage, the first phase need not be hurried provided the fetal heart rate gives no cause for concern. The mother need not be exhorted to push unless she has an overwhelming urge to do so. Progress is monitored by the descent of the fetal head through the vagina; normally it should have reached the pelvic floor within 30 minutes and should have rotated. If this progress has not been achieved (perhaps because of deteriorating quality of contractions), or if rotation is not complete, there may again be an indication for augmentation of contractions with intravenous oxytocin infusion, initially 2 units in 500 ml dextrose/saline at the rate of 30 drops/minute. Only when the fetal occiput has reached the pelvic floor should the mother be encouraged to make maximum expulsive effort and only when this proves insufficient to achieve delivery should intervention by means of episiotomy or low forceps application be considered. Operative interference before this point is the realm of the specialist obstetrician and not of the general practitioner.

INDUCTION OF LABOUR

The need for induction of labour usually implies a complication of pregnancy for which the mother would be better transferred to the care of a consultant obstetrician. However, there are two particular instances where the procedure may be undertaken by the experienced general practitioner obstetrician working with specialist support in the favourable environment of the integrated or alongside general practitioner maternity unit. The first example is when spontaneous rupture of the membranes has occurred at around term and when, if labour does not ensure spontaneously within a few hours, there could be a risk of intrauterine or neonatal infection. The second instance is uncomplicated postmaturity. Spontaneous labour occurs in 80 per cent of women within 2 weeks of term, but as Butler and Bonham (1963) showed, delivery at 42 weeks carries a 50 per cent increase in the risk of perinatal death which at 43 weeks doubles and at 44 weeks trebles when compared with delivery at term. Presumably this increased risk is largely the result of fetal hypoxia due to deteriorating placental function and, until specific indices of continuing fetal wellbeing (Manning *et al.* 1982) are more generally accepted, there would appear to be an obligation to ensure delivery before the end of the 42nd week.

Before embarking upon induction however, the general practitioner obstetrician should ensure that the following criteria are fulfilled:

(i)   the duration of gestation is not in doubt;
(ii) the presentation is cephalic;
(iii) there is no suspicion of cephalopelvic disproportion;
(iv) the woman has given her informed consent;
(v)   the cervix is favourable.

In respect of the last criterion Bishop's method (Bishop 1964) of assessing the state of the cervix can be recommended. A points system (Table 22.1)

Table 22.1   *Cervical assessment system (after Bishop, 1964)*

	0	1	2	3	Score
Cervix:					
dilatation (cm)	<1	1–2	3–4	>4	
length (cm)	>3	2–3	1–2	<1	
consistency	firm	average	soft	–	
position	posterior	central	anterior	–	
Presenting part:					
level*	−3	−2	−1,0	+1,+2	
				Total	

*Centimetres: above (−), at (o) or below (+) ischial spines.

based on dilatation, effacement, consistency, and position of the cervix is related to the station of the presenting part and gives a good indication of cervical readiness. Patients with a high score will labour easily after minimal intervention whereas those with lower scores will present increasing difficulty.

Methods of induction

OBE

The traditional OBE (castor oil, hot bath, and enema) is mentioned merely as an anachronistic affront to female dignity that should be relegated to history.

Sweeping the membranes

When the cervix is favourable, digital dilatation and gentle sweeping of the membranes away from the lower segment of the uterus will in many cases provoke labour within a short space of time. The mode of action is considered to be due to the release of endogenous prostaglandin (Mitchell *et al.* 1977).

Artificial rupture of membranes (ARM)

Perhaps the best established technique for induction of labour, this method should nevertheless be employed with caution since it commits a woman to delivery and increases risks of genital and neonatal infection. In the general practice unit it should only be performed if the cervical score is greater than 5 and if the fetal head is well engaged in the pelvis to avoid the possibility of umbilical cord prolapse.

Oxytocin infusion

Intravenous infusion of oxytocic drugs is normally employed as an adjunct to artificial rupture of the membranes if the cervix is initially unfavourable or if labour does not ensue within (say) 6 hours. Indeed, it should not be used if the membranes are intact owing to the potential hazard of amniotic fluid embolism. The method has the advantage that the dose can accurately be titrated against response and suitable regimes have been described above in connection with acceleration of labour. Oxytocin infusion is the method of choice in cases where spontaneous rupture of the membranes has occurred but labour has not become established within 12 hours.

Intravaginal prostaglandin (PGE$_2$)

A more recent innovation in induction technique has been the development of a prostaglandin E$_2$ vaginal gel initially designed to promote cervical ripening (MacKenzie and Embrey 1977) in women with low cervical scores prior to amniotomy. It subsequently became clear (MacKenzie and Embrey 1978) that, when the cervix was already ripe (Bishop score greater than 5) the need for oxytocin infusion was avoided in as many as 65.9 per cent of nulliparae and 87.5 per cent multiparae. Other interventions in labour were reduced and complications were rare. The gel has now been superseded by 2.5 mg PGE_2 vaginal pessaries which are simple to administer and aesthetically very acceptable to the mother. This non-invasive technique seems particularly appropriate to general practitioner obstetrics and the protocol, based on that proposed by MacKenzie, Bradley and Embrey (1981) is illustrated in Table 22.2.

Table 22.2 *Induction of labour—prostaglandin protocol*

Indications	1. Induction of labour in favourable cases to avoid amniotomy and/or oxytocic drip. 2. Preconditioning of unfavourable cervix prior to amniotomy, etc.

Assessment of cervix: Use Bishop's score method.
        6 or more—'favourable'
        5 or less—'unfavourable'

Dose:	Nulliparae:	5.0 mg PGE_2 pessary
	Multiparae:	2.5 mg PGE_2 pessary

Method:	Favourable cervix—insert pessary at 0600. Amniotomy at 0900; oxytocic drip at 1400 if labour not established by then.
	Unfavourable cervix—insert pessary the evening before formal induction.

CAUTION	The pessary should be inserted into the posterior fornix, NOT into the cervical canal.
	Do NOT use this method to accelerate patients already in desultory labour.

OTHER INTERVENTIONS IN LABOUR

In general, one might expect the practising general practitioner obstetrician to continue to perform such procedures as he/she was trained to undertake during his/her postgraduate hospital appointment in that specialty. Apart from the measures outlined above, he/she might well undertake such tasks as the application of a fetal scalp electrode for continuous monitoring, delivery by low forceps application, control of haemorrhage, repair of the perineum, and so on. Nevertheless, bearing in mind the trend towards defensive obstetrics (Singer 1978) even now pervading these shores, he/she would be wise not to exceed his/her acknowledged limitations or act hastily without due consultation or assistance except in the emergency situation.

REFERENCES

Bishop, E. E. (1964). Pelvic scoring for elective induction. *Obstet. Gynaecol.* **24**, 266–8.

Brinsden, P. R. S. and Clark, A. D. (1978). Postpartum hemorrhage after induced and spontaneous labour. *Br. Med. J.* **2**, 855–6.

Bull, M. J. V. (1982). The general practitioner obstetrician in the delivery room. *Update* **25**, 785–94.

Butler, N. R. and Bonham, D. G. (1963). *Perinatal mortality.* E. and S. Livingstone, Edinburgh.

Curzen, P. and Mountrose, U. M. (1976). The general practitioner's role in the management of labour. *Br. Med. J.* **2**, 1433–4.

Friedman, E. A. (1967). Cervical dilation pattern. In *Labour clinical evaluation and management.* Appleton-Century-Crofts, New York.

Hendricks, C. H., Brenner, W. E. and Kraus, G. (1970). Normal cervical dilatation patterns in late pregnancy and labour. *Am. J. Obstet. Gynecol.* **106**, 1065–82.

Hobbs, M. S. T. and Acheson, E. D. (1966). Perinatal mortality and the organisation of obstetric services in the Oxford areas in 1962. *Br. Med. J.* **1**, 499–505.

MacKenzie, I. Z. and Embrey, M. P. (1977). Cervical ripening with intra-vaginal prostaglandin E_2 gel. *Br. Med. J.* **2**, 1381–4.

MacKenzie, I. Z. and Embrey, M. P. (1978). The influence of preinduction vaginal prostaglandin E_2 gel upon subsequent labour. *Br. J. Obstet. Gynaecol.* **85**, 657–61.

MacKenzie, I. Z., Bradley, S., and Embrey, M. P. (1981). A simpler approach to labour induction using lipid-based prostaglandin E_2 vaginal suppository. *Am. J. Obstet. Gynecol.* **141**, 158–62.

Manning, F. A. *et al.* (1982). Antepartum determination of fetal health: Composite biophysical profile scoring. *Clin. Perinatol.* **9**, 285–96.

Mitchell, M. D. *et al.* (1977). Rapid increases in plasma prostaglandin concentrations after vaginal examination and amniotomy. *Br. Med. J.* **2**, 1183–5.

O'Driscoll, K. and Meagher, D. (1980). Active management in labour. In *Clinics in obstetrics and gynaecology: supplement 1.* W. B. Saunders, Eastbourne.

Philpott, R. H. (1972). Graphic records in labour. *Br. Med. J.* **4**, 163–5.

Singer, A. (1978). Towards defensive obstetrics. *Lancet* **2**, 1373–4.

Studd, J. (1973). Partograms and nomograms of cervical dilation in management of primigravid labour. *Br. Med. J.* **4**, 451–5.

23 Intervention in labour: machines in labour

K. A. Godfrey

Too often at present, the mother-to-be may feel that a machine and not a midwife is entrusted with her care during labour. Using cardiotocographic monitors it is possible to record the fetal heart continuously throughout labour and also estimate the frequency and magnitude of uterine contractions. The fact that the machine may faithfully record misleading information is often overlooked. A second machine may be programmed to administer an oxytocic agent and the two machines may converse to calculate the exact dose necessary. Intermittent visits from the attending midwife and/or doctor may largely be spent in checking the tracings produced by the machine. No wonder that some potential patients feel that intrapartum care is becoming impersonal. A vociferous minority, revolted by such stereotyped care, turn to the opposite extreme of home confinement. There can be little doubt, in any experienced and honest clinician's mind, that the safest place for childbirth to occur is in a hospital. This must be properly staffed and equipped to deal with the complications that can and do frequently arise unexpectedly. To advise otherwise would be irresponsible. However part of our responsibility as obstetric attendants must be to assist parents-to-be and baby through an essentially physiological process with as little interference as is absolutely necessary. In this context it is salutory to realize that no controlled study to date has demonstrated that continuous fetal heart rate monitoring of the low-risk obstetric population during labour significantly improves perinatal mortality or morbidity. However most of these studies do indicate that electronic fetal heart monitoring as opposed to old-fashioned auscultation does increase the likelihood of operative delivery either by forceps, ventouse or caesarean section. So there are potential hazards to a policy of continuous electronic heart monitoring which must be borne in mind. Consideration of which pregnancies to monitor should not, therefore, be confined to the logistical problems of machine and trained staff availability but should take into account risk categories and last, but by no means least, patients' wishes.

HIGH-RISK POPULATION

There is little doubt that certain groups of the obstetric population have identifiable risk factors which make fetal asphyxia in labour much more likely (Table 23.1). These risk factors are fairly sensitive though not perfectly so, but have a poor degree of specificity.

Scientific evidence

In this high-risk group fetal heart rate monitoring continuously during labour with electronic equipment is mandatory. A number of studies (Renou *et al.* 1976) have shown a reduction in the stillbirth rate and first-week deaths with such a policy. However it remains contentious to extrapolate this improvement to monitoring in the low-risk population. A study comprising many thousands (>10 000) of patients would be necessary to demonstrate a significant difference in mortality rates in the low-risk obstetric population. Perinatal mortality is the crudest of indices to use to evaluate monitoring practices; but many of the other indices are extremely subjective and imprecise. This is true of Apgar scores, admission rates to special care units or neonatal neurological abnormalities. Although fetal scalp or cord blood pH estimation are more objective there is still a problem of inadequacy in correlating these parameters to long term paediatric follow up of survivors. Many more studies are required to clarify this situation. In four (Haverkamp *et al.* 1976, 1979; Kelso *et al.* 1978; Wood *et al.* 1981) of the five recent controlled trials of fetal monitoring, in the low-risk obstetric population there were no differences in perinatal death rates between monitored and unmonitored groups. Fetal monitoring appeared to have no influence on cord blood pH values, rates of admission to special care nurseries, the frequency of abnormal neonatal neurological signs or in the frequency of convulsions. The fifth study (Renou *et al.* 1976) however did show an improvement in all these parameters in association with fetal monitoring of a high-risk population. All the studies exhibit a significant increase in the incidence of operative delivery. Some of the benefits conferred by continuous monitoring of fetal heart rate will result from earlier operative delivery of a compromised hypoxic baby by caesarean section, rather than later delivery per vaginam, of an asphyxiated baby, which may be more difficult and traumatic. But the converse is also true: the disadvantage may be the expeditious delivery, traumatic to either mother or baby, in response to an erroneous diagnosis of fetal distress.

Deficiencies of the technique

Continuous fetal heart rate monitoring by modern instruments will permit the identification of a number of heart rate characteristics. These are the baseline heart rate (normally 120–160 beats/min), heart rate variability (5–15 beats/min), and rate changes with uterine contractions (normally no change or acceleration). Deviations from normality in any of these components of fetal heart rate may have prognostic significance in terms of fetal condition at birth (Table 23.2). In order to interpret periodic heart rate

Table 23.1 *Risk factors for intrapartum fetal asphyxia*

General history	Antenatal	Intrapartum
Previous stillbirth/bad obstetric history	Bleeding during pregnancy (early or late)	Preterm labour
Primigravidae age 30 or over	Pre-eclampsia and hypertension	Meconium-stained liquor
Multigravidae age 40 or over	Intrauterine growth retardation (IUGR)	Induced/augmented labour
Grand multiparity	Diabetes mellitus	Fetal heart rate more than 160 beats/min or less than 120 beats/min
Significant maternal cardiac or respiratory disease	Multiple pregnancy	Fetal heart rate decelerations or loss variability
	Rhesus isoimmunization	Prolonged labour
	Breech presentation	Epidural anaesthesia
	Abnormal antenatal fetal heart rate	

Table 23.2 *Correlation of fetal heart rate and acidosis at birth*

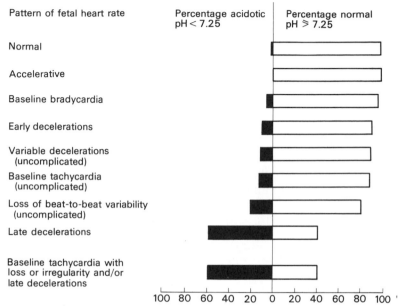

| Pattern of fetal heart rate | Percentage acidotic pH < 7.25 | Percentage normal pH ⩾ 7.25 |

changes, it is important to have a reliable indicator of uterine activity. This may be an experienced midwife's hand or a modern intrauterine pressure transducer. Decelerations are classified as early or late, depending upon whether or not the nadir of the heart rate deceleration occurs within 20 seconds of the peak of the uterine contraction. Falsely normal heart traces are uncommon but can occur due to misapplication of the electrode to maternal rather than fetal tissue. However as Fig. 23.1 illustrates, falsely abnormal heart traces are much more common. It is generally accepted that the most sinister fetal heart pattern is one showing late decelerations, loss of baseline irregularity and baseline tachycardia; even this pattern when correlated to Apgar score and fetal scalp blood pH is associated with fetal acidosis in less than 60 per cent of cases (Table 23.2). A number of factors can introduce confusion, such as maternal drug administration, maternal hypotension, uterine overactivity, maternal pyrexia etc. Even the attainment of full cervical dilatation affects interpretation. The accurate identification of fetal hypoxia may be improved if fetal scalp pH measurement is combined. The latter can help to reduce the erroneous diagnosis of fetal distress which occurs when fetal heart rate alone is employed. The local risks of fetal scalp blood sampling are small, even if repeated (Tutera and Newman 1975). Deficiencies exist as in the case of fetal heart rate in relating scalp pH to any index of perinatal wellbeing. Long-term paediatric follow-up studies are lacking. The enigma of how accurately fetal condition can be inferred from fetal heart rate and scalp blood pH was unresolved by three of the studies already discussed, which included fetal–acid–base balance in the monitoring programme. There are inherent difficulties in the technique of scalp sampling with most of the methods used to measure pH on such small samples (60 μml +) (Lumley *et al.* 1971) which may mislead.

TOCOGRAPHY

The author does not see any significant benefit in using the electronic monitor to demonstrate uterine activity routinely. Other than in very specific circumstances, such as intrapartum research, evaluation of fetal heart rate abnormalities, trial of labour, breech labour, and labour with a scarred uterus, an experienced midwife merits no comparison.

FUTURE POSSIBILITIES

As intermittent scalp blood sampling can only provide an indirect indication of fetal oxygenation a number of other techniques are under evaluation. Both continuous pH and P_{O_2} monitoring are possible using specially designed scalp probes but the accuracy and reliability of these methods require much improvement and evaluation (Huch and Huch 1981; Young 1981).

Continuous fetal electroencephalography (EEG) during labour in theory should be a better indicator of cerebral hypoxia. Technical difficulties and storage space for the voluminous tracings limit this to a research technique at present.

CONCLUSION

Continuous fetal heart rate monitoring is expensive not only in financial terms, and not yet available for all labours. Impartial examination of the available scientific evidence does not show conclusively that fetal heart rate tracing is valuable or desirable in low-risk obstetric populations. On the contrary, an unnecessary iatrogenic hazard exists with a non-selective policy.

However, continuous heart rate monitoring has provided an improved appreciation of heart rate changes occurring during labour and as a result dictates that intermittent auscultation should be performed during and immediately after uterine contractions which may necessitate use of a doppler device. The evolution of intrapartum care will probably result in a number of complementary techniques being utilized for the surveillance of the high-risk fetus. However the low-risk fetus will most benefit from greater personal interest in, and improved standards of, intrapartum care.

REFERENCES

Beard, R. W., Filshie, G. M., Knight, C. A., and Roberts, G. M. (1971). The significance of the changes in the continuous fetal heart rate in the first stage of labour. *J. Obstet. Gynaecol Br. Commonw.* **78**, 865–81.

Haverkamp, A. D., Thompson, H. E., McFee, J. G., and Cetrulo, C. (1976). The evaluation of continuous fetal heart rate monitoring in high risk pregnancy. *Am. J. Obstet. Gynecol.* **125**, 310–20.

Haverkamp, A. D., Orleans, M., Langendosser, S., McFee, J., Murphy, J., and Thompson, H. E. (1979). A controlled trial of the differential effects of intrapartum fetal monitoring. *Am. J. Obstet. Gynecol.* **134**, 339–412.

Huch, R. and Huch, A. (1981). Physiological insights based on fetal monitoring. *J. Perinat. Med.* **9**, 184–8.

Kelso, I. M., Parsons, R. J., Lawrence, G. F., Arora, S. S., Edmonds, D. K., and Cooke, I. D. (1978). An assessment of continuous fetal heart rate monitoring in labour. *Am. J. Obstet. Gynecol.* **131**, 526–32.

Lumley, J., Potter, M., Newman, W., Talbot, J., Wakefield, E., and Wood, C. (1971). The unreliability of a single estimation of fetal scalp blood pH. *J. Lab. Clin. Med.* **77**, 535–9.

Renou, P., Chang, A., Anderson, I., and Wood, C. (1976). Controlled trial of fetal intensive care. *Am. J. Obstet. Gynecol.* **126**, 470–6.

Tutera, G. and Newman, R. L. (1975). Fetal monitoring: its effect on the perinatal mortality and caesarean section rates and its complications. *Am. J. Obstet. Gynecol.* **122**, 750–4.

Wood, C., Renou, P., Oates, J., Farrell, E., Beischer, N., and Anderson, I. (1981). A controlled trial of FHR monitoring in a low risk obstetric population. *Am. J. Obstet. Gynecol.* **141**, 527–34.

Young, B. K. (1981). Continuous fetal tissue pH monitoring in labour. *J. Perinat. Med.* **9**, 189–94.

FURTHER READING

Hobel, C. J. (1977). Identification of the patient at risk. In *Perinatal medicine management of the high risk fetus and neonate.* (eds R. J. Bolognese and R. J. Schwarz). Williams and Wilkins, Balitmore.

Parson, R. J., Brown, V.A., and Cooke, I. D. (1981). Second thoughts on routine monitoring in labour. In *Progress in obstetrics and gynaecology.* (ed. J. Studd), vol. 1. pp. 139–48.

24 Intervention in labour: episiotomy

Rhiannon Walters

INTRODUCTION

How is the general practitioner obstetrician to assess the 'patient-led' call for fewer episiotomies? On the one hand, there are articulate and no doubt unrepresentative groups of women quoting cases of episiotomies stitched with little local anaesthetic, and never a sympathetic word, resulting in dyspareunia lasting over a year. On the other hand specialist obstetricians point to the lack of statistics to justify any major change in practice, the availability of analgesics for post-episiotomy pain, and warn of the third-degree tears and prolapses that would result from fewer episiotomies.

In a study done for the National Childbirth Trust the experiences of women who had an episiotomy were compared with those who had lacerations, and those with an intact perineum (Kitzinger and Walters 1981). The comparisons led to some striking conclusions, but sometimes, while going through the responses, the statistics had to be put aside while the horror of a few individual cases were perceived. There was the woman who, before she was stitched, 'lay for four hours in a pool of blood in an unheated labour ward waiting for the doctors to come on duty'. There was one who was told 'No, it doesn't!' when she complained that the stitching hurt. There were incompetent repairs that had to be laboriously undone and restitched, and 'dissolving' sutures that never dissolved and had to be 'dug out' by the domiciliary midwife days or weeks after the woman's return home. There were women who felt that pain in their perineum in the weeks following birth had damaged their relationship with the baby. They had been unable to sit and hold or feed their baby comfortably. Perhaps worst of all, there were those few women who felt their relationship with their sexual partner disintegrating as intercourse continued to be painful for months after the birth.

It is obvious that many episiotomies were badly done, but that in itself is not an argument against the operation. Since it will always be of benefit in some circumstances, consideration as to how to manage an episiotomy, while avoiding the pain and distress that can be the outcome of its performance and repair, is of paramount importance. It was clear from the study that some women found the idea of episiotomy distressing in itself, writing of feeling 'violated' quite apart from painful side-effects. For this reason, the evidence supporting the claims made for episiotomy needs careful scrutiny.

General practitioners will hear first of any problems with the healing of the episiotomy, since they look after all aspects of a woman's health, including her emotional wellbeing; and because of the need to preserve her good will for the future they have more incentive than other medical practitioners to ensure a trouble-free episiotomy. They are likely to have the medical view of episiotomy that is closest to the woman's own.

MAKING THE CUT

Sometimes the cut itself can be painful. Few obstetricians still support the view that the local anaesthetic is unnecessary, and Hoult (1981) stresses the need for good sharp scissors and a cut made with a single clean action. Some cuts reported in the NCT study had clearly been done before the perineum was distended to its thinnest, resulting in a difficult, painful cut, and unnecessary blood loss (House 1981). Sometimes this seemed to be the result of a time limit put on the second stage of labour, so that an episiotomy was performed before the woman had really had time to push effectively (see Chapter 20). Of the women who had episiotomies 62 per cent reported that they were done within 45 minutes of the onset of the second stage, and 44 per cent that they were done within half an hour.

STITCHING

Waiting for stitching was a frequent cause of distress. It means the mother may be anxious by the time she is stitched, and so may feel pain more intensely. The NCT study found an association between a wait of over an hour and subsequent wound infection; 37 per cent waited over half an hour to be stitched, and 13 per cent over an hour. Women's comments suggested that long waits occurred because the midwife who attended the delivery and performed the episiotomy was not the person to do the stitching; a doctor had to be found. The study also found that when midwives *did* stitch, the stitching was more likely to be painful than if it was done by a doctor or medical student. This last finding was puzzling, and there was no data against which to check any hypothesis for its cause, but it could be that midwives lack practice and confidence in stitching. (Only 4 per cent of episiotomies were stitched by midwives). The ideal would be for the delivery attendant, be they doctor or midwife, to be competent and confident about repairing the cut as soon as possible after the birth.

Pain during the stitching was a common complaint, and 22 per cent said that stitching was 'painful' or 'very painful'. Sometimes women believed that local anaesthetics had not been given time to take effect. Stitchers' responses to complaints that the stitching hurt were sometimes inadequate–the woman's complaint was ignored (11 per cent of those who complained) and sometimes she was just offered reassurance, distracting conversation, or a promise that it would not take long (32 per cent). So the message seems to be: 'Give the local anaesthetic time to work, and be attentive to the woman's feelings'. Several women mentioned that having the baby to hold at this time was a sufficient distraction. Conversely, anxiety about an absent baby can make the stitching a more distressing experience.

PAIN IN THE FIRST WEEK

Some pain during the week following birth is almost inevitable as the episiotomy heals. Assuming all has been done that can be to ensure that it is not more painful than necessary—that stitches are not too tight, that infection is avoided—it is important that any pain is considered seriously. The woman is forming a relationship with her baby, learning or relearning unfamiliar skills, coming to terms with a new status, usually in a strange environment. She may well feel incompetent, lonely or resentful. To find that she cannot sit comfortably when feeding or holding her baby, and possibly to be told, as some mothers in the NCT study were, that she may not feed in bed or standing up either, can be the last straw. It is simply not acceptable to be told, as one mother was: 'What do you *expect* after having a baby?' Sometimes simple remedies are all that are necessary—warmth from a heat lamp or even a hair-drier, a rubber ring to sit on, a diet that avoids constipation. Some are not as easy to arrange—low beds, enough baths or bidets to go round. Painkillers can be welcome, though a few women may not be happy to take them. All women, however, will welcome the knowledge that those who care for them take their post-episiotomy pain as seriously as they do themselves.

DYSPAREUNIA

Beischer (1967) in a study of the long-term outcome of episiotomy repair, found that 6 per cent of his sample had pain on intercourse lasting over 3 months, and 39 per cent found intercourse painful over a shorter period. He attributed the persistent type entirely to episiotomy repair, and the shortlived type mostly to this. House finds Beischer's 'persistent' figure of 6 per cent 'rather high'—'but it may well be that in hospital practice we do not see quite a lot of the long-term problems that we cause' (House 1981) General practitioner obstetricians have no such protection. They may, nevertheless, find that some women are reticent about reporting pain on intercourse—the NCT study figure for women reporting dyspareunia lasting longer than 3 months was much higher than Beischer's, very probably because of the safety of an anonymous questionnaire sent by an organization likely to be sympathetic. It would be sad indeed if women were not reporting treatable dyspareunia. One simple way of avoiding this would be to change the traditional advice to refrain from intercourse until 6 weeks after the birth, and instead encourage the woman to resume intercourse as soon as she feels comfortable. Any problems could then be discussed after a tactful enquiry at the postnatal examination (see Chapter 27).

Munsick (1980) has suggested that the decline in incidence of post-episiotomy dyspareunia in the United States is due to the use of the midline episiotomy, rather than the mediolateral, and several writers have advocated its use here (Beynon 1974; Coates 1980; Gordon 1981). It is not possible to draw on the experiences of women in the United Kingdom since so few midline episiotomies are done in this country. The advantages of the midline are less blood loss and less painful healing with fewer complications, but the occasional extension, with a third-degree laceration into the anal sphincter, may make it more suitable for hospital than home or general practitioner unit birth.

COMMUNICATION

While 99 per cent of the NCT sample knew what an episiotomy was before their labour started, only 33 per cent had discussed it with a doctor or a midwife during pregnancy, and communication seemed frequently to be a problem. Sometimes discussion was blocked with replies such as 'doctor knows best'. While the hurried, impersonal atmosphere of the hospital antenatal clinic, or the rather public forum of an antenatal class, may not encourage communication, the general practitioner's surgery should offer a woman the opportunity to discuss episiotomy with someone who is, it is to be hoped, a familiar and trusted figure.

But what are the alternatives to saying 'doctor knows best' to a woman who would prefer not to have an episiotomy? The doctor must either be able to justify his usual practice to the woman, or be willing to change in response to her preference. Let us consider the reasons given to women for performing an episiotomy.

REASONS FOR PERFORMING AN EPISIOTOMY

Laceration

The most usual reason given to women for having an episiotomy is that it is preferable to a laceration or a badly bruised intact perineum. When a woman's perineum is painfully distended, and she fears she is about to tear, an episiotomy may come as a relief. However, it is not certain that an episiotomy is preferable to a tear. In the NCT study, women suffered less pain in the first week, and were less likely to have pain on intercourse if they had a laceration than if they had an episiotomy and those with an intact perineum suffered least of all. (Women who had forceps deliveries were omitted from the episiotomy group, to avoid attributing pain to episiotomy that was actually due to an instrumental delivery.)

It is also not certain that episiotomy prevents laceration. Episiotomy rates as high as 90 per cent have been reported in some units (though rates for home births are much lower). If these figures represent the number of women who would have torn, this has worrying implications for the management of the second stage. It is not uncommon for a woman to have a laceration in addition to an episiotomy—16 per cent of the NCT episiotomy group, and 22 per cent of Harris' (Harris 1970) sample of primigravidae had a double wound. What is disturbing is that episiotomy is used to protect against tears instead of other methods—antenatal teaching in relaxing the pelvic floor (Montgomery 1981), careful management of the second stage (Fisher 1981; Willmott 1981)—whose aim is to avoid any perineal injury. If episiotomy were to be abandoned, and management of the second stage unchanged, neither mothers nor their birth attendants would welcome the crop of third-degree tears that would be the result. But building the skills in doctors, midwives and mothers that will help to avoid both episiotomy and laceration is preferable to relying on episiotomy to protect against tears, and dealing with the consequences.

Prolapse

It is frequently asserted in obstetric textbooks that episiotomy prevents prolapse of the vaginal wall—cystocele and rectocele—by shortening the second stage (Donald 1979; Dewhurst 1976). The evidence for this is simply absent. Intuitively it sounds likely, but so does this hypothesis: cystocele and rectocele are caused by a rapid second stage such as occurs when the woman is urged to push harder and longer. Neither assertion seems to have been tested. Anatomy does not suggest any link between uterine prolapse and pressure on the perineum, although this is another condition that episiotomy is sometimes said to prevent.

Episiotomy and the fetus

Performing an episiotomy to shorten the second stage is said to be in the interest of the fetus. Obviously this is true in some cases, for example where there are signs of fetal distress, or malpresentation, or a premature baby. It is hard, however, to justify accelerating the second stage, with continuous urges to 'push', and an episiotomy, as a prophylactic measure in a normal labour. Caldeyro-Barcia (1979) has compared babies born to women who were instructed to bear down for long periods with those who were allowed a long second stage using only uterine contractions and the woman's involuntary urges to push. He found that the Apgar scores of babies were no lower after long second stages, and that the breath holding involved in prolonged bearing down could actually cause fetal distress. It seems that a hurried second stage actually creates the need for an episiotomy, with all its possible complications, when both the fetal distress and the episiotomy could be avoided by allowing the woman to push at her own pace. This confirms the experience of midwives such as Fisher (1981) and Willmott (1981). Fisher has written, 'it is possible, in fact, to manage a second stage without ever using the word "push"'.

CONCLUSION

Naturally, general practitioners will want to do all they can to avoid any painful outcome of episiotomy by careful performance and stitching, and sympathetic aftercare. At the same time they may well suspect that the high rates of episiotomy found in many hospitals are not necessary. The incidence of episiotomy has increased with increasing rates of hospital delivery, and greater levels of technology in the labour ward. Research papers and textbooks are written by hospital obstetricians, who see an exceptionally high proportion of complicated births, and who see the woman only as an obstetric patient. Episiotomy rates are much lower for home births, and it is likely that this is also true of births in general practitioner units. General practitioners may well wonder whether obstetric findings are relevant to them, or whether they take full account of their broader experience. Now some senior hospital obstetricians (House 1981) are beginning to say what many general practitioners must have suspected for some time—that too many episiotomies are done with too little consideration for the risks of blood loss and complicated healing. With their high proportion of normal deliveries, and with the chance to build a close team of midwife and doctor with a common approach, general practitioners are ideally placed to rebuild the traditional pride in an intact perineum.

REFERENCES

Beischer, N. A. (1967). The anatomical and functional results of mediolateral episiotomy. *Med. J. Aust.* **2**, 169.

Beynon, C. L. (1974). Midline episiotomy as a routine procedure. *J. Obstet. Gynaecol. Br. Commonw.* **81**, 126.

Caldeyro-Barcia, R. (1979). The influence of maternal bearing-down efforts during the second stage on fetal well-being. *Birth Fam. J.* **6**, 17–21.

Coates, P. M. (1980). A comparison between midline and mediolateral episiotomies. *Br. J. Obstet. Gynaecol.* **87(5)**, 408–12.

Dewhurst, C. J. (1976). *Integrated obstetrics and gynaecology for postgraduates.* Blackwell Scientific, Oxford.

Donald, I. (1979). *Practical obstetric problems*. Lloyd-Luke, London.

Fisher, C. (1981). The Management of labour: a midwife's view. In *Episiotomy: physical and emotional aspects*. (ed. S. Kitzinger). National Childbirth Trust, London.

Gordon, Y. (1981). The midline episiotomy. In *Episiotomy: physical and emotional aspects*. (ed. S. Kitzinger). National Childbirth Trust, London.

Harris, R. E. (1970). An evaluation of the median episiotomy. *Am. J. Obstet. Gynaecol.* **106**, 660–5.

Hoult, I. (1981). The management of labour: an obstetrician's view. In *Episiotomy: physical and emotional aspects*. (ed. S. Kitzinger) National Childbirth Trust, London.

House, M. J. (1981). To or not to do an episiotomy. In *Episiotomy: physical and emotional aspects*. (ed. S. Kitzinger). National Childbirth Trust, London.

Kitzinger, S. with Walters, R. (1981). *Some women's experiences of episiotomy*. National Childbirth Trust, London. The study was based on questionnaires given to all women attending the classes of 40 National Childbirth Trust antenatal teachers across England and Wales, over the period March 1979 to March 1980. Of 2300 questionnaires distributed, 1795 were returned.

Montgomery, E. (1981). Teaching women about the pelvic floor. In *Episiotomy: physical and emotional aspects*. (ed. S. Kitzinger). National Childbirth Trust, London.

Munsick, R. A. (1980). Introital operations for dyspareunia. *Clin. Obstet. Gynecol.* **23(1)**, 243–71.

Willmott, J. (1981). Too many episiotomies. In *Episiotomy: physical and emotional aspects* (ed. S. Kitzinger). National Childbirth Trust, London.

FURTHER READING

Reading, A. E. *et al.* (1982). How women view post-episiotomy pain. *Br. Med. J.* **284 (6311)**, 243–6.

Section D
Postpartum care

25 The puerperium and breast feeding

Chloe Fisher

INTRODUCTION

The puerperium is the culmination of all the professional care that the woman received during her pregnancy and her labour. She has at last become a mother of a totally dependent newborn baby. If this is her first child, she is completely without experience and has to learn everything about caring for it. If she has had another child her memories of her first experience will have been dimmed by all that has occurred since, so she will also need advice and support. She differs from the first time mother only because she is more confident—she has done it before and survived!

Should there be any doubt about the importance of the provision of care to the postpartum woman in the community, the size of the task is revealed by the following figures. Only 12 per cent of mothers returned home before the seventh postpartum day in England and Wales in 1958. Data for England was collected separately from 1970, when the corresponding figure was 48.7 per cent. By 1978 this had riscn to 64.9 per cent (OPCS 1982). Those working in this field know that this trend has continued steadily since then. Apart from this increase, there are various patterns of maternity care in which the general practitioner is medically responsible for the whole of the puerperium, as in a general practitioner unit—or almost the whole of it, as in a Domino delivery scheme.

There are many advantages to the family which come from the mother being cared for in her home from, or shortly after, birth. The father can choose to have as much involvement as he wishes. Siblings, especially if they are very young, are much happier with their mother in the house and with access to her and the baby much freer than could be possible if she were in hospital. Finally, the mother can be in control of her environment. She can eat when she wants and what she wants, and she is not nearly so likely to become sleep-deprived at home. For others outside the immediate family, a new baby provides an excuse for warmth and love and this is much easier to demonstrate in the home.

But there are problems about the provision of the necessary support, because expertise in child rearing in the community is much scarcer than it was 20 or 30 years ago. Families have become smaller and comparatively few babies have been successfully breast-fed. More and more women return home soon after birth and they now have to rely on the health professional to fill the role previously held by experienced relatives and friends. It is important that these people—the midwives, doctors and health visitors—should understand the major influence they can have on the family at this time. Though they will be concerned about monitoring the physical state of the mother and her baby, they need also to assume that role of '*doula*'—that is, the person who mothers the mother (Raphael 1976). The greatest share of this role will be taken by the midwife, but the mother will be receptive to the influence of the family doctor and later to the health visitor.

The community midwife has had a corresponding increase in responsibility for mothers and babies in the home. This has given her a renewed sense of the importance of her role in the maternity service. Most members of the medical profession are not aware that her sphere of responsibility is defined in a professional Code of Practice (UKCC 1983).

She meets the woman at least once during the pregnancy. 'The midwife should visit by arrangement the place(s) where postnatal care is to be provided after transfer home.' This occasion provides an opportunity to educate the mother, especially about the need to make adequate provision for domestic support during the early days after her return home. The woman frequently has unanswered questions which she had not considered important enough to 'bother' the midwives or doctors with at a routine antenatal visit, but which the midwife can answer at this time. Frequently these questions revolve around infant feeding. Together the woman and the midwife can decide on the most appropriate time for her return home with the baby, providing both are well, and this information is then shared with the midwife's hospital colleagues.

The role of the community midwife in the puerperium is clearly defined

The midwife is responsible for the care of the mother and the baby during the post-natal period. The assistance of a registered medical practitioner must be sought in all cases of illness of the mother or baby or any abnormality occurring during the post-natal period. The midwife should promote breast feeding but in the event of artificial feeding of the baby being necessary, must give advice and guidance on the preparation of artificial feeds. She must also ensure that the woman has information on how to obtain advice from or call a midwife if necessary.

Of the duties that are particularly relevant to care of the baby in the home:

A midwife must call in medical aid without delay if there is any sign of infection or abnormality in the baby. Routine screening must be carried out while the midwife is in professional attendance. A midwife must bear in mind the possibility of danger to the baby through cold, and should take steps to see that the means are available for keeping the room warm by day and by night.

The largest proportion of time that this new mother will be spending with her baby will be concerned with feeding. This frequently takes more than 6 hours in every 24. As the majority of women now wish to breast-feed their babies, most of this chapter will be devoted to the establishment and maintenance of lactation. It seems important to share as much useful information as possible because it has been almost impossible for the medical profession to learn much about the subject in recent years. As recently as 10 years ago breast-feeding rates were very low, and of the few mothers who started very few maintained lactation for very long (Sloper, McKean and Baum 1974).

However, there are other problems which specifically pertain to the care of the newly delivered mother and her baby in the home and a few will be discussed.

CONTINUITY OF CARE

Though there will inevitably be a great reduction in the number of care-givers, the mother will almost certainly still have a variety of people coming to her home, because of off-duty, rotas etc. Therefore the only was that there can be a semblance of continuity is if all these meet regularly to share ideas and agree to a common approach in dealing with some of the more common problems.

MONITORING PATHOLOGICAL CONDITIONS

Good laboratory facilities are necessary for the many investigations which may have to be carried out, and there should be an efficient system for transporting the specimens and for getting the results back quickly. Monitoring bilirubin levels requires such a service, if neonatal hospital admissions are to be prevented.

THE MOTHER

Physiotherapy

Early discharge home after delivery can mean women do not have the benefit of early treatment by a specialist physiotherapist (in other words, a member of the Association of Chartered Physiotherapists in Obstetrics and Gynaecology). In the first 36 hours after delivery ultrasound and ice are most effective in dealing with the effects of trauma to the perineal area. Also during this period diastasis of the abdominal recti (more than 5 cm separation) needs assessment, support (tubigrip) and early re-education.

Some 3–5 days after delivery some perineal suture lines separate, incomplete breakdown can often be prevented by infrared irradiation twice daily. Would it be best to delay discharge for women who need these treatments? Restoration of the levator muscles to full function to avoid stress incontinence and vaginal slackness needs a minimum of 3 months' accurate exercise

(Harrison 1980; Sleep *et al.* 1983). If there is no contact with an obstetric physiotherapist extensive teaching programmes will have to be instituted for midwives and general practitioners to enable them to instruct women and check their progress by digital examination.

The most satisfactory answer can lie in using accurate instructional leaflets of the do-it-yourself type (to include self-testing of the pelvic floor muscle function) written and supervised by an obstetric physiotherapist. These leaflets should offer direct self-referral back to the obstetric physio-therapist by phone and then personal appointment as soon as difficulties arise. Women will seek this specialist help quickly if they can make the con-tact easily. Pelvic floor weakness, backache due to faulty positioning and activity, diastasis of the abdominal recti and dyspareunia due to contraction of perineal scars are the most likely referral subjects. The latter responds speedily to treatment by ultrasound.

Weekly postnatal exercise and advice groups should be available for women to join when their babies are about 10 weeks old. It is essential these are conducted by physiotherapists who specialize in obstetrics and gynae-cology as the content of the class will be directed at prevention of the com-mon conditions of women related to childbearing as well as the promotion of general fitness. It is only by close cooperation and communication between the midwives, general practitioners and obstetric physiotherapists that the best interests of these women will be served.

Perineal toilet

In poor home conditions, perineal toilet can be carried out by using a shower attachment on the taps, or warm water in an old 'squeezy' bottle—a tolerable substitute for a bidet.

Perineal discomfort

Friction and tugging of sutures can occur if vulval pads are not firmly secured. This may happen with modern self-adhesive pads. The mother should be advised to use normal pads or invent a way of reducing the fric-tion.

Bright red lochia

Frequently the lochia have diminished to a scant pinky-brown loss by the 8th day—particularly if the mother is breast-feeding—and she may imagine it has almost stopped. Therefore she may become very concerned if she starts to lose bright red blood on about the 9th day. This occurs so frequently as to be normal, but warning the mothers beforehand may prevent un-necessary calls to the midwife or doctor.

Breast engorgement in women who are not breast-feeding

Though this condition does not occur very often it can cause much distress and pain. A simple solution is to express sufficient milk to relieve the discomfort. This also speeds up the resolution of the engorgement so that the mother may not need to express again (Page 1980).

THE BABY

Sticky eyes—moderate discharge

This condition often occurs because there is some degree of blockage of the nasolacrimal duct, and often seems to manifest itself at weekends or bank holidays! If the baby is being breast-fed, there is a simple treatment which could be tried. After feeding, the mother should swab the eyes clean and instil a few drops of her milk. Many eyes will clear up with this simple treatment.

THE ESTABLISHMENT OF LACTATION

The following description of the early days of the puerperium provides a link with the remainder of this chapter, which will be devoted to the establishment of lactation.

The patient should be kept in bed, but after the 3rd day, if she is strong enough, she should be propped up in bed for a short time, perhaps during the time she is having her meals. This raising of the shoulders allows a thorough drainage of the uterus and the vagina. About the 7th day, unless the patient is too weak, she should be lifted out of bed on to a couch or easy chair, long enough to have her bed made. This should be repeated each day, and by the 10th day she may be allowed to sit up for a short time and in a few more days she may move about the room a little (Jardine 1920).

In the light of modern medical knowledge this advice is unquestionably out of date and could be the cause of serious complications. Unfortunately advice about the management of breast-feeding which also had its origins at this time has not been recognized by many as being equally out of date.

During the first quarter of this century little was known of the physiology of lactation, and there had been hardly any study of the physiology or psychology of infants. Hence writers could speculate at will! Because there was a great interest in infant care at this time much was written and this found its way into the textbooks where it survives essentially unchanged until the present day. Is this 'classical' teaching still of value now that the majority of women once again wish to breast-feed their babies, or does it hinder the fulfilment of such wishes? Before we look more closely at the origins of this teaching, let us have a quick look at the situation now.

In England and Wales only 51 per cent of mothers started to breast-feed in 1975 (Martin 1978). By 1980 the rate had increased to 67 per cent (Martin 1982). But in 1975 33 per cent of those who had started to breast-feed had given up after 2 weeks, and in 1980 the corresponding fall was still 19 per cent.

These figures suggest there is scope for improvement and also illustrate the vital importance of the early period when lactation is being initiated. This takes place during the time midwives, whether in hospital or at home, have full responsibility for the day to day care of the woman and her baby—and when general practitioners will be still involved if problems arise. That there is insufficient knowledge to deal with such problems is illustrated by the fact that frequently the mother who has problems during this period is advised to stop breast-feeding. This is undoubtedly the surest way of preventing further breast-feeding problems!

CLASSICAL ADVICE—ITS ORIGINS

By the turn of this century it was believed that 'nature' could be improved upon in almost all respects, and this becomes obvious when one looks at the new 'science' of infant feeding which had its origins at this time. Because there was much concern about infant feeding, the heyday of medical intervention into breast-feeding occurred between 1900 and 1920. A multitude of theories led to many beliefs. For instance, feeds were to be absolutely regular and given at precise intervals (Pritchard 1914). Few, or no feeds, were to be given at night (King 1913). The duration of the feed was to be precisely timed and on no account to exceed 10 minutes at each breast (Pritchard 1914). Both breasts were to be used at each feed (King 1924). The most severe intervention was that of limiting the time allowed at the breast in the first few days to a matter of a few minutes in the belief that this would prevent nipple pain and damage (King 1913). No wonder it was stated that 'the clock is the most important item of furniture in the nursery' (Langmead 1916).

These practices have become so firmly established that they are recommended in the firm belief that they are soundly based. This becomes apparent when one looks at modern medical and midwifery literature. A paper published in a major medical journal contains the following description of early breastfeeding management:

Standard feeding schedule—the breast-fed infants were put to the breast within 4 hours of birth and then fed 4 hourly for 5 feeds, starting with 3 minutes at each side on the first day and increasing daily to 10 minutes on each side on the 5th day. They were given a night feed of 5% dextrose until the 5th night when the mothers were asked if they wished to be woken for night feeds' (Culley *et al.* 1979).

A modern midwifery textbook, designed for use in a developing country states: 'Feeding time . . . 1st day—2 minutes at each breast. 2nd day—5 minutes at each breast. 3rd day—7 minutes at each breast. 4th day onwards —10 minutes from each breast, making 20 minutes feeding time. 20 minutes altogether is the maximum time from then on' (Ajayi 1980).

One of the earliest references to the practice of limiting sucking time is 'allowed to suck for 2 or 3 minutes' (Vincent 1904). This was accompanied by some interesting statements. The author says that the amount of colostrum would inevitably be limited by this practice but 'in anything but a small amount colostrum seriously disturbs the infant—a fact that is not at all surprising when its chemical constitution is considered'. Then, on the effect of suckling on the uterus '. . . though in regard to this, the author must confess that his experience does not lead any support to the theory'. Significantly, he recommends a substitute food made from cow's milk 'until its mother is able to nurse it'. Surely it is of great importance that this early reference to limiting sucking time recognizes the problem thus being created by recommending complementary feeds?

In the same year another expert was saying 'Now it is clear that we cannot have the same control over the chemical constitution of maternal milk that we possess in the case of cow's milk which can readily and at pleasure be modified to the varying needs of the child'. Regretting this lack of control he asks how breast-feeding can be made 'scientific and exact'. The answer to this question is simple. 'Although we must leave to nature the qualitive modification we can on the other hand control the quantity' (Pritchard 1904). By 1916 he was so convinced of the superiority of artificial feeding that he was saying 'In the artificial feeding of infants we can take particular and individual necessities into account. We can give the active child a full proportion of protein, the quickly growing child his due portion of sugar and the infant who lives in the Tropics a different quantum of cream to that which we give to the Esquimaux baby who lives in the Arctic regions' (Pritchard 1916). These last two authors provide some insight into the limited knowledge that existed in this subject at that time. What is surprising is that their theories remained unquestioned and untested for so many years.

CLASSICAL AND MODERN ADVICE—SOME COMPARISONS

The initial duration of feeds

Classical

The duration of early feeds was severely restricted in the belief that this prevented sore nipples from occurring (King 1913). That this objective was not achieved should have been obvious, because sore nipples continued to occur. But this belief is still so firmly rooted that it may take many years to eradicate.

Modern

Observation of feeding practices in the few remaining societies where there is no medically based advice available during the puerperium (Lozoff *et al.* 1977) and research carried out in the developed world, shows that not only is no benefit demonstrated by limiting feeding time but that complications may actually be caused (Harvey and Slaven 1981; Illingworth and Stone 1952; Newton 1952). In reality, the first feed may last from 10 to 45 minutes and may be from one or both breasts. The duration of feeds varies greatly over the first week, often becoming considerably shorter than in the first day or two. Each mother–baby dyad is unique, so there can only be guidelines, not rules.

Ultimate duration of feeds

Classical

The mother was forbidden to feed her baby for longer than 10 minutes on each breast, though the reasons for this advice varied. The three used most frequently were:

(i) that there was a risk of a condition called 'over-feeding';
(ii) that most of the milk had been taken in the first 5 minutes;
(iii) that both breasts must be used.

Modern

Observation of baby-led breast-feeding suggests that the neonate has the ability to control its intake of milk. This may be influenced by the change in the composition of the milk that occurs as the feed proceeds; the proportion of fat increases to at least twice the initial value (Hall 1975). Some babies will be satiated after one breast, some will always require both breasts and some will vary from feed to feed. Evidence that there is a great variability in the length of time that it takes babies of the same age to consume similar amounts of milk now exists (Fig. 25.1). This research also suggests that each mother–baby dyad has a pattern of milk transfer which is specific to them. The pattern will almost certainly change as the baby becomes older and the mother's milk ejection reflex becomes more efficient. This could lead to the duration of a feed becoming considerably shorter. Unfortunately the influence of classical teaching is so strong that feeds which last less than 10 minutes can cause concern to the mother because she may believe that the baby will be inadequately fed! If, during the first week, the mother is told that the feeds are more likely to become shorter, not longer, as the baby grows older, considerable anxiety may be prevented. On the other hand, unduly prolonged feeds—not easy to define but probably lasting more than 20 minutes at each breast after the first week—may be an indication of inadequate milk transfer stemming from poor feeding technique.

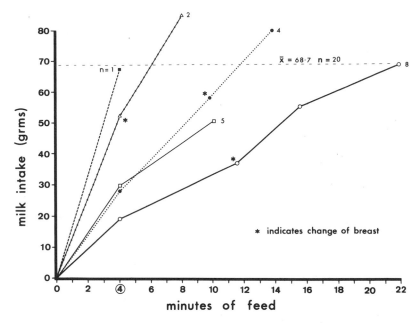

Fig. 25.1. Pattern of milk intake at a feed for 20 6-day-old babies, divided into five groups depending upon the length of time for which they fed. All babies were weighed after 4 minutes of feeding on each breast, and at the termination of feeding (determined by mother or baby) on each breast. On the extreme left, one baby, with a high rate of intake, took sufficient milk in just 4 minutes from one breast only. At the other extreme is the pattern of intake for eight babies feeding for a full period from both breasts (that is, greater than 4 minutes on each), completing their feed after a mean of just under 22 minutes. The remaining eleven babies have intermediate rates of intake and finish after intermediate periods of time. (From Woolridge, Baum and Drewett 1982).

Frequency of feeds

Classical

Rigid timetables were laid down prescribing specific times for feeds and specific gaps between them though, curiously, the recommendations changed very rapidly during the first 20 years of this century. These ranged from every 1½ hours at the turn of the century to every 4 hours by 1920. Whatever the interval between feeds, it was considered that absolute regularity was essential (King 1913).

Modern

With the resurgence of medical interest in breast-feeding that occurred in the early 1970s, research which had been published 20 years earlier was reassessed (Illingworth and Stone 1952; Newton 1952). This indicated that an important contribution to improving the initiation of lactation would result from removing any restrictions on the duration or frequency of feeds. Though these ideas have been accepted slowly and reluctantly they have already been shown to be beneficial (Martin 1982). Hopefully this approach will be universally practised when the next national survey is undertaken.

What has been less well described is the evolving pattern of feeding times which occurs during the first week of life. At the beginning, if the duration of the feed is unrestricted, there may be long gaps between feeds—6–8 hours or even more being common. By the third day the frequency increases and the feeds become shorter, but by the fifth day frequency may have been reduced to six or seven feeds in 24 hours, and the duration will vary between one breast-feeding pair and another. This behaviour is contrary to that described by many authors, in particular those whose writing is aimed directly at mothers, for they commonly describe the early feeds as being 'frequent and short' (*Breast feeding* 1983). The explanation for this discrepancy is that the shortness is imposed, so of necessity the feeds have to become more frequent. By the second week of the baby's life it often happens that feeds occur more frequently during one part of the 24 hours and less frequently at another. The longer gaps often occur during the night and this is pleasing for the parents. But some mothers may interpret the short gaps as an indication of an inadequate milk supply and they may need considerable reassurance.

THE NEED FOR CHANGE

It is not surprising that the result of the 'classical' restrictions on feeding time often led to an inadequately fed baby. This deficit was met by giving the baby cow's milk complementary feeds. This is one of the reasons why the confidence of health workers in human lactation reached its nadir in the 1960s—for by that time almost all women in Great Britain gave birth in hospital and that is where these long established practices continued to flourish.

Understanding the background may help health workers to start afresh and may enable them to learn to trust the new well-founded information that is becoming available. They might be spurred on by the conclusion to a history of infant feeding which said 'When this regime (baby-led feeding) becomes universally adopted, as surely it will, so the last chapter in the history of infant feeding will be concluded' (Wickes 1952). It is disturbing to realize that this was published more than 30 years ago and that some parts of the country are still a long way from concluding this last chapter.

A COMMON CAUSE OF FAILURE

The majority of women who chose to breast-feed but failed either to establish lactation or to feed their baby for as long as they had intended were genuinely motivated—and they very much regret their inability to achieve this objective. It is important to realize that positive action can be taken to prevent many of these failures. One of the reasons why so many women have problems arises from the fact that there is much ignorance among health workers about how a baby feeds at the breast. They are very familiar with the mechanisms of bottle-feeding and imagine that breast-feeding is the same. When a baby breast-feeds it does not take only the nipple into its mouth, in the same way that a bottle-fed baby takes the teat, but part of the breast as well. In fact, if the baby 'nipple sucks' instead of 'breast-feeds', failure is inevitable—though the timing and reason for the failure will vary.

BREAST-FEEDING TECHNIQUE

An excellent description of the mechanism of breast-feeding, based on cine-radiographic studies in the 1950s, includes clear diagrams to illustrate the text (Ardran, Kemp and Lind 1958). Fig 25.2 shows how the baby makes a teat out of the breast and the nipple. The nipple forms about one-third of this teat and lies far back in the baby's mouth, where it cannot be trauma-tized. Note that the mouth is not centrally positioned, so that the lower lip is further from the base of the teat than the top lip. Because of this, more areola will be visible above the breast than below. Unfortunately, mothers are frequently instructed to try to get all of the areola into the baby's mouth and because they can only see the top of the breast, they misalign the baby. This brings about the incorrect position shown in Fig. 25.3, with the baby 'nipple sucking', not breast-feeding. As so many problems arise from this error it is helpful to observe the baby at the breast before giving advice.

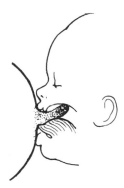

Fig. 25.2. Correct method. A teat is formed from the nipple and the breast; the tongue is inserted between the lower gum and the teat.

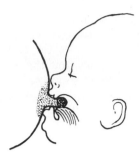

Fig. 25.3. Incorrect method. The nipple is resting just within the gums; the tongue is rubbing the tip of the nipple.

PREFERRED SIDE

Confirmation that many of the early feeding problems derive from poor feeding technique comes from the fact that a large proportion of the physical problems—sore or cracked nipples, overfull breasts, engorgement, mastitis and even abscesses—occur in the right breast. The majority of women normally hold their baby in their left arm when not feeding—for cuddling, or winding, for instance. They may find feeding the baby the 'wrong' way around—on the right breast—awkward and fail to achieve a satisfactory position for the baby. For the minority who naturally hold their babies on the right arm the situation is reversed. Mothers are very grateful to be given this explanation because it may be all that they need to sort out their problems and they can move away from believing either that the baby is rejecting that breast or that the breast has an inherent flaw. Switching the baby around, so that its feet point backwards under the arm, will allow that mother to handle the baby using her hands in the same way that she uses them on the 'good' side.

PROBLEMS RELATED, DIRECTLY OR INDIRECTLY, TO BREAST-FEEDING TECHNIQUE

Early nipple pain or nipple damage

Since 1980 the following information has been given to the majority of pregnant women in Great Britain: 'Breastfeeding should not hurt at all. If one of your nipples hurts as the baby starts to feed, do ask for professional help to get it better' (Gunther 1980). The current problem is that there is not enough skilled professional help available to enable the mothers to 'get it better', because the best possible way to prevent these problems from occurring at all is to provide supervision for the early feeds with help in repositioning the baby if pain does occur, and few people know how to do this.

When the cause of this problem is universally understood more health workers will want to develop these skills.

If the nipple has already been damaged—either at the tip or at the base—it will heal very quickly if no further trauma occurs. The use of ointments, creams or sprays have never been proven to be beneficial, but unfortunately, they continue to be recommended instead of encouraging the development of the skills that would provide the real solution.

Mastitis

There is much confusion about this condition because many people believe that it occurs directly as the result of infection, and treat all cases with an antibiotic. Sometimes the mother is told to stop feeding from the breast, or to stop feeding altogether, either of which may lead to abscess formation. The greatest proportion of cases originate from stasis of milk in one or more segments of the breast which causes milk to leak from the alveoli into the surrounding tissue. This may cause pain, lumpiness or erythema—and may be accompanied by pyrexia, general malaise and aching limbs. Continued breast-feeding with a special effort made to ensure good positioning —to encourage a good milking action—may quickly resolve the problem. It may help to suggest that the baby feeds from the affected breast first for the next two feeds. It has been recommended that antibiotic cover should be given in case the mastitis does not resolve and a bacterial infection supervenes (Gunther 1973), but where close supervision is available it may be reasonable to withhold antibiotics for 6–8 hours to see if the condition resolves spontaneously—which it often will. This type of mastitis has been called 'acute intramammary' and it is probable that lumpiness and blocked ducts are less serious manifestations of the same condition. 'Superficial mastitis' is much rarer and is due to infection. It occurs in women whose nipples have been damaged or when breast shells are worn continuously. The inflammation is near the areola and may resolve if antibiotic treatment is started quickly—otherwise pus formation occurs and the abscess has to be incised. It is recommended that breast-feeding from the affected breast should continue if at all possible because this leads to quicker healing (Benson and Goodman 1970). The position of the incision may make direct breast-feeding impossible and expressing may prove to be difficult. Breast-feeding can continue on the unaffected breast. As is the case with twins, one breast is capable of providing sufficient milk for one baby. (Many women have fed from only one breast. They may have had a mastectomy, or have insoluble physical problems on the other side).

Feeding problems after a previously successful lactation

It is normally assumed that a mother who has breast-fed previous babies requires no assistance with her new baby. But the initiation of lactation differs greatly from established lactation, and no mother should ever be considered an expert in the first few days. Problems may arise. The mother's nipples may have become longer or larger or she may have a totally different type of baby—it could be smaller, or it might be premature. If she has not previously experienced problems she may not know how to solve them and may require help urgently.

Postural problems

An observation made in the home, and which relates to achieving a good feeding technique, is that 'modern' furniture, with its deep, backward sloping seats, is not conducive to good breast-feeding. The mother is forced to lean back and her lap is not parallel with the floor but tilted, with her knees higher than her hips. A move to a chair of an appropriate height, or even sitting on the edge of the bed, will allow the woman to lean slightly forward comfortably. With the baby placed on a pillow to bring it into the correct level, the mother will be in the ideal position to place her baby correctly on to the breast. Once the mother and baby have learnt the technique they can be quite adventurous about where to feed.

COMMON PROBLEMS AND UNCERTAINTIES IN THE MOTHER

Demand feeding

Unfortunately the term 'demand feeding', which is most commonly used to describe baby-led feeding, conjures up an image of a 'demanding' baby for many people—whereas in reality the baby may be very amenable, probably having become confident that its hunger will be assuaged whenever it occurs. Probably for these same people the idea of letting the baby control when it should be fed implies a chaotic situation which they believe could be resolved by making the baby adhere to a rigid timetable. The difficulties that this approach can create are beautifully illustrated by the following

If he wakes at 4 am instead of at 3 am after having taking his 10 p.m. feed at midnight, and water does not satisfy him, the 6 a.m. feed may be given an hour earlier. If this is done, it may also become necessary to give the 10 am feed half an hour earlier than usual if the baby wakes and cries for it, but the balance of the day's feeds should be given at their customary hours of 2 pm and 6 pm (Halpern 1945)!

We should surely be endeavouring to encourage the mother to learn how to respond to her baby's needs, in the belief that this will foster a closer relationship with her baby. And with this should go an easy and abundant lactation.

How much should the mother drink?

Lactating women have an increased thirst and providing it is quenched the extra fluid requirement will be met. The thirst frequently manifests itself at the beginning of a feed so it is helpful to suggest to the mother that she should have a drink easily available before she settles down with the baby. Health workers should refrain from suggesting that the mother should drink a specific amount because she might take this to imply that an increased fluid intake would directly affect milk production and it does not (Illingworth and Kilpatrick 1953)! This could lead a mother who is anxious about her milk supply to drink excessively. Some people will remember that in the early 1960s mothers were urged to drink 3 litres of water in the first 48 hours in order to *suppress* lactation. As a corollary, limiting fluid intake because the breasts are overfull is equally unphysiological (Gunther 1973).

Should both breasts be used?

Since early this century English-speaking countries have recommended that both breasts should be used at every feed (King 1913). This can be difficult because the mother will be worrying about the length of time she should allow the baby to have on the first breast if she is to persuade it to have the second breast. She may also deprive it of high fat hind milk if she terminates the feed artificially. Curiously, in Europe and in Scandinavia, mothers were urged to restrict their babies to one breast only at a feed, and only recently have accepted that the baby might want to feed from the second breast! These 'foreign' practices suggest that no harm will come to the unused breast, but it would be sensible to start the next feed on that side.

Having too much milk

If the initiation of lactation gets off to a good start the amount of milk initially available will be in excess of the baby's need. Indeed, the mother could be reassured that she starts with enough for at least two babies. Provided that the baby is allowed to control the length of the feed, and to feed from one breast only on some occasions, the supply quickly adjusts to the amount required by that particular baby. But if the mother has been told that she should use both breasts, she may inadvertently prolong excessive lactation. This problem responds in about 24 hours when the appropriate advice is given.

Dripping from the other breast

A high proportion of lactating women drip from one breast when the baby feeds from the other side, particularly when demand feeding from birth is the rule. This may occur only during the first week or two but in about 15 per cent it may continue and become a nuisance (Gibbs *et al.* 1977). If a leakproof breast shield is placed over the nipple during a feed the problem is greatly reduced. On the other hand, shells should not be worn regularly between feeds because this tends to encourage dripping and may also make the nipples soggy.

Anxiety about the volume and quality of breast milk

Many mothers have been persuaded into believing that their milk is deficient in either amount or quality—or sometimes both—because almost all of the remaining folklore surrounding breast-feeding is negative and concentrates on the innumerable signs which are purported to indicate these deficiencies. Mothers could be helped to resist these pressures if, in the early days, they received instruction on the changes which normally occur but are frequently misunderstood. The most common are alterations in the baby's behaviour; breast becoming softer or stopping dripping; and colour changes in the milk. They might also benefit from being told that attempting to change the baby's behaviour by changing to artificial feeding may not bring about the desired result. Recent research showed that 56 per cent of mothers who did change the method of feeding reported that the baby's behaviour remained the same or became less settled (Houston 1983).

Late onset sore nipples

Thrush is the commonest cause of sore nipples occurring after a period of pain-free feeding. The baby often develops a sore bottom at the same time, and occassionally has evidence of oral thrush as well. If both mother and baby are treated, the condition slowly but steadily improves. A less common cause is from skin sensitivity which has developed from the use of a topical application—it maybe a cream, ointment or spray.

COMMON PROBLEMS AND UNCERTAINTIES IN THE BABY

Does the baby require 'extra' fluids?

To quench the baby's thirst

An advertisement for a baby feeding bottle says that it is 'essential for those thirst quenching drinks between feeds'. However there is no evidence that breast-fed babies need anything other than their own mother's milk, or that thirst is separate from hunger and cannot be met by human milk. Recent research in the Sinai desert led the authors to conclude: 'Urine osmolarity under hot and dry climatic conditions remains within the expected physiological ranges and thus shows that supplementary water for breastfed infants is not necessary' (Goldberg and Adams 1982). Previous research had already led to the conclusion that supplementary water was not required in hot and humid climates (Armelini and Gonzalez 1979). Perhaps the origin of the widely held belief that 'extra' fluid is required arose from the need to deal with the hypernatraemia that commonly occurred in bottle-fed infants before the advent of the modified formulas of more recent years.

To prevent or treat jaundice

It has been suggested that jaundice occurs in breast-fed babies because of the 'low intake of milk' (Valman 1980). Unrestricted feeding may go a considerable way towards removing this cause. Another suggestion is that absorption of bilirubin from retained meconium contributes to a raised serum bilirubin level and that unrestricted feeding increases intestinal motility and so reduces the possibility of jaundice from this cause (Carvalho, Merkatz, and Klaus 1982). There is no evidence that giving 'extra' fluids prevents jaundice from occurring, nor that giving 'extra' fluids to term babies in any way alters the course of jaundice if it has already occurred (Carvalho, Hall, and Harvey 1981).

Can a breastfed baby be overfed?

This is really a health worker's anxiety, but it is readily transmitted to the mother. The original description of a condition called 'overfeeding' which led to the limitation of total feeding times was of a baby who initially grew well but following 'serious digestive disturbances' ceased to grow. It is difficult to recognize the phenomenon which is being described, and there is now a totally different description of 'overfeeding'. This is a breast-fed baby who is thriving and growing rapidly. There is no evidence that this is harmful, and indeed it may be genetically determined.

Crying and colic

Crying which occurs immediately *before* a feed is most likely to be due to hunger—it will be intermittent, especially if the mother has always been quick to respond, and is easily quieted for short periods by picking up and holding the baby until it can be fed. Under these conditions the baby may soon wake for a feed without crying. Mothers can be encouraged to respond quickly to their babies by telling them that research has shown that babies whose crying is ignored tend to cry more in the first year (Bell and Ainsworth 1972). It will probably take some time for our society to move away from the belief that picking up a crying child will spoil it or that 'A baby who cries simply because he wants to be picked up must be left to cry it out' (King 1934). One of the most common times for a new baby to cry is after a feed, and this can be most disconcerting for the mother. The crying is often accompanied by behaviour which suggests hunger—the baby 'roots' frantically, turning towards anything that makes contact with its face including its own fist. However, hunger is the least likely cause of the crying that occurs *after* a feed. Babies who behave like this are usually growing well and it may help to console the mother if this is explained to her. Holding or giving a short suck at the breast may be all that is needed to comfort the baby.

If the situation develops into prolonged crying, often with behaviour which suggests pain—such as the baby's knees being drawn up—it is called colic. For the more fortunate mother this condition occurs only once a day between two of the feeds, and usually in the evening when she may well have an extra pair of hands available to help comfort the baby. This time is usually when the baby was most active *in utero* and a suggestion that this pattern of behaviour may have been set before birth may make it a little easier to tolerate. The cause is not understood but because the condition rarely continues for more than 3 months it has been suggested that it may be due to immaturity of the nervous and digestive systems. More recently it has been suggested that prostaglandins excreted in the breast milk may be the cause (Anon. 1981*a*). Dicyclomine hydrochloride syrup has been marketed in the United Kingdom for about 30 years and has been liberally prescribed as a treatment for infant colic (12 million doses for babies in 1984). Reports of possible adverse effects have been published (Williams and Watkin-Jones 1984). One manufacturer has now deleted infant colic as an indication for its use, also stating that its use in infants under 6 months of age is contraindicated. Another manufacturer has stated that it is no longer indicated for infants under 3 months of age.

A much more difficult situation exists when the baby cries after almost every feed. It is possible that the most common cause for this is distension arising from air swallowed during the feed, occurring when the milk flows rapidly from the first breast as the result of the let-down reflex. The mother may be missing the signals from the baby that suggest it has a problem—it may pause unduly, or may start wriggling (babies feeding happily are still) or even let go of the breast. If she can cause the baby to bring up wind at that point, it is unlikely that it will have any more to bring up later. This situation may be exaggerated if the baby is not correctly positioned at the breast for then milk may be swallowed in an untidy and noisy fashion.

Only when these mechanical causes have been eliminated and the problem persists should the possibility of sensitivity to food in the mother's diet be considered. Although cow's milk has frequently been implicated (Whichelow and Greenfield 1980) other foods such as oranges, strawberries, eggs or chocolate could be the cause. More rarely, wheat, apple, banana, coffee and tomato have been found to be responsible (Evans *et al.* 1981; Gerrard 1980). Provided that the other causes have been excluded, the mother should be asked to observe if her baby reacts to specific foods she has eaten. Only if there is no recognizable pattern should the mother reduce or remove cow's milk from her diet.

Breast-fed babies' stools

Recently this question was asked: 'An infant passes loose motions after breastfeeding but when articially fed produced *normal* motions. Why should this be?' (Anon. 1981*b*) This reveals another aspect of our familiarity with bottle feeding and it may take some time for breast-feeding and all that appertains to it to be accepted as normal again. Breast-fed babies stools *are* loose, often quite liquid. The colour is mustard yellow, occasionally tinged with green, and the smell inoffensive. The baby may pass a stool at every feed and this is quite common in the early days, but as the baby gets older the gap may increase so that a stool is passed every few days. Once a week is not uncommon, and once a fortnight has been reported by several mothers. It is important to accept that breast-fed babies do not become constipated—and to understand that the baby who has long gaps between stools may be uncomfortable for an hour or two before having its bowels open. Disposable nappies were not originally intended for breast-fed infants and they often leak, causing much washing. If they have to be used, tucking cotton wool between the nappy and the thigh may help.

How fast should the baby grow?

The growth curves on existing weight charts were based on the rate of growth of artificially fed babies and of breast-fed babies whose intake was restricted. In practice, well-fed breast-fed babies often grow rapidly initially and then slow down at about 3 or 4 months. It is unfortunate that mothers are told that both these patterns are unacceptable, especially as it is impossible to control intake at the breast.

Insufficient breast milk?

The commonest reason given for stopping breast-feeding, at the age of up to 9 months, is 'insufficient milk' (Martin and Monk 1982). However, it seems unlikely that this was the real reason in many instances because a variety of reports indicate that almost all women are capable of providing an adequate milk supply for their baby. One of the most dramatic of these reports came from an internment camp in Singapore—20 babies were born, 20 were breast fed and all 20 survived (Williams 1947).

Some of the anxieties and problems which lead people to believe that there is an inadequate supply—the crying baby, the frequency of feeds and the duration of feeds—have already been discussed. In almost all of these cases the baby's satisfactory growth can be used to reinforce the reassurance that is given.

Failure to thrive at the breast

When the baby fails to grow at a reasonable rate the conclusion most frequently reached nowadays is that this is the direct result of inadequate lactation. The following case illustrates a common problem, but with a resolution that occurs very infrequently:

Case history

First baby. Born 2 June. Weight: 8lb 2oz (3.69 kg)

21 June. Attends general practitioner because of painful haemorrhoids. He weighs the baby, is concerned because the birth weight has not been regained. Test weighing recommended, but no advice given about what to do with the information.

24 June. Health visitor comes to home and suggests that the mother gives cow's milk feeds after every breast-feed.

27 June. Different health visitor comes to visit. She suggests building up breast milk supply by increasing the frequency of the feeds and stopping the complementary bottles.

1 July. First health visitor returns. The baby's naked weight is 8lb 1oz (3.66 kg). The mother is urged to resume complementary feeds.

5 July. Baby seen by general practitioner. The clothed weight of the baby was 8lb 12oz (3.97 kg). The mother is now told that she must limit the time at each breast and give more cow's milk at each feed. She returned home in a distressed condition. Her doctor husband was so concerned about her state that he contacted the general practitioner that evening. A reassuring and concerned locum was on call that night who promised to try to obtain expert advice for them.

6 July. The promised expert adviser observed a breast-feed, and it was obvious that the baby was only nipple sucking. The baby was gently repositioned and the mother commented almost immediately on the difference in her baby's behaviour because the sucking had become both slower and deeper. The mother was shown how to help the baby to feed like this. Complementary feeds were stopped from this time but the mother was encouraged instead to feed the baby whenever an opportunity arose.

11 July. The baby's naked weight is now 8lb 12oz (3.97 kg). The mother's confidence rises.

During the following 7 weeks this now fully breast-fed baby gained 2lb 10oz (1.19 kg) and has continued to thrive ever since.

Several points for discussion arise from this case:

(i) If the midwife did not discharge breast-fed babies until they had regained their birth weight more thought might go into discovering the causes. In this case the solution might have been found much earlier.

(ii) The baby's failure to thrive was almost certain evidence that it was not obtaining sufficient milk. Test weighing only added to the mother's anxiety, particularly unfortunate because it was almost certain to be inaccurate. Recently, researchers into the accuracy of test weighing concluded: 'We have found test weighing, using standard baby scales, in the routine clinical context, to be a poor indicator of feed intake in small babies. The reliability of the results depends on the magnitude of the test weight and to a lesser degree on body weight. An inaccuracy around 20 per cent can be expected in babies weighing over 2.5 kg taking about 60 g per feed' (Steven and Whitfield 1980).

(iii) Some of the professional advice illustrates the loss of confidence in breast-feeding that currently exists. It may take many years to change this.

Failure to thrive—another variation

In this case the baby's initial weight gain is satisfactory for the first 2 or 3 weeks and then begins to fall off. This may be a nipple-sucking baby but the problem has been disguised because the mother's let-down reflex has enabled sufficient milk to be transferred into the baby initially, but without a good breast-feeding technique the supply will almost inevitably diminish and this becomes evident when the weight begins to alter. Teaching the mother how to position the baby correctly may well resolve the problem. This pattern of failure to thrive might be the origin of the belief, held by many, that the mother's milk supply frequently fails when she resumes her domestic duties.

Failure to thrive—other causes

(i)   The advice the mother has received may lead her to restrict the frequency of the feeds, or the duration. Doing either of these may cause the baby to fail to thrive.

(ii) Again, following common advice, the mother may believe that she must make the baby feed for equal lengths of time from both breasts at every feed. In certain circumstances, this could lead to the baby obtaining a high volume of low fat foremilk. In one such case the baby started to grow again as soon as the mother allowed it to finish the first breast spontaneously.

(iii) Illness in the baby—poor feeding or vomiting might be caused by illness in the baby, so that investigation for infection and other causes of vomiting should be carried out (Davies 1979).

Failure to thrive from a genuine inadequacy of breast milk

It seems probable that some women are unable to produce enough milk to promote adequate growth in their babies, but many fewer than is commonly believed. There is no reason why these women should not continue to breast-feed if they so wish, making up the deficit with artificial feeds. Some people believe that 'nipple confusion' occurs if the baby has bottle-feeds while breast-feeding (Franz 1983). In practice, many babies appear to be able to do both without any difficulty.

It has not been possible to include the management of lactation when special problems occur in either the mother or her baby. However, as knowledge about normal lactation increases that information can be adapted and applied to a variety of abnormal situations.

Many factors have been implicated in the high rate of breast-feeding failure which is occurring at the present time. Contributory factors include the influence of family and friends, social class, the woman's own experience and the quality of professional support. All of these should change for the better if breast-feeding once again becomes accepted as the normal way to feed the newborn baby. In spite of all the problems, a surprisingly high proportion of women wish to breast-feed. Surely it is the responsibility of those health workers who are directly concerned with the mother and her baby at this important time to make absolutely certain that the information they give is up-to-date, well-founded, and useful.

REFERENCES

Ajayi, V. (1980). The normal infant. In *A textbook of midwifery*, p. 145. Macmillan International College Editions, London.

Anon. (1981*a*). In answer to a question about colic. *Br. Med. J.* **282**, 1445.

Anon. (1981*b*). In answer to a question about babies motions *Br. Med. J.* **282**, 459.

Ardran, G. M., Kemp, F. H., and Lind, J. (1958). A cineradiographic study of breast feeding. *Br. J. Radiogr.* **31**, 156.

Armelini, P. A. and Gonzalez, C. F. (1979). Breast feeding and fluid intake in a hot climate. *Clin. Pediatr. (Philadelphia)* **18**, 424–5.

Bell, S. M. and Ainsworth, M. D. S. (1972). Infant crying and maternal responsiveness. *Child Develop.* **43**, 1171–90.

Benson, E. A. and Goodman, M. A. (1970). An evaluation of the use of stilboestrol and antibiotics in the early management of acute puerperal breast abscess. *Br. J. Surg.* **57**, 258.

Breast feeding (1983). B. Edsall and Co. Ltd., London, p. 15.

Carvalho, M. de, Hall, M., and Harvey, D. (1981). Effects of water supplementation on physiological jaundice in breast-fed babies. *Arch. Dis. Child.*, 568.

Carvalho, M. de, Merkatz R. and Klaus M. (1982). Frequency of breast-feeding and serum bilirubin concentration. *Am. J. Dis. Child.* **136**, 737.

Culley, P., Milan, P., Roginski, C., and Waterhouse, J. (1979). Are breast-fed babies still getting a raw deal in hospital. *Br. Med. J.* **13 October**, 891.

Davies, D. P. (1979). Is inadequate breast-feeding an important cause of failure to thrive? *Lancet* **10 March**, 542.

Evans, R. W., Fergusson, D. M., Allardyce, R. A., and Taylor, B. (1981). Maternal diet and infant colic in breast-fed infants. *Lancet* **20 June**, 1340.

Franz, K. (1983). Slow weight gain. In *A practical guide to breast-feeding* (ed. J. Riordan) The C.V. Mosby Company, St Louis, p. 218.

Gerrard, J. W. (1980). Adverse reactions to foods in breast-fed babies. In *International symposium on breast feeding, Tel Aviv* (eds. S. Freier and A. I. Eidelman) Excerpta Medica, Amsterdam, p. 170.

Gibbs, J. H., Fisher, C., Bhattacharya, Goddard, P., and Baum, J. D. (1977). Drip breast milk: its composition, collection and pasteurization. *Early Hum. Develop.*, **1/3**, 229.

Goldberg, N. M., and Adams, E. (1983). Supplementary water for breast-fed babies in a hot and dry climate—not really necessary. *Arch. Dis. Child.* **58(1)**, 73.

Gunther, M. (1973). Difficulties in breast feeding. In *Infant Feeding*. Penguin Handbooks, Harmondsworth, p. 106.

Gunther, M. (1980). Thinking ahead about breast feeding. In *You and Your Baby Part 1*. British Medical Association, London. p. 24.

Hall, B. (1975). Changing composition of human milk and early development of an appetite control.

Halpern, L. J. (1945). From two weeks to six months. In *How to raise a healthy baby*. Medical Publications Ltd., London, p. 46.

Harrison, S. M. (1980). Study of patients with stress incontinence treated with muscle re-education. In *Incontinence and its management*. (ed. D. Mandelstam). Croom Helm, Beckenham.

Harvey, D. and Slaven, S. (1981). Unlimited suckling time improves breast feeding. Correspondence, *Lancet* 1, 392.

Houston, M. (1983). *Requirements for successful breast feeding*. Doctoral thesis, p. 170.

Illingworth, R. S. and Stone, D. G. (1952). Self-demand feeding in a maternity unit. *Lancet* 1, 683.

Illingworth, R. S. and Kilpatrick, B., (1953). Lactation and fluid intake. *Lancet* **5 December**, 1175.

Jardine, R. (1920). The normal puerperium. In *Text-Book of Midwifery*, Henry Kimpton, London, p. 137.

King, F. T. (1913). *Feeding and care of the baby*, Society for the Health of Woman and Children, London, p. 36.

King, F. T. (1924). Normal breast-feeding. In *The expectant mother and baby's first month*. Macmillan and Co. London, p. 33.

King, M. T. (1934). Progress and development. In *Mothercraft*. Whitcombe and Tombs Limited, Sydney and Melbourne, p. 168.

Langmead, F. (1916). Breast-feeding. In *Mothercraft*. The National League for Physical Education and Improvement, London, p. 74.

Lozoff, B., Brittenham, G. M., Trause, M. A., Kennell, J. H., and Klaus, M. H. (1977). The mother–newborn relationship: limits of adaptability. *J. Paediatr.* **91**, 6.

Martin, J. (1978). *Infant Feeding 1975*. OPCS, HMSO. London.

Martin, J. and Monk, J. (1982). *Infant Feeding*. OPCS, HMSO, London.

Newton, N. (1952). Nipple pain and nipple damage. *J. Paediatr.* **41** 411.

OPCS (1982). *Health and personal social service statistics for England*. Government Statistical Service. HMSO, DHSS, London.

Page, M. (1980). In *Puerperal mastitis and breast abscess*. A paper given at the London Conference of research and the midwife.

Pritchard, E. (1904). Breast feeding. In *The physiological feeding of infants*. Henry Kimpton, London, p. 16.

Pritchard, E. (1914). Breast feeding. In *The family encyclopaedia of medicine no. 4* (ed. by H. H. Riddle) Amalgamated Press Ltd., London, p. 290.

Pritchard, E. (1916). Artificial feeding. In *Mothercraft*. The National League for Physical Education and Improvement, London, p. 94.

Raphael, D. (1976). *The tender gift: breastfeeding*. Schoken Books, New York.

Sleep, J., Spencer, J., Grant, A., *et al.* (1983). West Berkshire Perineal Management Trial. *23rd British Congress of obstetrics and gynaecology Birmingham*.

Sloper, K., McKean, and Baum, J. D. (1974). Patterns of infant feeding in Oxford. *Arch. Dis. Child.* **49**, 749.

Stevens, S. and Whitfield, M. F. (1980). How accurate is clinical test weighing of the newborn? In *Midwives Chron. Nurs. Notes* **93**, 148.

UKCC (1983). *Notices concerning a midwives code of practice for midwives practising in England and Wales*. United Kingdom Central Council for Nursing,

Midwifery and Health Visiting. Spottiswoode Ballantyne Ltd. Colchester and London.

Valman, H. B. (1980). Jaundice in the newborn. In *The First Year of Life. Br. Med. J.* 23 February, 543.

Vincent, R. (1904). Lactation. In *The Nutrition of the Infant.* Baillière, Tindall and Cox, London, p. 36.

Whichelow, M. J. and Greenfield, M. (1980). Coping with colic in the breast fed Baby. *Health Visitor* **53**, 6.

Wickes, I. G. (1953). A history of infant feeding: V. *Arch. Dis. Child.* **128**, 151.

Williams, C. D. (1947). Nutritional conditions among women and children in internment in the civilian camp in Singapore. *Proc. Nutr. Soc.* **5**, 127.

Williams, J. and Watkin-Jones, R. (1984). Dicyclomine: worrying symptoms associated with its use in some small babies. *Br. Med. J.* 24 March, and correspondence 21 April.

Woolridge, M. W., Baum, J. D., and Drewett, R. F. (1982). Individual patterns of milk intake during breast-feeding. *Early Hum. Develop.* **7**, 269.

26 Supervision of mother and baby from 2 to 6 weeks

Sandy Tinson

The short period from the 2nd week of a child's life to the postnatal examination at 6 weeks is a significant one for both mother and her child. It is a time of adjustment for the entire family, and there is usually a need for support, help and guidance. The health visitor's role should provide all of those things.

THE ROLE OF THE HEALTH VISITOR

As a profession, health visiting has changed dramatically over the past 50 years, as the health and social needs of society have also changed. The role of 'well-baby nurse' has gradually progressed to 'family visitor' (Owen 1977). The NHS Act 1972 states that she (or he—so great is the change) was 'a person employed by a local health authority to visit people in their homes or elsewhere for the purpose of giving advice as to the care of young children, persons suffering from illness, and expectant and nursing mothers . . .'. This vague definition forms the basis of the health visitor's work. Each geographical area has a variable social and economic structure and she must adapt to those needs.

The Court report highlights the value of preventive medicine, and the importance of the health visitor's role in this. The trend in the past 10–15 years has been towards health visitor attachment wherever practicable. Large city areas, and some rural areas are usually still visited by health visitors working within a geographical area. Successful health visitor attachment to a general practitioner's surgery can only work if each member of the primary care team is aware of the role and expertise of their colleagues. If a member works in seclusion it can lead to confusion, not only for the patient but for other agencies involved. Decisions should also be made within the team regarding confidentiality and the availability of records. Regular liaison between general practitioner, health visitor, midwife and sometimes social worker is essential if the team is to function successfully (see Chapter 12). Personalities may clash but the needs of the patient should come first! However, such an arrangement may not prove successful for several reasons. If the general practice is a large one, the number of individuals involved may be too great for any purposeful liaison. In many cases the health visitor is based at a clinic, a distance from the surgery and this can cause problems with communication. It has been suggested that 'if one person had the complete knowledge held by . . . three people, then a completely different course of action would have been followed' (Emery 1981).

The health visitor is a trained nurse, with additional midwifery experience, who has undergone a specific training enabling her 'to play an important part in the positive promotion of health' (HMSO 1972). She will be working closely with general practitioners and other medical and non-medical staff. She should be able to offer the mother and baby the guidance, help and support they need.

THE ANTENATAL PERIOD

The care and screening offered to the pregnant woman has been discussed fully in previous chapters but this period before birth has a significant bearing upon the health visitor's role, and the subsequent health and welfare of mother and baby in this postnatal period.

All too often the health visitor's role in antenatal care is described as 'the provision of parentcraft classes'. These classes are usually attended by those of the population who need them the least. There is a need to provide classes to attract those who would not normally attend. Generally such classes need a change of image. This may be achieved by better local and nationwide publicity, easier accessibility and a provision of evening classes and crêche facilities. Perhaps the professional should go out to the public, and meet their needs in this way. A mobile clinic may prove more acceptable than an efficient, well-run health centre or hospital. Those involved in running classes should be trained to do so and provide a service that is valuable and meaningful to all.

Formal, well-run classes cannot replace the value of a visit to a family at home. The basis of sound postnatal supervision is dependent upon a good relationship between the health visitor and the family. If she visits a family for the first time after the baby's birth she must begin to establish that relationship then. How much easier and worthwhile it would be to meet the family during the important antenatal period.

It is essential that all members of the team decide upon a policy for antenatal care. This ensures that each says the same thing and their roles complement each other. This should provide reassurance to the mother-to-be. Those mothers attending large maternity hospitals sometimes feel confused and anxious. It is they who will benefit from such an approach.

Preparation for a home visit may be time-consuming but is essential. The sooner the health visitor makes contact the better, and the topics she may cover will be relevant during the first months of pregnancy. This inevitably means that the midwives' and health visitors' roles will overlap but with an agreed approach this should not matter.

The value of these visits is important to all, regardless of social class, but it does enable the health visitor to identify high-risk groups and those of special need. Practical help as well as health education is offered to ensure the entire family are 'physically, mentally and emotionally' prepared for the birth of the baby. Such ante-natal preparation by the health visitor enables her to know the family she is to visit and for them to know her, and thus are the foundations laid for the future visits. The health visitor's involvement with a family can and should continue past school age where the need arises.

THE PATTERN OF VISITING

Each health authority has a responsibility to inform the health visitor of any new births, and each baby is the responsibility of a health visitor even if the child is not registered with a doctor.

The first visit to a family usually occurs on the 10th–14th day following delivery, and may overlap with the midwife's visit. Close liaison is needed here to prevent any undue pressure upon the family. The health visitor has no statutory right of entry and it is only the health visitor *service* that is required by statute. Her visits to a family are largely determined by their needs and her own ability to meet them. The demands of a high case load, unfortunately may also control the frequency of home visiting. Recommended case loads have been discussed in the past but they still vary considerably from area to area. Regular routine visiting following this first visit is important as a mother is more likely to turn to someone she has seen regularly for help and guidance (Council for the Education and Training of Health Visitors (CETHV) 1977). It is reassuring to know the health visitor will visit at times of 'non-crisis as well as crisis'.

The birth notification is usually a computer-printed card and the information recorded varies from area to area. Standardization of this information would be desirable to provide a more efficient system of record keeping.

A national child health system has been designed and made available since 1977, but only 60 per cent of districts actually use this system. At present, committee meetings are held routinely to advise on content, design, and development of such a system.

The details given usually include:

(i) Surname
(ii) Date and place of birth
(iii) Sex
(iv) Birth weight
(v) General practitioner

Additional information may be received from the general practitioner, midwife or social worker. The health visitor must rely upon her own knowledge of the family to complete the picture. Any congenital abnormalities, handicap, or special problems may be recorded but this is not always the case. Close liaison with all workers will prevent and distressing visit to the home. This mistake can be detrimental to any relationship the health visitor may have with the family.

THE PRIMARY VISIT

This visit is an important one for the health visitor and one she enjoys. It is a high priority visit (Health Visitors Association (HVA) 1975) that requires time and consideration. Good preparation before a visit will ensure that she is aware of the current situation within the home.

The objectives of a primary visit can be described thus:

(i)   For the health visitor to introduce herself, explain her role, and establish a basic working relationship (this may already have been carried out during the ante-natal period).

(ii)   To generally examine the condition of the baby.

(iii) To assess social and environmental conditions.

(iv)   To identify attitudes within the family.

(v)   To advise generally on services available locally.

(vi)   To assess the emotional, mental, physical and social needs of the family.

(vii) To assess the mother's ability to manage and advise if necessary.

(viii) To discuss feeding.

(ix)   To give a card with all the applicable information.

Hopefully, she may be able to carry out all of these objectives at the primary visit, but it is important that they are achieved within the next few weeks.

Following the primary visit, subsequent visits are made to the home as a matter of routine, or at the request of the mother. Mothers are encouraged to contact their health visitor if they become anxious or unsure, and no problem is considered too small or trivial. The professional should not only give advice, but work with the mother to meet both her needs and those of her baby. As with all members of the team the health visitor should be aware of her limitations and refer to appropriate agencies where necessary.

The most frequent problems arising during those first few weeks relate to feeding. It is in this area that the health visitor comes into her own. She is the one with the expertise and it is important that other members of the team realize this! Once again an agreed approach to feeding is desirable, without forgetting the individual needs of the mother and baby. Frequently, a feeding problem is masking some other underlying worry and the health visitor should be able to identify this.

The method of feeding chosen is determined by several factors: age, social class, social pressure among them (Newson and Newson 1965). Increased media coverage of the advantages of breast-feeding has led to a growing trend towards it being the chosen method of feeding (Brimblecombe and Cullen 1977). Whatever method is chosen the professionals must support the mother and her family in these crucial first few weeks. The needs and demands of a breast-feeding mother and baby differ slightly from those of a bottle-fed child, and indeed a mother's expectations of the health visitor's role vary also. Breast-feeding mothers seem to have a more positive attitude to the postnatal role of the health visitor, particularly in the 8 weeks following delivery (Foxman *et al.* 1982). Certain problems and queries arising during this period are common to both groups of mothers and babies but it will be convenient to deal with them separately.

VISITING THE BREAST-FEEDING MOTHER AND BABY

The arrival of a first baby always constitutes a crisis point in the family (Hunt and Hilton 1975) and requires an adaptation to a new way of life. The confidence a new mother has in breast-feeding her baby is of the greatest importance. A mother who has successfully breast-fed a first child will be more likely to succeed in feeding the subsequent child (Cullen *et al.* 1978). The first-time breast-feeding mother will therefore need additional support and encouragement. Certain publications for 'the new parent' still exist to perpetuate the myth that the 'average, normal baby' feeds 4-hourly, and apart from being bathed and changed, sleeps for the rest of the day! It sometimes comes as a great shock to new parents to realize this may not be the case.

The most valuable function the health visitor can carry out is one of *listener*, and be able to interpret any fears or anxieties the mother may or may not express. Her advice must be sound, as problems may arise when certain explanations cause more confusion than clarification (Clayton, Clement, and Finch 1980).

Common complaints of breast-feeding mothers

'She doesn't sleep much, and she's always hungry'

The terms 'demand' or 'unrestricted' feeding do not mean that a baby will not cry. The fears a mother may have about her milk 'not being rich enough' or 'drying up' should be countered by positive advice and encouragement. These fears may mask an underlying lack of confidence in a mother's ability to care for her child and Cartwright (1979) has found evidence of 'nerves' or 'depression' in 45 per cent of women following discharge from the maternity ward. The most common reasons given for giving up breast-feeding in the first 6 weeks are fears of the baby being underfed, the poor quality of the milk, and the discontentment of the baby (Brimblecombe and Cullen 1977). The health visitor must offer positive advice, encouragement and support to help the mother regain her confidence. There are several ways she can do this:

(i)   Show the mother that her baby is thriving, that is, the general condition, weight gain.

(ii)   Introduce her to other breast feeding mothers; postnatal support groups can be invaluable at such times.

(iii)   Stress the normality of the situation and encourage her to play with and amuse her baby; help her to understand why her baby is crying.

The reduction of any anxiety the mother feels may in itself result in a peaceful solution.

'He wakes each evening, and cries until his last feed'

Often, to be forewarned is to be forearmed and the primary or subsequent visit may be an ideal time to mention this 'common' pattern of behaviour in a young baby. It is important to listen to the problem and ascertain what the 'problem' really is, by asking a few questions:

(i)   What is he like for the rest of the day?

(ii)   When do you prepare the family meal? (Usually this is a time of increased anxiety for the mother.)

(iii)   Does he settle well at other times?

To show concern and interest and reassure the mother that she is not being 'silly' is important. Asking questions may underline this approach.

Whatever advice and guidance the health visitor offers the family with a new baby, it is given with due regard for the emotional and financial standing of that particular family. She can offer suggestions to help or improve the situation but she is never dictatorial. This would only ensure the families' lack of cooperation. She has to strike a happy balance between friend and professional. Some mothers welcome advice on management and in some way, using her skills, the health visitor can persuade a mother to rest and maintain a reasonable diet. Practical help may be the answer in some cases and the health visitor may be able to help here, for example, organizing a home-help (each area varies with availability).

Certain suggestions may be appropriate:

(i)   Prepare the meal earlier; eat a cold meal; eat earlier in the day?

(ii)   Does the baby enjoy a ride in the pram? Go for a walk or perhaps a car journey (only recommended in the summer months!)

(iii) Bath him in the evenings; if he is going to cry, it is always less traumatic for the parents to cope with a baby crying in the bath than for no apparent reason.

(iv) If he wants to suckle, let him as he may require comfort.

A health visitor must retain her sense of reason as well as humour, because invariably the next-door neighbour provides the solution.

'My nipples are sore, and he is becoming very restless'
The mother who manages well in hospital with constant midwifery support may have problems at home. It may be helpful to observe a feed at home and ensure the baby is 'fixing' correctly. She should not feel that another expertise would not be relevant and may call for support from the midwife, or a breast-feeding counsellor if appropriate.

'He's not gaining enough weight'
The obsession with weight gain seems to be lessening and it is interesting to note that Cullen found that breast-fed babies do not gain weight at the same rate as bottle-fed babies if fed on a 4-hourly regime (Cullen *et al.* 1978). However, monitoring is important during this period and the result is to strike a happy balance between concern and reassurance. A detailed history of the feeding pattern should be noted and any concern or significant weight loss be referred to the general practitioner. An explanation of 'average weight gain', the range of 'normality' and the possibility of 'growth spurts' may be appropriate at this stage. Relatives and friends seem to be preoccupied with the child's weight gain and the professional can support the mother and her method of feeding, if this causes concern.

'I'm very tired, and my husband feels he cannot help'
There are several factors to consider here, and it is important that the health visitor does not cause any antagonism between the two partners. The father's role within the family is dependent upon several factors, social class and local cultural patterns being two of them. The health visitor must assess the needs of each family and offer advice accordingly. Contact with the father antenatally will certainly help her to give the best guidance to the family. She should stress the need for rest, and a good diet. Her partner may feel unable to help and practical advice of ways to help may be useful. He may be able to give a feed of expressed breast milk if this is acceptable. If, however, they decide to discontinue breast-feeding, no guilt should be attached to their decision. Advice and supervision should then be offered to enable a smooth transition to an alternative method of feeding.

'He keeps being sick, and I can't bring his wind up'
Paediatrician Hugh Jolly (1977) marvels at the preoccupation we have for 'winding' babies in this country. A baby will usually pass the wind out of his

body in one form or another! This can be a real concern to a mother and practical advice on the positioning of the baby following feeds may help. A posseting baby can be very distressing, as well as antisocial, and a mother needs a tremendous amount of reassurance if her baby develops this habit. Once again, constant reassurance of 'normal' progress is desirable. The new mother, particularly, is more susceptible to advice from friends and relatives. Mixtures of homemade and purchased medication may be given to alleviate the 'problem'. A knowledge of local customs may prove useful. The health visitor must use her personality and professionalism to great advantage here.

'His stools are loose' or 'He hasn't had a dirty nappy for two days'

Bowel habits seem to feature prominently in discussions during the first few weeks. Descriptions of content, colour, and consistency are numerous! Once again the health visitor must stress the normality of the condition and any aperients or medication must be discouraged. She may find it helpful to see a specimen or advise the mother to see her general practitioner.

'When will he drop his night feed?'

The health visitor knows there is no answer to this type of question but conversely some women have been shown to require firm advice (Foxman *et al.* 1982). The statement above is usually prompted by a comparison with another baby. The health visitor needs all her skills as counsellor and adviser to reassure the mother that the pattern is 'normal' and she is managing well.

Most common problems encountered in the postnatal period can be discussed antenatally; the value of home visits to the mother and baby is immense (Bax, Hart, and Jenkins 1980). A survey carried out in 1982 to test 'consumer satisfaction' of the service found that 56 per cent of breast-feeding mothers and 44 per cent of bottle-feeding mothers found home visiting valuable (Foxman *et al.* 1982).

VISITING A BOTTLE-FEEDING MOTHER AND BABY

The number of routine home visits to a mother who is bottle-feeding her child should not be any less than to breast-feeding mothers. The choice of this method may be due to past experience or an unsuccessful attempt to breast-feed (Cullen *et al.* 1978). A mother may experience guilt feelings if she feels she has 'failed' in some way. This is associated with the erroneous methods commonly used by lower social classes and also faulty utilization of western methods of feeding by Asian and other immigrant families.

Special attention must be given to ensure that feeds are made up correctly and equipment has been effectively sterilized (Taitz 1971). The habit of thickening a feed and adding one scoop 'for the pot' is still prevalent. It may be appropriate here to discuss the danger of 'assuming everything is fine'. Appearances may be misleading and the health visitor cannot assume that feeds are made up correctly, or that sterilizing is efficient. Many people are still illiterate or do not understand sufficient English, so leaflets and instructions on boxes are of no help. Once again close liaison with colleagues may prevent any assumptions being made and the problem can be handled sympathetically.

The introduction of modified milks following recommendation in 1974 (DHSS 1974), has resulted in a greater increase in the incidence of green stools. Careful advice must be given to explain that 'green does not mean danger' (Jolly 1977). A healthy contented baby is a perfect example that all is well. However, some parents may need to have additional support from the general practitioner.

Common complaints of bottle-feeding mothers

'He is constipated'

Very often what is considered to be constipated by parents is not; careful questioning may show that infrequent stools are the concern. General advice may be offered regarding additional fluids. This may provide an opportunity to dissuade the use of sweet additives.

'She's very sick, and seems colicky'

The nature of the sickness really must be discussed before anything else. If the health visitor has observed a feed in the home and remains worried, she should contact the general practitioner. If the problem lies with the way the child is being fed, this may easily be dealt with, in other words, change of teat, position of baby during and after feeds. The constant concern for bottle-feeding mothers is that a change of milk may result in a more settled baby. The health visitor can only discourage this but it is better to offer advice than to forbid such action as it could only result in secrecy and mistrust.

The pattern of health visiting depends upon numerous factors. Each area, town, and street has its own characteristics and customs. The health visitor has her training and knowledge as a basis for all her visits, but she cannot have rigid rules, when visiting the families. Each family's needs are different, as are their expectations. In the first 6 weeks following delivery feeding seems to be the main topic of conversation. Each query is dealt with individually with regard to the needs of that family. Common feeding problems, however, all too frequently mask some underlying problem. The health visitor can try to establish the real need of the family and act accordingly. She may need to refer to her colleagues for advice and guidance, and may decide to refer to the appropriate agency.

COMMON MINOR PROBLEMS

Besides being physically accessible it is also important the health visitor be approachable (Foxman *et al*. 1982). A home visit provides a relaxed and informal setting in which the mother can ask any questions about which she feels anxious. There is a danger, however, that the parents may become totally reliant on the advice and guidance of others. The health visitor should endeavour to develop the parents' own confidence and help the family to become self-reliant in decisions concerning the care and management of their child.

Parents and mothers in particular are bombarded by high-pressure advertising on television and in the press. To a certain extent, their own peer group also presents certain pressures. They believe their baby should look and behave in a certain way. They are also encouraged to use certain brands of baby goods otherwise they may be 'failing as a parent'. Financial pressures notwithstanding, it can be a tremendous strain on a family. The health visitor should be aware of this. This pressure is also present in popular medications for certain common minor ailments and up-to-date knowledge of new products really is essential.

The most common areas of concern are as follows.

Sticky eyes

A discharge may be present in the first few weeks after discharge. It may be helpful to explain the cause, when appropriate, if it is a blocked tear duct and to recommend expressing the lacrimal sac (Modell and Boyd 1982). Bathing and hygiene can be discussed and the general practitioner informed if necessary.

Colds and blocked noses

Problems usually arise when the baby cannot feed efficiently. Central heating tends to give a dry atmosphere in the home and humid conditions may relieve the condition. The use of baby 'cotton buds' is *strongly discouraged* to clear noses and ears. Any concern should be referred to the general practitioner.

Heat rash

A baby is rarely kept at a temperature below the 18°C (65°F) recommended by all baby books. The new parents are usually more anxious to keep him warm and may go to great lengths to cover him with warm clothes and blankets! General advice and guidance on the suitability of fabrics and amount of clothing is usually helpful.

Nappy rash

Bottle-fed babies are more likely to have a nappy rash because of their alkaline stools. This can be a very emotive subject as it can be equated with cleanliness and general care of the baby. It must be dealt with sympathetically.

The way a nappy is washed is important and this will need to be discussed. Automatic washing machines and the practice of adding 'perfumed softness' may have added to the incidence of nappy rash. Frequent changing, the use of barrier creams and the advantages of exposing the area to the air should all be mentioned. The increased use of disposable nappies may help the problem as they need to be changed more frequently than the more absorbant counterparts. However, the cost of this item may be prohibitive to many families. Any infection should be referred to the general practitioner for advice, as thrush infections are particularly related to bottle-fed babies (Cullinan and Treuherz 1981).

INTRODUCTION OF SOLIDS

There is still a tendency for mothers to introduce solids at too early an age. They should be discouraged until the child reaches 4 months as recommended by the HMSO report on infant feeding (DHSS 1974).

Once again rigid rules cannot be applied easily. The health visitor must use discretion in this area. A mother may be discouraged from introducing solids under 4 months but it may be necessary to advise a more acceptable cereal if she intends to introduce a highly undesirable one anyway.

DEVELOPMENT

Parents are anxious to know when a baby smiles, can see, can recognize his mother. Encouragement and reassurance can be given to help with the bonding process and to reassure them they can do all of those things (MacFarlane 1980). It has been useful in some antenatal programmes, as well as in schools, to discuss the achievements of a young baby. To show parents that babies can see, hear and respond to them in the first week of life can be rewarding.

SKIN CARE

Dry and peeling skin may cause some concern to parents and general advice on the use of creams and oils may be helpful. 'Cradle cap' can be avoided by advice on the use of shampoos and soaps. A family with a history of eczema may be advised on diet and particularly encouraged to breast-feed.

POSTNATAL ADVICE FOR THE MOTHER

The mother may seek advice for herself in the postnatal period. The health visitor can ensure that all mothers are aware of the postnatal care they would follow. Advice on *family planning* and *postnatal exercises* are vital. The mother may want to discuss various methods of contraception and their suitability. This means a knowledge of services available in the area and a good liaison with other workers, in other words, obstetric physiotherapists, family planning clinics, general practitioner services etc.

SUPPORT FOR THE MOTHER

The image of the family group has changed and more young couples move away from their families and start life as parents in a new neighbourhood. A new mother may feel isolated, as she loses the social contacts of work and lacks the company of other adults during the day. Motherhood is portrayed as a fulfilling role and great store is put on the mother–child relationship. Blurton-Jones (1974) has suggested that 'maternal behaviour is improved, by contact with other adults'. In the early weeks following the baby's birth the mother feels increasing strain and responsibility and this may be highlighted if she has a crying, fretful child. Her apprehension about feeding and general care of the child may be increased. Brown (1978) found that one-quarter of women with young children in London suffered from depression.

Other mothers may remain in close contact with parents and friends. This pattern can be reflected in social class, age and culture. The mother's dependence upon her own mother may be essential to the family. The health visitor must be aware of the importance of such support and give advice and guidance accordingly.

Home visiting may help a depressed mother or it may require help from other professionals. A health visitor should be aware of the signs of increasing anxiety and depression within a family and take appropriate action where necessary. Health visitors are in an ideal position to help an isolated or anxious mother as they know the facilities available in their area. Help can take several forms and it is important to stress the 'normality' of such support groups. They do not suit everyone's needs and no pressure should be applied suggesting such groups.

Postnatal support groups
These may be locally run groups of mothers. They may offer a relaxed setting where mothers of very young children can meet and get to know each other. The National Childbirth Trust and La Leche League form such groups nationwide and give particular help and support to breast-feeding mothers.

Mother and toddler groups

These may be a group of mothers with young children who meet for coffee on a regular basis, or they may be run by a health visitor at a health centre and may provide certain relevant health education input, with guest speakers, etc.

Child health clinics

The first place mothers are likely to meet is at the clinic and mothers of young babies can gain much from seeing others at different stages and hearing of the kind of 'problems' that may arise later.

A crying baby service

Health visitors are ever aware that they have an important part to play in crisis intervention (CETHV 1977) and a persistently crying baby can create anxiety and stress in new parents. An on-call system has been devised in several areas (Huddersfield in Yorkshire and Kingston and Richmond in Surrey) and has proved to be of invaluable support to anxious parents (Beech 1981; Greenwood 1979).

SPECIAL GROUPS

It has been stated previously that identification of high-risk groups at an early stage is desirable. A single parent, an unwanted pregnancy, poor housing conditions are all factors that contribute to possible problems once the baby has arrived. The needs of these families are multiple and they may require the additional support of a social worker and other agencies. The health visitor will need to resist the temptation to 'fulfil all the necessary roles herself' (Owen 1977).

In Bradford, social workers have shown that child abuse can be reduced by spotting high-risk groups at an early stage. The health visitor will be one of several people visiting such a family and the importance of good liaison is obvious. Her 'normal' visiting pattern to a mother and baby will still be followed.

Those with obvious problems are not the only group needing special attention. The middle classes have the less obvious problems of high mortgages, high pressure at work, and a standard of living they wish to maintain. They are as susceptible as the other more obvious groups and it may prove more difficult to expose the problem and then offer help. A 'team effort' with such families can aid the family as well as support each team member. This type of visiting can be very stressful and the needs of the health visitor and her colleagues should not be ignored.

Parents needing special attention by the health visitor, particularly during those first few weeks are those with a handicapped child. The parents' reaction to a handicapped child may be unexpected and difficult to assess. The health visitor must use all her skills to help the parents wherever possible. In such a case, antenatal contact is such a help. These may be practical advice on feeding and general management to discuss. It is essential the health visitor acquire some knowledge of the condition to be aware of 'the limits of her own knowledge'. Special support groups may be appropriate and she may contact them on behalf of the parents, if they so wish. Home visiting should provide the help by parents both emotionally and on a practical level.

A tragic group of parents that may need the health visitor's support are those whose baby dies within the first weeks of life. Emery (1981) has researched the role of the health visitor in such cases and sees her role as being one to provide practical advice and emotional support. Follow-up visits to such a family are invaluable.

Parents whose child is in a special care unit may appreciate contact from the health visitor. The mother will be feeling distinct lack of identity. Hospitals are well aware of the problems of early bonding in such cases, and welcome the mothers into the units. A health visitor should show concern and interest for the child and be able to share the information with the mother. This can only help the relationship between mother and her health visitor when she returns home.

In conclusion, the health visitor as 'key figure in the preventive services' (Court 1976) is in a unique position to observe all mothers and their babies at home. She can make assessments of parental skills in mothering and mothercraft, and be aware of possible crisis situations. Good health visiting is based upon the professional understanding of the needs of the mother and her baby.

REFERENCES

Bax, M., Hart, H., and Jenkins, S. (1980). *The health needs of the pre-school child.* Thomas Conran Research Unit, London.

Beech, C. P. (1981). A new service for parents with crying babies. (Kingston and Richmond AHA). *Nursing Times* 77, 245–6.

Blurton-Jones, N. G. (1974). *Biological perspectives on parenthood. The family in society.* HMSO, London.

Brimblecombe, F. S. W. and Cullen, D. (1977). Influence on a mother's choice of method of infant feeding. *Public Health* 91, 117–26.

Brown, G. W. (1978). *Depression. A sociological view. Basic readings in medical sociology.* (eds. D. Tuckett and J. M. Kaufert) Tavistock Publications, London.

Cartwright, A. (1979). *The dignity of labour, a study of child bearing and induction.* Tavistock Publications, London.

Clayton, S., Clement, J., and Finch, J. (1979). Breast feeding: time for subtle changes. *Nursing Mirror* 148(22), 18–20.

Clayton, S., Clement, J., and Finch, J. (1980). Response and initiative: breast feeding in the community *Midwives Chron.* 93, 272–5.

Court, S. D. M. (Chairman) (1976). *Fit for the future*. Report on Committee on Child Health Service. HMSO, London.

Council for the Education and Training of Health Visitors (CETHV) (1977). *An investigation into the principles of health visiting*. CETHV, London.

Cullen, P., Milan, P., Raginski, C., and Waterhouse, J. (1978). Are breast fed babies still getting a raw deal in hospital? *Br. Med. J.* 851–93.

Cullinan, T. R. and Treuherz, J. (1981). *Born in East London 1979–1980*. Department of Environmental and Preventive Medicine, St Bartholomews Hospital. G. W. Beamond and Son, London.

DHSS (1974). *Present day practice in infant feeding*. HMSO, London.

Emery, J. L. (1981). Cot deaths: the current situation of role of the health visitor today. *Health Visitor* **54**, 318–20.

Foxman, E. *et al.* (1982). A consumer view of the health visitor at 6 weeks post partum. *Health Visitor* **302**, 304–6, 308.

Greenwood, G. (1979). A cry in the night and help is immediate. *Nursing Mirror* **148**, 24–7.

Health Visitors Association (HVA) (1975). Health visiting in the seventies. *Health Visitor* **48**.

Health Visitors Association (HVA) (1979). *Feeding children in the first year*. B. Edsall and Co. Ltd., London.

Hunt, S. and Hilton, J. (1975). *Individual development and social experience*. George Allen and Unwin, London.

HMSO (1972). *The report of the committee on nursing*. (Cmnd 5115) HMSO, London.

Jolly, H. (1977). *Book of child care*. Sphere Books, London.

MacFarlane, J. A. (1980). *Child health*. Grant McIntyre, London.

Modell, M. and Boyd, R. (1982). *Paediatric problems in general practice*. OUP.

Newson, J. and Newson, E. (1965). *Patterns of infant care*. Pelican, Harmondsworth.

Owen, G. M. (1977). *Health visiting*. Baillière Tindall, London.

Taitz, L. S. (1971). *Br. Med. J.*, 315–16.

Welsh Health Technical Services Organization (1979). *Child health system*. Cardiff.

FURTHER READING

Gilmore,M. *et al.* (1974). *The work of the nursing team in general practice*. CETHV, London.

The Black Report (1980). *Inequalities in health* (eds. P. Townsend and N. Davidson). Penguin, Harmondsworth.

27 The final postnatal examination

D. C. Morrell

This chapter is concerned with examining the content of the postnatal examination and the ways in which it may contribute to the continuing care of a young family.

In a survey of postnatal care in Hertfordshire (Cranfield 1983) reported that 96 per cent of mothers received a postnatal examination about 6 weeks after delivery, the vast majority of these being carried out by the general practitioner. The fact that such a high proportion of mothers took advantage of this service indicates that, to the mothers at least, it is seen as an important event. Where the postnatal examination is arranged at the hospital as opposed to the general practice, there is evidence that the response rate is lower (Zander *et al.* 1978). This is not surprising as it is very much easier for a mother to visit her general practitioner, whose surgery is usually close to her home, who is likely to provide facilities for her pram and to encourage the attendance of accompanying siblings, where waiting is likely to be minimal and where other members of the primary care team are usually in attendance. When the doctor has played a full part in preparing the mother during pregnancy for delivery, she will also see the postnatal examination as relevant to the continuing medical care of her growing family.

Even with proper prenatal advice however, some mothers fail to attend for a postnatal examination. Very often these are the patients with inadequate family and community support who are most in need of counselling at this time. Fortunately, in general practice the attached midwife and health visitor will often have identified these patients in advance and through their continuing relationship with them will be able to persuade them to attend. In a few patients, particularly those with a large number of small children, a home visit by the doctor may be desirable and may prevent further unwanted pregnancies and nutritional problems which some of these mothers experience.

REVIEWING AN IMPORTANT EVENT

It is easy for doctors to underestimate the importance of childbirth to the family. The creation of a new individual by parents is probably the most momentous event in their lives. At the same time, it is an event which can make or break the relationship between husband and wife. The general practitioner must try to ensure that childbirth positively contributes to the loving relationship between husband and wife and establishes a firm base from which the new family can develop. The doctor's role in the case of second or subsequent births will differ in some ways from his role for the firstborn, but is nonetheless important.

The first objective of the postnatal visit should therefore be to review with the mother her experiences in pregnancy, labour, and the immediate postnatal period. Hopefully this will have been happy and she will be able to share this with the doctor. On some occasions the happiness will have been marred by anxiety, unsympathetic care, or physical trauma. In such cases the mother should be encouraged to describe her experiences and to try to put them in perspective in relation to her achievement in producing a healthy infant. If there is any bitterness towards her medical attendants it should be explored and, where possible, explained so that she can look back more positively to her experience. Enquiry should extend to her husband's experiences of pregnancy and labour, the contribution he did or did not make and his role in the immediate postnatal period. This is indeed the beginning of preconception counselling for the next pregnancy, for it is an ideal opportunity for the parents to identify shortcomings in the recent pregnancy and delivery which may be remedied in the future (see Chapter 4).

At the same time as the mother's subjective impressions are reviewed, the doctor should also review objectively the medical record. Did she suffer from urinary tract infection during the pregnancy or pre-eclamptic toxaemia or anaemia? Was she immune to rubella, and if not has she been immunized in hospital? Was there evidence of rhesus incompatibility and has this been managed appropriately?

A few minutes of relaxed discussion at the beginning of the postnatal visit will also usually indicate how the patient is responding to her new role as mother, how this is influencing her relationship with her husband, and in the case of a second or subsequent pregnancy, how the children are responding to the new competition for maternal attention.

A REVIEW OF PHYSICAL SYMPTOMS

Pregnancy and labour are demanding physical experiences and it is important to establish at the postnatal visit that the mother is functioning physically at a normal level. In general terms, how does she feel? Is she energetic, vivacious, and enjoying her new baby? Is she sleeping well, and if not is this due to nights disturbed by her baby or is she experiencing a sleep disturbance which might suggest a depressive illness? Specific questions should be asked about her bowel and bladder function and in particular, whether or not she wets herself if she laughs or coughs. If she is breast-feeding she will almost certainly not have had a period since delivery, but does she have any persistent bleeding or discharge? If she is not breast-feeding, she may have had a period and enquiry will be made as to its character and the presence of any other vaginal discharge. It is important to determine if she has any persistent perineal discomfort, and if she has had intercourse, whether this was comfortable. She should be encouraged to talk about her sexual feelings since the birth of the baby and her attitude to resuming sexual intercourse and it is important to ascertain her husband's attitude.

If the mother is breast-feeding she will be asked about her perceptions of this. Does she enjoy it, has she any breast discomfort or problems with her nipples? Does the baby enjoy it and appear satisfied? How is it affecting her domestic and social life? In the context of the primary care team, good communications between doctor and health visitor will often have drawn attention in advance of the postnatal consultation to any special problems that should be explored at this time.

THE PHYSICAL EXAMINATION

This is usually much less important than the opportunity which the postnatal visit presents for an assessment of the impact of childbirth on the mother's perception of herself, her baby and her relationships in the family. To the mother it is, however, an important ritual at the end of which she can hopefully be reassured that all has returned physically to her prepregnancy state. The mother should be weighed, blood pressure recorded, and if there has been excessive blood loss in labour or if she comes from a deprived background, the haemoglobin measured. Examination of the abdomen affords an opportunity to congratulate her on a return of normal abdominal musculature or encourage her to persist in carrying out abdominal exercises. The vulva is inspected and palpated to ensure that there are no areas of tenderness. A vaginal examination confirms that two fingers can comfortably be accommodated. A speculum examination is then carried out to inspect the cervix to exclude any tears or identify a cervical erosion as a possible cause of persistent abnormal discharge. If a cervical smear has not been carried out in the preceding 3 years, this may be undertaken at this time and an excessive discharge should prompt the doctor to take a high vaginal swab. The uterus is then palpated to ensure that it is returning to normal size and there is no tenderness in the fornices.

A REVIEW OF THE PHYSICAL STATUS

Following the physical examination, the mother should return to the consulting room where the doctor can review his findings. In the vast majority of cases he will be able to reassure her that she has returned to normal. In the minority, abnormalities may have been detected which merit specific advice.

Persistent hypertension

A very small number of mothers who have suffered from toxaemia of pregnancy will be found postnatally to have a raised blood pressure. They should be told about this finding but reassured that it will almost certainly return to normal and be asked to return for a check in 3 months' time. Very rarely the hypertension will persist and at 3 months further investigation by urinalysis, renal function tests and possibly an intravenous pyleogram may be desirable. Persisting mild hypertension in the absence of any evidence of renal disease should be reviewed at annual intervals. If there is any evidence of renal functional impairment, reference to a specialist is indicated.

Excessive weight gain

This is a more common problem and the postnatal visit presents an opportunity for the doctor to counsel his patient about this. The patient should be invited to discuss the cosmetic and medical problems which may arise from excessive weight and she should be encouraged to seek dietetic advice. The doctor should take a very positive stance in regard to this problem because many women accept a weight gain of 1 or 2 stone (6 or 12 kg) as an inevitable result of childbearing and spend the rest of their lives regretting this disfigurement. The importance of exercise may be stressed to both parents and it should be pointed out to them that this is no time to 'hang up their boots' but they should rather be preparing for the new demands which will be made upon them by their new offspring.

Stress incontincence

A few women experience this disturbing symptom following childbirth and may be shy to complain about it; this is why mothers should always be specifically questioned about it. In most cases it will respond to perineal exercises which the general practitioner can prescribe, but in the rare case which fails to respond, early referral to a gynaecologist is desirable.

Perineal tenderness

Scar tissue formed during healing from an episiotomy or perineal tear in labour may remain tender for some time after delivery. This may then cause dyspareunia. In most cases the tenderness will disappear if a little more time is allowed for healing and the patient should be advised to postpone resuming intercourse until it is comfortable. This is important because persisting with painful intercourse may lead to vaginismus which may then be difficult to cure. Gentle stretching of the scar tissue by the patient herself and the use of a lubricant, such as KY jelly when intercourse is resumed will lead to resolution of the problem in most cases. It is sometimes helpful for the doctor to see husband and wife together when this problem arises and he should always arrange a follow-up visit 4–6 weeks later to ensure that all has returned to normal.

Fissure in ano

This may rarely complicate delivery and persist into the postnatal period. In most cases the fissure will heal spontaneously if the bowels are kept regular and well lubricated by taking Emulsion of Liquid Paraffin 10 ml each night and applying a simple lubricant to the anus before defecation. If spontaneous healing does not occur, surgical treatment will be necessary.

Haemorrhoids

These quite commonly develop during pregnancy and may be troublesome. They almost always settle down spontaneously in the puerperium and use of a high-fibre diet may be helpful in ensuring this.

Uterine abnormalities

A retroverted uterus is quite commonly found at the postnatal examination, which 20 years ago was treated by antiversion and introduction of a Hodge pessary. Retroversion is now accepted as a normal variation and no treatment is required.

Problems due to retained products of conception usually present within the first 3 weeks of delivery as secondary postpartum haemorrhage (PPH) with or without pelvic pain, uterine tenderness, and fever. If these have been dealt with expeditiously the uterus should be returning to normal by the postnatal visit. In such cases it is well to ensure that this is so and that there is no tenderness on manipulating the uterus or in the fornices.

Cervical erosion

A large proportion of patients are found to have a cervical erosion 6 weeks after delivery. Most of these heal spontaneously without producing symptoms. If symptoms in the form of an excessive discharge are present, it is usually sufficient to explain the cause, reassure the patient and review the situation 4–6 weeks later. If the symptoms continue at 3 months, then cauterization of the cervix using a cryocautery or electric cautery is within the competence of the general practitioner and a painless procedure.

Urinary tract infection

If there has been evidence of urinary tract infection in pregnancy, a midstream specimen of urine (MSU) should be collected and sent to the laboratory to ensure that the infection has resolved.

Follow-up

Where important abnormalities are identified at the postnatal examination or laboratory tests are conducted, it is important to ensure that these are followed up. The patient should be asked to make a future appointment with the doctor or the practice nurse to ascertain that any abnormality has resolved and any abnormal laboratory test has been adequately treated.

REVIEW OF RELATIONSHIPS

The postnatal visit provides an opportunity for the doctor to review with the patient the way in which the arrival of the new baby is influencing the relationships within the family. Although husbands are becoming increasingly involved in pregnancy and childbirth, it is still fairly common to encounter situations where the new baby is absorbing all the mother's time and affection to the exclusion of her husband. This can lead to animosity which is very destructive of family life. As in most marital problems, prevention is easier than cure and if difficulties are occurring they should be fully discussed if possible, by bringing the husband into the consultation. Sometimes the new mother may experience a loss of libido during the postnatal period and this may lead to suspicion and jealousy in the husband which can be resolved by explanation from the doctor.

Good antenatal care providing the patient with plenty of time for discussion will anticipate many of the potential problems in the postnatal period and good team work between midwife, health visitor and general practitioner should ensure that they are dealt with if they arise. Psychological problems in the puerperium are described in more detail in Chapter 29.

THE NEONATE

Some doctors like to carry out the 6-week examination of the neonate at the same time as the postnatal consultation. Others prefer to conduct this on a separate occasion during a well-baby clinic. The detailed care of the new baby is discussed elsewhere in Chapter 28. The postnatal consultation does however, offer opportunities to talk to the mother about the effect of environment on the new baby's development in terms of parental relationships, sibling rivalry and such physical factors as parental smoking habits.

FAMILY PLANNING

Some patients start taking a progestogen-only contraceptive within a week or two of delivery, but many prefer to refrain from taking pills and intercourse until after the postnatal visit. This visit then provides the opportunity to discuss family planning and provide appropriate care. Most patients who are breast-feeding at 6 weeks can commence taking low oestrogen combined contraceptives without interfering with the flow of breast milk. Some however, may prefer to use a progestogen-only pill. Patients who wish to use rhythm methods of family planning such as the 'mucothermal' method will need to use some other precautions until at least three normal menstrual cycles have occurred. In such cases a barrier method is best as it will not interfere with the return of natural cycles. Some mothers still believe that breast-feeding protects them from further pregnancy. Although a mother fully breast-feeding her first child is very unlikely to become pregnant during the first 3 months, this cannot be completely depended upon.

CONCLUSIONS

Enthusiasm for a 6-week postnatal examination has diminished among doctors in recent years although, as has been demonstrated in Cranfield's (1983) survey, it is still popular among mothers. For the general practitioner it presents an excellent opportunity to review an important life event and open a new chapter in the care of the family. The chance to provide health education and preventive care is probably more important than the physical aspects of the consultation.

Antenatal and postnatal care form an integral part of the continuing care which a general practitioner provides for his patients. They are but part of the continuity of care represented by family planning, preconception counselling, well-baby care and family and sexual counselling. Most patients welcome this continuity in the context of a developing relationship between themselves, the doctor and other primary care professional staff, in which communication about the expectations and objectives of medical care can flourish. It is into this setting that the postnatal consultation fits so comfortably.

REFERENCES

Cranfield, F. C. (1983). Survey of postnatal care. *J. Roy. Soc. Med.* **76**, 41–4.
Zander, L. I., Watson, M., Taylor, R.W. and Morrell, D. C. (1978). Integration of general practitioner and specialist antenatal care. *J. Roy. Coll. Gen. Practit.* **28**, 455–8.

28 The neonate

S. R. Burne

CARE OF THE BABY DURING NORMAL BIRTH

Most deliveries which occur under the care of general practitioners will be normal in every respect, but during birth and the time immediately afterwards the infant should be carefully observed to detect the earliest sign of respiratory or circulatory difficulty and it should be remembered that even careful monitoring during labour may fail to give advance warning of birth asphyxia.

Physiology

Those attending a delivery should have an understanding of the normal processes involved in the transition from intrauterine to extrauterine life. A normal baby is likely to be born in a stage of primary apnoea (Table 28.1) during which he can respond to the sensory input of delivery by intermittent strong gasps. If these gasps succeed in expanding the lungs then normal spontaneous respiration will be established. Sometimes, due to asphyxia or delay in the second stage of labour the child will have already passed this stage by the time of delivery and reached terminal apnoea. In this case the child will be pale, hypotonic and unresponsive, he will not gasp spontaneously or in response to stimulation and he will have a bradycardia. Unless effective resuscitation is performed this state will lead to death (Davies *et al.* 1972).

Table 28.1 *Primary and terminal apnoea*

	Primary apnoea	*Terminal apnoea*
Colour	Cyanosed becoming pink	Pale
Tone	Normal	Floppy
Movements	Spontaneous and in response to stimuli	Lies still
Heart rate	Greater than 100 accelerating	Less than 100 decelerating
Respiration	Gasps spontaneously or in response to stimuli	Will not gasp

These respiratory adaptations are accompanied by profound cardiovascular changes in which cessation of placental blood flow and reduction in pulmonary vascular resistance result in functional closure of the foramen ovale and subsequent gradual closure of the ductus arteriosus.

Normal delivery

Immediately the baby's mouth and nose are clear of the perineum any blood or mucus should be gently wiped away with a cottonwool swab. In the absence of complicating factors such as asphyxia or maternal sedation most babies will gasp spontaneously and start breathing quietly as soon as the thorax has been released from constriction. Where the child has already established respiration nasopharyngeal aspiration is unnecessary, but it should be carried out if the child has not gasped by 30 seconds or where excess secretions are present. In primary apnoea gentle stimulation is usually sufficient to initiate gasping but a gentle flick on the sole of the foot, a stream of facial oxygen or use of the sucker may also result in reflex gasping.

The baby may be delivered quietly and smoothly on to his mother's abdomen at which stage many parents prefer to discover the sex of the child for themselves. During this process a rapid assessment of the baby will be made by the attendants to detect any indication for immediate intervention.

The baby should be covered with a warm dry wrap. If urgent resuscitation is required the cord should be divided between clamps without delay but otherwise it is reasonable to wait for a few moments after delivery while spontaneous cord pulsation dies down before the cord is divided. As soon as the immediate procedures surrounding delivery have been completed the baby may be put to the breast. Most mothers seem to find this a natural and enjoyable part of the delivery and early suckling is associated with a high success rate for subsequent breast-feeding.

After delivery a plastic cord clamp should be applied, and the baby will be labelled, cleaned, weighed and dressed.

The midwife should carry out these procedures in the presence of the mother. If the baby has to be taken to a separate nursery this should only be for essential activities following which it should be returned to its mother (Valman 1980).

Immediate assessment at birth

During delivery a careful assessment of the child's state should be made. This assessment need not cause any interference in the normal sequence of events which has already been described. A formal record of the child's condition should be made within the first minute of life. This may be as an Apgar score (Apgar 1953; Table 28.2) although some units have now discarded this, preferring to make a separate record of the various signs observed. In either case the purpose is to detect all babies in need of resuscitation (Table 28.3). It is also necessary to look at the child during the delivery to check for obvious congenital abnormalities which may require immediate care. This rapid assessment should be repeated 5 minutes after birth.

Table 28.2 *Apgar score for the newborn*

Apgar score	0	1	2
Appearance	central cyanosis or pallor	peripheral cyanosis	completely pink
Pulse	absent	below 100	above 100
Grimace (response to stimulation)	no response	grimace	cry or cough
Activity (muscle tone)	limp	some flexion in extremities	active movements
Respiration	absent	weak irregular	strong regular

Table 28.3 *Indications for resuscitation of the newborn*

Terminal apnoea
Thick meconium in liquor
Heart rate less than 100/minute (at any time)
Respirations not established by 1 minute

RESUSCITATION OF THE NEWBORN

An infant who is diagnosed as being in primary apnoea will normally respond to the simple methods of stimulation which have already been described. Failure to respond or presence of any of the indications for resuscitation listed in Table 28.3 means that the baby requires intubating in order to start intermittent positive pressure respiration (IPPR).

The infant is placed on his back with his head towards the examiner, the head is extended on the neck and a straight-bladed laryngoscope passed gently over the infant's tongue until the epiglottis comes into view. The tip of the laryngoscope can then gently lift the epiglottis bringing the slit-like glottis into view. Gentle external pressure on the cricoid cartilage by an assistant may help in case of difficulty. Any mucus should be aspirated under direct vision before a suitable-sized endotracheal tube is introduced. A fine tube should then be used to suck out the trachea down the endotracheal tube before this is connected to a source of oxygen when IPPR is applied at the rate of about 30/minute. The oxygen supply circuit must include a water manometer or pressure release valve which ensures that the pressure cannot exceed 30 cm of water. In domiciliary practice a supply of oxygen should normally be available but in case of emergency the doctor may apply IPPR using only the volume and pressure of air available from his cheeks.

The examiner should auscultate both lung fields to ensure that they are expanded and that the endotracheal tube has not been inserted into the stomach by mistake. If undue difficulty is experienced in intubating the child the lungs may be expanded using a well-fitting face mask and inflatable bag before a further attempt at intubation is made.

If a pulse is not detected or in case of profound bradycardia (less than 30/minute), external cardiac massage should be applied to the upper sternum with two fingers. A satisfactory response to resuscitation should be quickly apparent. The heart rate will accelerate, the colour and tone will improve and spontaneous respiration will become established. The endotracheal tube may then be removed but the baby should be kept under close observation until the doctor is fully satisfied that his condition is stable and satisfactory.

Meconium in the liquor

The presence of thick meconium in the liquor indicates fetal asphyxia prior to delivery and a paediatrician should be called to all such deliveries. In addition to the risks of asphyxia there is a considerable risk of respiratory problems (meconium aspiration syndrome) should the baby inhale meconium. For this reason such babies should have their pharynx carefully sucked out under direct vision followed by intubation in order to suck out the trachea before they are stimulated to breathe. After clearance of meconium these babies are likely to require reintubation with a clean tube and IPPR.

Maternal drugs

The baby's respiration may be depressed by drugs which have been administered during labour and this possibility should always be considered. If pethidine or morphine is thought to be responsible for respiratory depression then naloxone 10 μg/kg body weight should be administered intravenously or intramuscularly.

Hypothermia

All newborn babies are at risk of hypothermia but this risk is especially marked in the case of asphyxiated and low birth weight babies. The baby should be quickly and gently dabbed dry and wrapped in a warm dry blanket leaving only the minimum area exposed compatible with the needs of safe and effective resuscitation. Following resuscitation the rectal temperature should be checked.

Reassuring the parents

The parents will have been silent but anxious and frightened witnesses to these procedures. The needs of the baby will of course take immediate priority but it is usually possible to give a simple and very brief commentary on what is happening and how the baby is responding to resuscitation. Following resuscitation the baby should be given to his mother for a cuddle; this is usually possible even when the baby requires transfer to a special care baby unit. Attendants should also remember that the parents may wish to hold or see a stillborn baby or one who has died despite attempts at resuscitation.

In all cases the parents should be given a full explanation of the resuscitation and any further treatment that may be required. Usually the baby may remain with the mother and she should be told that babies often need help with their breathing at birth but that in itself this is not a cause of any continuing problem. Only in the case of prolonged or continuing failure to respond to resuscitation should the baby need to be transferred to a special care unit. If this is necessary the parents should be told the reasons, where the unit is situated and the arrangements for visiting the baby.

EXAMINATION OF THE NEWBORN

A newborn baby requires a full examination and assessment to detect any significant deviations from normality, to act as a baseline for future assessment, and to reassure the parents about the child's physical health. The examination usually takes only a few minutes. It should be undertaken by a doctor who has been appropriately trained. For women delivered in general practitioner care this will normally be the general practitioner obstetrician who has attended her although in some practices the baby will be seen by another partner who has special responsibility for child health. In the case of women delivered under consultant care and also where significant deviation from normal is detected by the general practitioner a specialist paediatrician will have this responsibility. The administrative arrangements of the maternity unit should be such that the parents are always able to be present to witness the examination and discuss the findings with the doctor immediately.

One fairly common routine is for the doctor to check the basic functions of the baby immediately after birth—colour, movement, heart, lungs, and orifices—and carry out a more systematic and comprehensive examination at about 5 or 6 days of life.

Examination of the newborn should follow an ordered sequence. It is convenient to start the examination with the baby's head and work gradually down the body finishing with the feet. This systematic examination should take place in a warm well-lit room. The child should have all clothes removed.

General observation

General observation forms an important part of the neonatal examination and should include the following:

Colour

The normal infant will have a healthy pink colour with possibly some slight peripheral cyanosis. Any pallor or central cyanosis which may have been present immediately after birth should have fully responded to the initial resuscitation and persistence of these signs is of considerable significance and should be further investigated. Jaundice is unlikely to be present at this examination, but if detected will always require referral. Assessment of a child's colour is always more difficult in a child of Asian or African origin when special attention will need to be paid to the colour of the mucous membranes (Tarnow-Mordi and Pickering 1983).

Tone and movement

Much information about the central nervous system may be obtained by general observation and the child's response to handling during examination. The child's tone may be conveniently assessed if the doctor removes the clothes himself and at the same time spontaneous symmetrical movements of the limbs should also be noted. Assessment of tone and motor activity depends greatly on the child's state of arousal; ideally the examination will be taking place while the child is awake but neither hungry nor overfull from a recent feed. This state may often occur an hour or two after delivery when both mother and child may be remarkably alert (MacFarlane 1977). A more detailed neurological examination including the various reflexes is an important part of detailed specialist assessment but adds little to the general initial examination. The examiner should always remember that both the limp, unresponsive, abnormally quiet child and the wide-eyed screaming, irritable one may have sustained damage to the central nervous system.

Birth trauma

Significant birth trauma may often be anticipated following a difficult instrumental delivery but a careful check should be made for any signs of trauma following every delivery.

Respiration

The child's respiration should be observed. The normal baby will be breathing quietly at a rate which should be below 60/minute and there will be no signs of respiratory difficulty such as rib retraction, flaring of the nostrils, or grunting.

Minor blemishes

There are a large number of possible superficial blemishes and abnormalities which may be noted during the general observation. The most common of these are discussed below.

The head and neck

The anatomy of the vault of the skull should be checked and the anterior and posterior fontanelles palpated. Separation of the cranial sutures or large fontanelles are not significant unless associated with increased tension of the anterior fontanelle. The head circumference should always be carefully recorded. Many babies seem to object to this procedure and it may conveniently be left as the final item in the examination.

Both eyes should be carefully examined and the red reflex elicited to exclude retinoblastoma or cataract. Many newborn babies will look at and follow a face and this should be demonstrated to the mother. Nose, ears and mouth should all be checked including a careful search for cleft palate by inspection inside the baby's mouth and gentle palpation of the palate with the little finger.

A caput succadeum may be present due to oedema of the presenting part, this is likely to be especially marked after prolonged labour. The parents should be reassured that this will resolve within 48 hours.

Thorax

Careful auscultation of the heart for murmurs must be carried out but detailed auscultation of the lungs is unnecessary beyond checking that both lungs are expanded. Crepitations in the lung fields are quite common in healthy babies immediately after delivery and need cause no concern.

Abdomen

The abdomen should be carefully palpated for masses and enlarged viscera. The liver edge may be palpated just below the right costal margin, the lower poles of the kidneys may often be felt and the spleen is occasionally felt.

The umbilical cord should normally have three vessels and this will have been checked at delivery. A single umbilical artery may indicate associated internal malformations.

Limbs

Normal tone and movement of all four limbs will have been noted during the examination. If there is any asymmetry a careful search should be made for the cause. The number of fingers and toes should be consciously counted as it is easy to miss an extra digit. The palms of the hands should be checked for a transverse palmar crease. Minor degrees of talipes may be due to intrauterine posture; if the foot can be easily manipulated through a normal range of movement the parents can be reassured that the condition will resolve spontaneously, but if there is any restriction of movement an urgent orthopaedic opinion should be arranged as splinting will be necessary.

Hips and genital region

The external genitalia should be inspected. In a boy both testicles should be descended, a small hydrocele would be a normal finding. The penis should be checked for hypospadias or other abnormalities. In girls the labia should be gently separated to inspect the introitus and exclude an enlarged clitoris. A mucous discharge and sometimes slight vaginal bleeding are normal findings, which are due to maternal oestrogens. With the hips gently abducted the femoral pulses are palpated with the index fingers.

Examination of the hips to exclude congenital dislocation should not be omitted from the examination of any child under 1 year of age. With the knees fully flexed and the hips flexed to 90 degrees the upper thighs are gently grasped with the examiner's thumbs on the infants lesser trochanter and the index and middle fingers on the greater trochanter. Using the minimum of force and testing one side at a time the hip is first adducted and then gently abducted. A 'clunk' may be felt either by lifting the already dislocated femoral head gently forward into the acetabulum or by gentle pressure from the thumb on the lesser trochanter pressing the dislocatable femoral head over the posterior lip of the acetabulum. Asymmetrical skin creases in the groin and buttocks and limitation of abduction at the hip may support a diagnosis of congenital dislocation, but neither of these signs is necessary to make a diagnosis.

Spine

The child may now be turned over and a careful check of the full length of the spine made, starting at the base of the nose, going back over the occiput and finishing at the coccyx, in order to detect any minor dermal sinus or spina bifida which may not have been immediately apparent at birth. Inspection of the anal passage then completes the examination.

Consultation with the parents

At the end of the examination the doctor should share his findings with the parents and give them an opportunity to ask any questions or discuss any worries they may have. It is important to remember that doctors and midwives may accept as normal blemishes such as moulding, bruising, or small birth marks which may be a cause of extreme anxiety to the parents who will take the first available opportunity to perform their own careful examination of the baby. Any further investigations or treatment which may be needed should be explained to the parents. When significant deviation from normal has been detected in a baby of any age communication with the parents is of special importance. The earliest possible opportunity should be taken to give the parents an authoritative statement of the child's condition. Any explanation should be clear, honest and accurate and include some guide as to prognosis although it is important to avoid idle speculation. The information may need to be repeated several times if the parents have difficulty understanding the condition. It is important to avoid medical jargon and explain the meaning of any specialized terms which cannot be avoided. It is helpful if the nurse or midwife looking after the mother can be present during this discussion as she will often be questioned later about 'what the doctor said'. If the general practitioner is not already aware of the circumstances he should be informed by telephone.

Examination at 1 week

A full examination should be repeated at the end of the first week of life either in hospital or by the general practitioner at home. On this occasion the physical examination is unchanged but greater emphasis should be placed on the detection of infection especially on the skin, eyes or umbilicus. Prolonged jaundice should be excluded and further time will need to be given for discussion with the parents.

Both the initial and 1-week examinations form invaluable opportunities to discuss feeding patterns and encourage the initiation and continuation of breast feeding.

Genetic counselling

After the birth of a child with a congenital abnormality the parents are likely to become anxious about the risk of recurrence in any future pregnancy. This may be an immediate anxiety or it may not be expressed for a considerable length of time. In any case where this question may arise the parents should be informed of the availability of specialized genetic counselling services to which they may be referred in due course.

Examination at 6 weeks

As part of the routine care of infants a formal examination should be conducted at about 6 weeks of age. This is a convenient opportunity to repeat the basic physical examination very much as it has already been described. Attention should be paid to the child's nutrition, the most useful measure of this will be weight gain compared with that recorded at birth. It is advisable, if these measures are to mean anything, that they be recorded on a standard chart showing the ranges of normal.

Various aspects of the examination have enhanced importance at 6 weeks. The hips must be rechecked with care to detect any case of congenital dislocation which may not have been recognized at birth. Even when the heart has previously been found to be normal, examination of the cardiovascular system should be carried out with care as serious congenital abnormalities may manifest themselves during the first 6 weeks.

Observation and handling of the child is again of great importance. Attention should be paid to the movements and tone of all limbs, the head and neck and trunk.

By 6 weeks all babies should be smiling, should fix their gaze on a face and follow it and should respond to a quiet conversational voice. Absence of any of these responses is of great importance and should always call for more detailed assessment.

A fixed squint, if present, would require early referral to an ophthalmologist and in boys the presence of both testicles in the scrotum should be recorded.

The 6-week examination also provides a good opportunity to observe mother–child interaction, to discuss any small problems or worries which may be present and to mention the normal programme of immunizations and checks (see Chapter 27). It is appropriate to ensure that the mother has had her postnatal examination and such contraceptive advice as she requires.

It is also important to ensure that the newborn child is registered with a general practitioner of the parent's choice and that the parents are aware of routine and emergency consulting arrangements. All these services which are provided for parents and children should be judged by the use which the least intelligent and most insecure patients are able to make of them.

SCREENING FOR METABOLIC AND OTHER DEFECTS

The newborn period is a good time to screen for treatable defects. In addition to those which may be detected during routine clinical examination every baby should have a capillary blood sample taken at the end of the first week to detect cases of phenylketonuria. A similar test is also available now to screen for hypothyroidism and this should rapidly become universally available.

SOME COMMON PROBLEMS

Minor blemishes

Caput and moulding

During most labours and especially when prolonged, the presenting part will become moulded and oedematous due to pressure. In the case of a vertex presentation the head will be moulded and elongated. A caput succadeum may be present due to oedema over the vertex. In a breech presentation the buttocks and genitalia may be oedematous and rather bruised. The parents should be reassured that all these changes will resolve rapidly.

Cephalhaematoma

This is a more pronounced but localized swelling over one of the bones of the vault of the skull. It is due to subperiostal haematoma and consequently the swelling does not cross the cranial sutures. Again the parents can be reassured that this will resolve spontaneously but that complete recovery will take some weeks.

Normal skin appearance

There are a number of normal skin appearances which may cause parents some surprise or even alarm. Perhaps the most common of these is the thick white greasy vernix present on most term and preterm babies. At the other extreme parents may need reassurance that the dry red scaly skin of the postmature or growth-retarded baby who appears old before his time will, in fact, rapidly return to the soft normal baby skin which all mothers expect.

Marks or blemishes on a child's face are especially important and are also exceedingly common. Most children have a number of tiny white vesicles across the nose and cheeks; these are known as milia, or 'milk spots' to most parents.

Erythema toxicum, or urticaria of the newborn, is a variable widespread blotchy erythematous rash sometimes surrounding white papules which may even appear septic. This condition is of unknown aetiology but is commonly known by doctors, parents and midwives alike as a 'heat rash'. It is of no significance.

Stork marks are livid red vascular marks on the forehead and the nape of the neck and also sometimes involving the eyelids. These are present in up to half of all newborn babies but fade rapidly. A portwine stain is an uncommon vascular malformation which will also be present at birth, but which is permanent. The lesions are flat, vary in size, colour, and distribution but are commonest on the face and may be very extensive.

Mongolian blue spots appear over the sacrum and lower back of babies with pigmented skin especially in those of African descent. The only importance is to recognize and record them as they may very easily be mistaken for bruises, but they become less obvious as the child grows older.

Seborrhoeic dermatitis may appear in the first weeks of life either as thick crusts on the scalp (cradle cap) or as a rather blotchy red eczematous rash on the forehead, cheeks and sternum. Occasionally it is necessary to prescribe limited quantities of a mild steroid cream such as ½ per cent hydrocortisone for seborrhoeic dermatitis, but usually it is sufficient to reassure the parents and give simple advice.

Breasts

Both boys and girls may have palpably enlarged breast tissue present at birth or soon after. This is due to maternal hormones and will resolve. Occasionally accessory nipples may also be present.

Jaundice

Most if not all newborn babies can be expected to show some sign of jaundice. This is a physiological condition which requires only observation and exclusion of any significant pathology. Standard works on neonatal paediatrics contain comprehensive lists of the causes of jaundice (Chiswick 1978). In practice the general practitioner may usually confine himself to recognizing those cases in which the jaundice is pathological and ensuring prompt referral to specialist care.

Physiological jaundice normally appears after the first 48 hours, reaches a peak in about 4 days and disappears within 10 days. Throughout this time the infant will feed well and remain otherwise healthy. The peak level of bilirubin does not normally exceed 200 mmol/l. Further careful investigation and examination, usually by a paediatrician is necessary if the jaundice does not remain within these limits, if the child is not feeding or appears in any way unwell.

The general practitioner will often be faced with the problem of a healthy, breast-feeding infant who is gaining a satisfactory amount of weight but who remains jaundiced after 10 days. This will usually be the harmless 'breast milk jaundice' but more serious conditions should be excluded. In most cases further investigations will be carried out including routine swabs and urine to screen for infection, urine testing for reducing substances to exclude galactosaemia and monitoring of serum bilirubin levels. In all cases serum thyroid stimulating hormone (TSH) or T4 should be measured to exclude hypothyroidism. Provided that investigations are normal and the serum bilirubin falls gradually no further action is needed and the mother should be encouraged to continue breast feeding.

Within the recent past haemolytic disease of the newborn due to rhesus incompatibility was an important cause of perinatal mortality and morbidity. This condition is now preventable with appropriate prophylactic use of antiD immunoglobulin. The general practitioner has an important role in ensuring that all rhesus negative women receive appropriate doses of antiD after delivery, miscarriage or termination of pregnancy.

Recognition of serious illness

The recognition of infants who are seriously ill is not always easy bu. it is of great importance due to the speed with which a serious or even life-threatening condition may develop. Three useful rules should always be rememered.

(i) The low birth weight child is at special risk whether it is preterm or small for dates.
(ii) The symptoms of illness in infancy are very commonly non-specific.
(iii) The child's mother is seldom wrong if she thinks her baby may be seriously ill.

Some symptoms are especially important and deserve urgent consideration. Altered behaviour may present as irritability, lethargy, crying or altered feeding or sleep patterns. Cyanosis, pallor or jaundice are likely to be quickly recognized though these signs will be less obvious in a black child (Tarnow-Mordi and Pickering 1983). In the newborn respiratory difficulty may present with rib recession, grunting, flaring of the nares and raised respiratory rate. Fits in childhood are universally recognized as being of great importance while diarrhoea and vomiting, if serious, may quickly lead to dehydration. Any signs of haemorrhage or bruising is likely to be serious in this age group.

Where any of these symptoms are detected, especially if more than one is present, then close observation and assessment is required, and this will frequently involve admission to hospital. An excellent card summarizing the symptoms and signs of serious illness in infancy and giving straightforward and practical advice is available from the Foundation for the Study of Infant Deaths for distribution to parents.

Crying

Babies cry for many different reasons. As well as being a sign of distress or discomfort, a baby's cry can be an effective form of communication. Parents quickly learn to distinguish different types of cry associated with certain common situations such as hunger or tiredness. A crying baby may be presented to a doctor because the crying is different or frightening to the parents or because they believe the cry to be a symptom of illness. Sometimes the crying will in fact be due to a simple everyday cause which the parents have overlooked in their anxiety and many general practitioners must have been asked to see infants who turn out to have no more the matter with them than hunger, thirst or a dirty nappy.

An abnormal cry especially if it is associated with other non-specific signs of illness should alert the general practitioner to the possibility of serious illness. A careful examination of the baby is necessary to detect the cause of the crying to exclude illness and to reassure the parents that their worries are being taken seriously. Often such an examination together with simple advice will solve the problem although very occasionally it may be necessary to give the baby a sedative such as promethazine hydrochloride.

Quite commonly babies from about 2 weeks of age until about 3 or 4 months exhibit a pattern of regular episodes of crying, often in the early evening which are associated with drawing up of the knees. This is commonly known as 'colic'. In the past, treatment with dicyclomine hydrochloride was advised, however this drug is now contra-indicated in children under six months. (Williams and Watkins Jones 1984). At present there is no obvious alternative.

Some babies seem to swallow excessive quantities of wind and regurgitation of this together with variable quantities of milk is sometimes associated with apparent discomfort and crying.

In considering the crying baby it is important to remember that the child who is abnormally quiet or who has a thin feeble cry may be in much more urgent need of help than the infant who is bawling lustily (Table 28.4).

Table 28.4 *Common causes of crying in small babies*

Feeding problems	Hunger
	Thirst
	'Wind'
	'Colic'
Social	Tiredness
	Loneliness
	Overstimulation
	Boredom
	Personality
	Family tension
Discomfort	Dirty nappy
	Overheating
	Cold
Illness	Drug withdrawal (such as pethidine)
	Infections
	Injury

Low birth weight

Infants of low birth weight are at special risk and even when every care is taken to ensure their delivery in specialist units a general practitioner will sometimes be called on to be responsible for the management of an unexpectedly small baby.

Preterm babies

A preterm baby is defined as one before 37 weeks' gestation. The term prematurity used to be used to refer to any infant weighing 2500 g or less at birth but this term has now fallen into disuse as it caused confusion between preterm and small-for-dates babies. Recognition and management of preterm babies is greatly assisted by accurate obstetric dating of the pregnancy which should enable identification of any women with preterm labour so that appropriate facilities for the child may be made immediately available. Estimates of the child's gestational age should also be made by observing neurological reflexes and physical characteristics of the baby (Dubowitz, Dubowitz and Goldberg 1970; Farr, Mitchell and Nelligan 1966). Due to their incomplete development preterm babies are vulnerable to a number of complications, the most important of which are listed in Table 28.5.

Table 28.5   *Complications of preterm babies*

Respiratory	Idiopathic respiratory distress syndrome
	Apnoea
Infection	
Hypothermia	
Jaundice	
Intracranial haemorrhage	
Gastrointestinal	Feeding difficulties
	Necrotizing enterocolitis

Management

The management of preterm babies requires a high concentration of specialist facilities. Whenever possible arrangements should be made for the baby to be delivered in a unit with specialist neonatal paediatric facilities. If this is not possible the baby should be transferred to such a unit as soon as possible. Many of these units can now provide a paediatric flying squad to ensure transfer of such babies in an incubator and under continuous expert supervision.

Small-for-dates babies

A small-for-dates baby is one whose birth weight is below the 10th percentile appropriate for his gestational age. By adopting this broad definition many normal babies will be included but it does ensure that all babies at risk of the complications of growth retardation will receive appropriate supervision (Table 28.6). The ideal time to detect these babies is as early as possible during pregnancy in order to anticipate and prevent the substantial risks of intrauterine death and birth asphyxia which are inherent. Unfortunately, however careful the antenatal care, children continue to be born with unsuspected growth retardation.

Small-for-dates babies are a diverse group of varied aetiology. Although a single cause can seldom be found various contributory factors have been identified (Table 28.7).

Table 28.6   *Complications of small-for-dates babies*

Intrauterine death
Birth asphyxia
Birth injury
Meconium aspiration
·Hypothermia
Hypoglycaemia
Congenital abnormalities
Intrauterine viral infections
Polycythaemia

Table 28.7   *Factors contributing to fetal growth retardation*

Smoking
Intrauterine viral infection
Alcoholism
Drug addiction
Maternal malnutrition
Congenital malformations
Severe pre-eclampsic toxaemia (PET) or hypertension
Multiple pregnancy

Management

The management of small-for-dates babies is largely concerned with the prevention and presymptomatic detection of hypoglycaema. Early feeding is established and regular capillary blood glucose estimation (Dextrostix) are taken. In very small-for-dates babies regular 3-hourly feeds are advised with Dextrostix tests before each feed. In less severely growth retarded babies routine feeding schedules and 8-hourly Dextrostix are adequate. These should be continued for the first 72 hours of life. Any baby with hypoglycaemia (blood sugar less than 1.1 mmol/l) will require a slow intravenous infusion of 10 per cent glucose if neurological symptoms are present and if the hypoglycaemia fails to respond to increased oral feeds in an asymptomatic baby.

Hypothermia

Newborn infants have a relatively large surface area and do not have the same capacity to conserve heat as adults. These facts are especially important in low birth weight infants who are also relatively deficient in subcutaneous fat. Thus all newborn infants, but especially those of low birth weight and those who are otherwise ill for any reason, are vulnerable to hypothermia. This must be constantly borne in mind when dealing with the newborn. A room which is uncomfortably warm to an adult may still allow an unclothed neonate to become rapidly hypothermic. After delivery all babies must be carefully and quickly dabbed dry and wrapped in a warm dry blanket. Resuscitation should be carried out under a radiant heater if possible with only the essential areas exposed. Even in an incubator it may be difficult to maintain a normal temperature and a perspex heat shield may be of great benefit. It is advisable to check the rectal temperature of all newborn babies about 1 hour after birth, as a temperature below 35 °C (95 °F) centigrade indicates hypothermia. Only babies at special risk should need further monitoring.

Prognosis for low birth weight babies

During the last few years improvements in intensive neonatal care have resulted in much better chance of survival for low birth weight babies. The improvements in prognosis may be due to the modern understanding of the need for proper warmth and nutrition and the energetic prevention and treatment of hypothermia, hypoxia, jaundice and infection. Unfortunately, although the benefits of modern intensive care are great so is the cost both in financial and emotional terms.

Undoubtedly further advances in intensive neonatal management will be made in years to come but the main hope for improvement in both mortality and handicap rates may lie firstly in a general improvement in standards of living and health and secondly in fundamental advances in obstetric care especially in relation to the prevention of preterm labour, growth retardation and congenital abnormalities.

Superficial infections

Systemic infections in the newborn are always likely to be serious and require specialist care; however, there are a variety of superficial infections which occur commonly and are readily treated in general practice. Although treatment of these infections with antibiotics may be relatively easy and safe it should be remembered that prevention by careful attention to hygiene and hand washing is always preferable.

Sticky eye

Simple sticky eye is a common symptom and often represents an accumulation of dry mucus which may be cleaned with sterile water. In the absence of pus or inflammation no further treatment is necessary. Where signs of infection are present then antibiotic eye drops are required (sulphacetamide 10 per cent). A profuse purulent discharge presenting within the first 48 hours may indicate a gonococcal conjunctivitis. This requires vigorous treatment with topical and systemic penicillin pending bacteriological confirmation of the diagnosis.

Umbilical infections

The healing umbilicus is especially vulnerable to infection. For this reason routine care of the newborn should include measures to ensure that this area remains clean and dry. Prophylactic use of a suitable antibacterial preparation (such as Ster-Zac Powder) is advisable.

Skin and nail folds

Bacterial infections of the skin may present as scattered pustules or as exfoliative lesions. Such infection is often associated with paronychia. Where the condition is minor and localized careful cleansing together with a topical antibiotic (such as fucidic acid) is usually effective. If oral antibiotic therapy is required in the home then a combination of ampicillin and flucloxacillin is suitable.

Thrush

Oral or perianal infections with *Candida albicans* are common especially after administration of antibiotics to mother or baby. Oral thrush is easily recognized by its white plaques adherent to an inflamed mucosa. The condition is intensely uncomfortable and may cause feeding problems and irritability. Treatment is with oral nystatin suspension together with topical nystatin cream to the nappy area if this is required.

Vomiting

All babies regurgitate a small amount of milk from time to time (see Chapter 26). This harmless and normal event needs to be carefully differentiated from pathological vomiting which may quickly lead to dehydration. Any vomiting which is forceful, prolonged or associated with other symptoms is likely to be abnormal. The occurrence of diarrhoea in association with vomiting is commonly due to gastroenteritis and requires rapid action to prevent dehydration. Bile-stained vomit is likely to indicate some intestinal obstruction while the presence of blood should be assumed to indicate haemorrhagic disease of the newborn although swallowed maternal blood from a cracked nipple may also present in this way.

REFERENCES

Apgar, V. (1953). Proposal for new method of evaluation of newborn infants. *Curr. Rese. Anaesth. Analg.* **32**, 260–7.

Chiswick, M. L. (1978). Jaundice. In *Neonatal medicine*, Chapter 7, pp. 40–55. Update Books, London.

Davies, P. A., Robinson, R. J., Scopes, J. W., Tizzard, J. P. M., and Wigglesworth, J. S. (1972). Birth asphyxia and resuscitation. In *Medical care of newborn babies*, pp. 32–9. Spastics International Medical Publications, London.

Dubowitz, L., Dubowitz, V., and Goldberg, C. (1970). Clinical assessment of gestational age in the newborn infant. *J. Paediatr.* **77**, 1–10.

Farr, V., Mitchell, R., and Nelligan, G. (1966). *Develop. Med. Child Neurol.* **8**, 507.

MacFarlane, A. (1977). The first minutes. In *The psychology of childbirth*, (eds. J. Bruner, R. Cole, and B. Lloyd) p. 55. Fontana/Open Books, London.

Tarnow-Mordi, W. O. and Pickering, D. (1983). Missed jaundice in black infants. A hazard? *Br. Med. J.* **286**, 463.

Valman, H. B. (1980). Mother–infant bonding. In *The first year of life*. pp. 25–7. British Medical Association, London.

Williams, J. and Watkins-Jones, R. (1984). Dicyclomine: worrying symptoms associated with its use in some small babies. *Br. Med. J.* **288**, 901.

29 Psychological problems from birth to the postnatal examination

B. M. N. Pitt

INTRODUCTION

Although most women cope with the puerperium as readily as they do with pregnancy, a significant minority are burdened with apparently incongruous depression, while a much smaller number are frankly psychotic.

Whereas pregnancy is a time of low psychiatric morbidity, the incidence of psychiatric disorder, leading to outpatient and inpatient treatment in the postnatal period, particularly the 6 weeks of the puerperium, is remarkably high. Childbirth therefore puts mental health at risk, but all the risk is post partum. Pugh et al. (1963) noted that the greatest risk for psychiatric hospital admission was in the first week after giving birth, and that the admission rate then declines week by week until by the 9th month after childbirth it is no greater than in women of like age who have not had a baby, or one as recently. Kendell et al. (1976) looked up Camberwell women on the Camberwell register of psychiatric contacts during the 2 years before and after they gave birth, and found as many referrals to a psychiatrist in the 3 postpartum months as in the previous 2 years. There were nine new psychotic episodes at this time, and only seven in the 2 previous years. Depression in particular, psychotic and neurotic, peaked in the postpartum trimester. In a later study in Edinburgh, Kendell et al. (1981) showed the psychiatric admission rate within the 3 months postpartum to be almost five times as high as the average over the previous 2 years, while the rate for admissions with a diagnosis of functional psychosis was no less than 16 times as high. According to Brewer (1978) psychiatric admissions following abortion are only a fifth of those following childbirth, so it follows that the ending of pregnancy, at or near to term, by the birth of the baby in some way constitutes the significant precipitating factor.

Nevertheless psychiatric admission follows no more than one in 500 child-births. Some moderately psychotic women may not require admission, but the total incidence of puerperal psychosis is unlikely to exceed 0.5 per cent. This obviously matters a lot to the women concerned, and their families, but milder, yet still troublesome 'neurotic' disorders, largely unrecognized until 20 years ago and still frequently undiagnosed are a much more common mental health hazard in the puerperium.

AFFECTIVE DISORDERS

Before discussing these it should be pointed out that almost all postpartum psychological problems are forms of *affective disorder*, major, moderate, or minor, and usually depression. Thus in the Edinburgh study already mentioned (Kendell *et al.* 1981) only nine of 71 women admitted to psychiatric units within 3 months after childbirth were not diagnosed as suffering from some form of affective illness, while no less than 49 (or 69 per cent) were considered to be depressed. Depression is the postpartum mental illness par excellence. Mania, though much less common, is also over-represented at this time. Other psychiatric states probably occur no more often than they do at other times.

A condition probably recognized by midwives and nursing mothers for centuries but only drawn to the attention of doctors by Hamilton (1962) in an important monograph on postpartum psychiatric problems was what he called the transitory syndrome, or third day, fourth day mother's, maternity or baby *blues*. This is a state of weepiness for no more than a day or two in the early puerperium and probably follows more births than it does not. It should not be confused (but frequently is) with *'neurotic' depression* post partum, a much more unpleasant and lasting disorder. This was first reported in the 1960s (Pitt 1965; Ryle 1964; Tod 1964) and is now confirmed by many other studies as following at least one birth in ten. It starts later in the puerperium and lasts for weeks, sometimes months and occasionally for longer than a year.

A CONTINUUM?

It is tempting to speculate that these various degress of emotional disturbance, psychotic and neurotic depression, lie along a continuum (Pitt 1975). Thus the same factor might produce little or no, moderate, or severe depression in different women according to different degrees of susceptibility. A genetic predisposition might very well predispose to psychotic depression (or mania), environmental factors, including the impact of the baby, to neurotic depression, and perhaps the quantity and rapidity of hormonal change post partum to the blues. This view may, however, be misleading. Stern and Kruckman (1983) have suggested that a biological aetiology is likely to be most important in the psychoses, whereas a failure of ritualization during the puerperium may account for the emergence of milder states of depression in western societies.

SEVERE POSTPARTUM MENTAL ILLNESS

As puerperal psychosis is relatively rare in general practice it will be dealt with only briefly.

Although some special features of these psychoses have been described, for example, confusion at the outset, a mixture of features of different clinical syndromes before the final picture emerges, and a tendency in major depressive disorder for puerperal patients to be more deluded, labile, and hallucinated than non-puerperal depressed controls (Dean and Kendell 1981), essentially puerperal mental illness resembles the same illness occurring at other times, but modified by the acuteness of the onset and the presence of the baby. There is equal evidence of genetic and constitutional predisposition. Protheroe (1969) found a previous, subsequent and family history of mental illness as often in puerperal patients as in their matched non-puerperal controls.

Severe or *psychotic* puerperal *depression* usually arises from a state of morbid anxiety (occasionally said to be apparent at the end of pregnancy, see Meares, Grimwade, and Wood 1976, and Chapter 7). This is rapidly replaced by profound melancholy, with impulses to suicide and infanticide, sometimes delusional guilt and despair, and the usual physiological disturbance of a severe endogenous depression—early waking, feeling worse in the morning, and loss of appetite, weight, and energy. There may be retardation to the point of marked inertia, or even stupor, or a harrowing agitation. Infanticide is fortunately less common than severe depression and is much more commonly the result of non-accidental injury. When it does occur it is more like a misguided act of euthanasia than a manifestation of psychotic aggression.

Mania and hypomania develop suddenly in the early puerperium. The subject shows a striking personality change towards buoyant optimism, self-confidence, garrulity and boisterous extroversion. The manic mother has too many other good ideas to give her baby enough attention. Her facetious good humour is brittle, and she may become suddenly angry or dejected. She feels erotic, may overspend, takes too little nourishment or rest, and makes wildly unrealistic plans. Sooner or later her state is likely to end in severe depression.

Severe depression and manic disorders are best treated in psychiatric wards. A mother and baby unit (Margison and Brockington 1982) is ideal, but these are not widely available. Still, most acute psychiatric wards are prepared to admit babies with their mothers, so that mothering is disrupted as little as possible by the illness and the admission. Open visiting by key family members and days and weekends at home as soon as seems sensible are encouraged. The appropriate *medication* (or ECT for the most severely depressed) is given. As it is desirable to sustain close contact between mother and baby (provided the mother is not overtaxed, nor the baby at undue risk) breast-feeding should be encouraged where it appears to be the mother's wish. Neither the major tranquillizers nor antidepressants are secreted in breast milk in more than minute quantities, but benzodiazepines and lithium carbonate which may be the preferred treatment in manic illness are, so if they must be used then breast-feeding should be stopped.

The psychological approach is a positive one of reinforcing the way in which the mother can still, or becomes able to, cope during her recovery from her illness. This does not mean denial of her anger, resentment, misgiving, or ambivalence. It may well be helpful for her to get such feelings, as far as possible, out of her system, specially if the ward is run as a therapeutic community (Martin 1968). There may well also be a place for some family therapy, but the immediate aim is to restore the mother's mental health and enable her effectively to assume or resume mothering. In the first instance, during her early return visits home, this is all that should be required of her. She should be relieved of other responsibilities, as much as possible, until later, by a rallying round of family, friends, and neighbours and the enlistment of a home help.

In her aftercare the primary health care team, notably the general practitioner, the health visitor, and the social worker, should be as involved as the psychiatric department, notably the psychiatrist and the community psychiatric nurse.

Medication may need to be continued for months but, unless there is a previous history of chronic or frequently recurrent mental illness, not usually for longer. The prognosis for puerperal mental illness seems to be better than for other like illness occurring at other times, probably because the disorder presents acutely, is quickly diagnosed and, not least for the baby's sake, there is a general drive towards a quick recovery. Affective illnesses in particular do well, and the rule is a complete remission within 2–3 months. This makes a depressive suicide or infanticide all the more tragic. There is a risk of relapse, especially after a subsequent childbirth, which far exceeds the general expectation of one in 200–500 births. Several studies (Foundeur *et al.* 1957; Martin 1958; Protheroe 1969) have shown the risk of psychiatric admission after a later delivery to be of the order of one in six or seven births. This is likely to be an underestimate of the true risk, firstly because there is very likely to be an avoidance of further childbearing in women who have suffered a serious puerperal mental illness, and secondly because not every woman who relapses will necessarily be admitted.

If a woman with a past history of serious mental illness postpartum badly wants another baby, she will need the fullest support from her partner, family, and general practitioner and psychiatrist and their respective teams throughout pregnancy, and the postpartum year, with prompt medication at the first signs of relapse or even in some cases prophylactically, from late pregnancy onwards.

NEUROTIC DEPRESSION

Having identified this disorder in 33 (10.8 per cent) of a random sample of 305 women having their babies in a London teaching hospital who were followed from the third or fourth month of pregnancy to 6–8 weeks post-partum, Pitt (1965) gave the following description of the clinical features:

This depression usually began mildly in hospital soon after delivery, at which time it was scarcely distinguishable from 'maternity blues' except, perhaps, by its longer duration. A few mothers, though, felt very well in hospital, all the time or apart from one to two days of the 'blues'. Others felt physically rather than emotionally unwell at this time, with such symptoms as fatigue, backache and perineal discomfort.

The depression was always most in evidence after the return home, though in one mother its onset was delayed until nearly 7 weeks after delivery. The depression was chiefly manifest in tearfulness, despondency and feelings of inadequacy and inability to cope, mainly in respect of the baby (one woman commented: 'Every other woman seems to be blooming'). Suicidal ideas were present only in two women admitted to a psychiatric hospital (who, as it turned out, were suffering from severe, not neurotic, depressive illness). Guilt was largely confined to self-reproach over not loving or caring for the baby sufficiently and falling short of an ideal of motherhood, and was not commonly expressed. Feelings of hopelessness were infrequent, but several mothers felt changed from their usual selves and many stated that they had never been depressed like this before. The mood, though predominantly depressive, was often labile; diurnal variation was occasionally described, the intensification of depression nearly always taking place in the evenings.

This depression was almost invariably accompanied, and in some instances over-shadowed by, anxiety over the baby. Such anxiety was not justified by the babies' health: none were seriously ill, and most were thriving. Feeding worries were the commonest. Babies which would not sleep and kept crying were found hard to love, with consequent guilt and anxiety. Two mothers had great difficulty in accepting that their babies were really theirs. Actual overt hostility to the baby, though, was rare. A few mothers could satisfy their babies' physical needs, but feared spoiling them. Multiparae tended to worry over their other children's jealousy of the new arrival.

Anxiety was also frequently manifest in hypochondriasis. Somatic symptoms abounded, and formed the basis of fears of ill health. One woman suspected (falsely) that her ovaries had been removed in the course of caesarean section, another feared tuberculosis, another regarded her thyroid as the root of her trouble, and another put her manifold disturbed sensations down to breast-feeding.

Unusual irritability was common and sometimes added to feelings of guilt. A few patients complained of impaired concentration and memory. Undue fatigue and ready exhaustion were very frequent, so that mothers could barely deal with their babies, let alone look after the rest of the family and cope with the housework and shopping. Sometimes there was a loss of normal interests. One woman felt imprisoned.

Anorexia, occasionally associated with nausea, was present with remarkable consistency. Sleep disturbance, over and above that inevitable with a new baby, was reported by a third of patients, taking the form of difficulty in getting to sleep and nightmares more often than of early morning waking. Seventeen patients lacked their normal sexual interest (as compared with nine of the puerperal controls who were not depressed—probably significant). In one patient the problem presented as puerperal dyspareunia which continued a year later despite the abatement of other depressive symptoms.

One mother described her feelings as rather like the premenstrual tension syndrome. In two, physical disorders—epilepsy and psoriasis—were exacerbated. Only a few lacked the support of relatives on their return home, but negative feelings towards the husband, who might be considered unsympathetic or unhelpful, were admitted by just under a quarter of the group.

It was possible to follow up 20 of these 33 women a year later: sixteen had fully recovered, taking from a few weeks to several months to do so; but the remaining twelve (that is, 40 per cent of the puerperal depressives followed up, or 4 per cent of the total sample of 305 women) had made little or no improvement, describing such symptoms as loss of sexual and other interests, irritability, fatigue, and ready depression.

While Kumar and Robson (1978) in another prospective teaching hospital study found a virtually identical incidence of postnatal depression—11 per cent, Neugebauer (1983) having studied Pitt's (1965) original data makes a good statistical case for believing that this is an underestimate, and that a truer incidence would be 19.7 per cent. Cox, Connor, and Kendell (1982) in yet another prospective teaching hospital study found that 16 per cent of 105 women assessed by Goldberg's Standardized Psychiatric Interview were mildly depressed, and another 12.4 per cent were more severely depressed; and in a retrospective study 20 per cent of Paykel *et al.* (1980) patients had developed postnatal depression. The prospective general practitioner study by Rees and Lutkins (1971) used the Beck scale, on which 3 per cent of their postnatal patients scored 25 points or more and were more depressed than those 7 per cent who scored between 17 and 24 points (the moderately depressed range), while 31 per cent scored between 10 and 16 points and were mildly depressed.

In Pitt's (1965) study there were a further nineteen postnatal patients (6 per cent of the total sample) who were judged doubtfully depressed and excluded from the study group, though they had developed such troublesome symptoms as unusual anxiety unaccompanied by depression, anxiety, and depression purely reactive to the baby's genuine ill-health, prolonged fatigue in the absence of obvious depression or anaemia, lessening of libido as a single symptom, and the development or reappearance of psychosomatic disorders such as rhinitis and migraine.

What all this means is that mild to moderate depression and anxiety are relatively common in the puerperium, are often a troublesome and distressing complication and can persist much longer than the facile misapplication of the label 'blues' to such states would imply. Only 10 per cent of Pitt's (1965) postnatally depressed patients appear to have had any treatment from their general practitioners. Kumar (1982) points out how easily the health visitor's home visit may miss postnatal depression. Cox *et al.* (1982) remarked that the four depressed women in their study who in their opinion required psychiatric help were not referred, and the two others who were referred were not suffering depression but from personality disorder.

Depression should be picked up at the postnatal examination(s) by simply asking all the women 'Have you been depressed since you had the baby?' This elementary enquiry allows women who had not thought to raise the matter themselves or felt too diffident to do so to answer in the affirmative and often weep with relief and as a release while talking of their feelings. This catharsis is the first step in treatment.

It is much more difficult to spot who is at risk for this disorder than for psychotic and severe illness. The term 'neurotic' simply contrasts the clinical form of the depression with that of 'psychotic' depression and does not necessarily imply that the subjects are neurotic women with low stress tolerance and a tendency to minor psychological illness. Of Pitt's (1965) 33 postnatally depressed subjects fourteen described neurotic traits, eight being anxiety prone, one obsessional, one shy, one hysterical, one frigid, one cyclothymic and one a regular user of hypnotics, but only three (compared with six of the puerperal controls who were not depressed) had a previous history of psychiatric illness. Dalton (1971) and Kumar and Robson (1978) also failed to find that postnatal depressives more often had a previous history of psychiatric disorder than controls, but 63 per cent of Paykel *et al.*'s (1980) depressed subjects had, compared with only 13 per cent of controls, a significant difference.

Table 29.1 lists some of the possible risk factors for postnatal depression identified in some of the more important and persuasive studies; none, how-

Table 29.1 *Factors predisposing to puerperal neurotic depression*

Predisposing factor	study
Maternal deprivation	
loss of mother before the age of 11	Frommer and O'Shea (1973)
limited contact with mother in childhood	Nilsson and Almgren (1970)
Previous psychiatric history	Braverman and Roux (1978)
	Paykel *et al.* (1980)
Ambivalance about pregnancy	Kumar and Robson (1978)
High anxiety in pregnancy	Tod (1964)
	Meares *et al.* (1976)
Lack of support	
unloving, unsupportive spouse	
lack of confidantes	
Poor housing	Paykel *et al.* (1980)
Life events	
four or more (unpleasant) shortly before or during pregnancy.	

ever, have been found by all. It will be seen that there is no mention of social class, the legitimacy or otherwise of the baby or its sex, or obstetric complications, because there is surprisingly little evidence that these have much bearing on postnatal depression. Cox (1979) found the postpartum psychiatric morbidity of Bugandan women much the same as in the United Kingdom. Lack of bonding seems to be a consequence, not a cause of depression (Robson and Kumar 1980). Clarke and Williams (1979) found that more women who had lost their babies were moderately depressed in the early puerperium as would be expected, but that time healed, and 6 months later there was no such difference. It would be nice to incriminate the major hormonal changes surrounding childbirth, but there is as yet no evidence.

It would appear that neurotic depression post partum is multifactorial, arising from various forms of predisposition and current stress, but frequently hard to predict or to explain. The best prevention at present is secondary. All who are concerned with women who have recently had babies should watch out for depression.

Treatment

The woman who has revealed her condition should be told that she has postnatal depression, a common but not trivial disorder, the cause of which is unknown but which is likely to get better, that medical treatment can be provided if necessary and that she will be seen regularly and supported until she has recovered. This information helps her to comprehend what is wrong with her (what woman after all, has not heard of postnatal depression these days?), may protect her from feeling freakish, inadequate, or unmotherly (postnatal depression is an affliction, not a failing, and no respecter of persons) and gives her hope.

Her husband and other key family members should be seen, heard, and counselled. It is not easy to live with a depressive, especially with a new baby in the home, and it is easy for the husband to become perplexed, dispirited, and resentful, while other children may feel neglected and play up. The health visitor in particular, a social worker, and a befriending organization like the Association for Postnatal Illness (whose members, having weathered postpartum depression, can help the sufferer to understand that there is a dawn after the dark) may all be involved in support, but the doctor should not opt out. There may be times when medication or referral to a psychiatrist are advisable.

If the depression and any associated anxiety are very distressing, persist for more than 2 months or if there is a previous history of depression which responded to medication, then an antidepressant and sometimes a benzodiazepine tranquillizer should be given. A generally well-tolerated tricyclic like dothiepin should be given in a dose of 75–150 mg at night. If there is no response after a month, a monoamine oxidase inhibitor (MAOI) (say, phenelzine 15 mg three times a day) should be considered, though many general practitioners would wish to refer to a psychiatrist before such a prescription was given. Diazepam 2–5 mg up to three times a day or lorazepam 1–2.5 mg up to three times a day, are useful tranquillizers, but are liable to be secreted in breast milk and there is a strong risk of habituation. Medication should be continued for 2 months after depression and anxiety have been relieved, and then gradually be reduced and stopped.

A psychiatrist's opinion will be sought if he or she is known to be particularly interested in postnatal depression, has access to group therapy for the disorder or if the patient's condition fails to improve or worsens.

It is important to appreciate that support may need to be continued in some cases well past the baby's first birthday. As has been indicated above, postnatal neurotic depression can be a lingering disorder, and while it persists it presents a mental health hazard not only to the subject but also to her family.

Wrath *et al.* (1983) interviewed a representative sample of 91 mothers who had given birth in an Edinburgh maternity hospital 3 years previously about their child's current behaviour. 27 of these women had originally suffered depression during their puerperium. Surprisingly, those in whom the depression has lasted less than 4 months reported disturbed behaviour in their child not only more than those who had been free from depression but than those who had been more lastingly depressed (who were significantly more neurotic than the rest of the group and cited other anxieties than those about the baby). This suggests that the bonding problems which arise even from a shortish postnatal depression may have prolonged effects.

The puerperium is a period of considerable psychological vulnerability, and it behoves all who may have to do with mother and baby at this time to be aware and watchful.

THE 'BLUES'

In Pitt's (1965) study already cited, 100 newly delivered mothers on maternity wards were chosen for interview at random, and 50 admitted to spells of tearfulness and depression since giving birth, lasting from barely an hour to most of the day, on 1 or 2–3 successive days, usually on the 2nd, 3rd, and 4th day post partum; (of seven subjects whose distress lasted longer two went on to develop definite neurotic postnatal depression). Anxiety, mainly over the baby, was present in 35 of this 'blues' group and in only sixteen of the controls without the 'blues', while mild cognitive impairment, manifest as poor concentration, forgetfulness, and slowness to learn, was present in just under a half of the 'blues' subjects and in just over a quarter of the controls. The causes advanced for their mild distress by the 'blues' group were classifiable as worries over the baby and themselves, concern over lactation and breast-feeding and homesickness. Nine of the fourteen women chiefly worried over their babies had some reason (compared with five of the controls) while five were mainly concerned that their babies kept crying. Of 40 breast-feeders in the 'blues' group fifteen compared with only seven of 40 breast-feeders in the control group were having difficulty with the feeding—a probably significant difference.

The condition was usually mild and transitory, though there was a probably significant tendency for women with postnatal neurotic depression to have experienced the 'blues'. With such fleeting symptoms it is surprising that estimates of the incidence of the 'blues' are so consistent, ranging from 50–66 per cent (Kane *et al.* 1968; Nott *et al.* 1976; Yalom *et al.* 1968).

Pitt (1973) argued that the absence of personality predisposition to the 'blues' and of any exceptional stress, together with the subjective cognitive impairment could justify regarding the condition as organically determined. The relative absence of infection and obstetric complications suggested that the most likely factor was the profound endocrine change which accompanies parturition. The occurrence of most cases within 4 days post partum was consistent with this organic hypothesis.

The main interest of the 'blues', then, is not its clinical importance which is relatively trivial, but its possible relevance to the puerperal psychoses. In other words, whatever occasions the 'blues' in every other newly delivered women may precipitate psychosis in those few who are peculiarly predisposed.

The current state of knowledge about the 'blues' has been comprehensively reviewed by Stein (1982) who lists progesterone, oestrogen, prolactin, cortisol, thyroxine, cyclic adenosine monophosphate (cyclic AMP), monoamines, monoamine oxidase, and changes in electrolytes and body weight as possible factors which have been studied in this context, without proving persuasively to be implicated. He also points out that the subjective feeling of mental impairment has not been confirmed by clinical psychological testing (Kane *et al.* 1968; Yalom *et al.* 1968) and that depression itself appears to blunt mental acuity (Weeks, Freeman and Kendell 1980).

It is very likely that research in this field will continue. Meanwhile all that needs to be said about the management of the 'blues' is that prospective mothers should be told that they may expect it and reassured if it occurs, and that if it persists it should be regarded as incipient postnatal depression.

OTHER PUERPERAL PROBLEMS

Bonding

Klaus and Kennell's research (1976) suggested that there is a sensitive period from the moment of the baby's birth when impediments to the mother's seeing and fondling her baby may impair her intense attachment to the child and affect her maternal behaviour weeks or months later. The case may have been overstated, but Robson and Kumar (1980), for example, found an unexpected but highly significant association between a lack of maternal affection immediately after delivery and the induction or acceleration of labour by forewater amniotomy, especially when the labour was perceived as very painful or if extra pethidine was prescribed. The literature on early maternal attachment is well reviewed by Robson and Powell (1982).

There is no doubt that bonding theory has caused much critical questioning of obstetric practices by consumers as well as the professions involved (see, for example, Kitzinger 1979) and this is doubtless healthy. Any dogmatic approach, however, which does not allow for the differences between one puerperal mother and another is going to cause some avoidable distress. For example rooming-in suits many but not all mothers, some of whom value a respite from maternal care in the early days until perforce they must take on the job for 24 hours a day.

It must be recognized, too, that not every woman will bond to her baby at once, and she is no more a failure if she does not than if, after having prepared for natural childbirth, she needs analgesia. It is certainly a great asset to feel enraptured with one's baby in the trying early weeks postpartum, but just as not all love is at first sight, so some normal women will take some time to get to know and love their babies.

Readjustment

It is perfectly normal to experience some stress and difficulty in coping with a new baby in the house, especially if it is a first child. Some anxiety and disorganization are almost inevitable. If the new mother is left alone for long periods, and feels stranded in a third-floor flat with no lift or *de trop* in her inlaw's home, her plight is the more intense. If no-one will share the care of her crying child at night she will easily become exhausted.

Although husbands, having usually been present at the birth, seem more supportive than they were, they may not be able or prepared to take time off work (if employed) to help their wives when they first come home, and as about 50 per cent of middle-aged women now go out to work, mothers and mothers-in-law may not be available. Home helps can be prescribed, but often are not.

Liedloff (1975) and Stern and Kruckman (1983) have pointed out how the failure of western developed societies to provide postnatal support comparable with antenatal care, may contribute to the relatively high morbidity for postpartum depression, and though their theories are unproven, it seems evident that too many young mothers are left suddenly to their own devices with too much on their hands.

Ideally the new mother should be relieved of duties other than the care of her baby until she has established (often with the advice of the health visitor or well-baby clinic) a sensible routine. After a fortnight most women feel that they are getting on top of their problems. Failure to do so, and especially the feeling of floundering, being in a panicky muddle, feeling exhausted, and getting nowhere, may well indicate postnatal depression.

Sex

In Pitt's (1965) study nine of 35 puerperal subjects who were not depressed (20 per cent) lacked their usual sexual interest; 51 per cent of puerperal depressives lacked such interest. Depression, therefore, is only partly responsible.

Masters and Johnson (1966) reported that half their sample of mothers experienced low levels of sexual interest during the 3 months postpartum. Anecdotally, one all too frequently hears that a wife has gone off sex, or become less keen, since she had the last, or even the first baby! Often there is a previous sexual maladjustment, now manifest as frank dysfunction (Hawton, 1982). Possible factors include:

(i) Continuing or only partly resolved puerperal depression.
(ii) Perineal soreness, say after an episiotomy; or slackness of the perineal muscles after pregnancy and delivery.
(iii) Vaginal dryness due to relatively low circulating oestrogen postpartum, especially in breast-feeders.
(iv) The fear of conceiving again.
(v) Resentment of the husband, perhaps for his lack of support during the pregnancy and subsequently; or even a feeling that, having procreated, he has served his turn!

Whatever the cause, good sex is associated with marital stability, which is good for mother and baby. Sexual malfunction is common in the puerperium, and very unlikely to be presented by the mother, nor even her husband until some months later. An enquiry about sexual feelings at the time of the postnatal examination with a view to appropriate counselling if necessary, is as appropriate as questioning about depression.

SUMMARY

Childbirth puts mental health at risk, but all the risk is postpartum and for affective illness, mainly depression, mild, moderate or severe. Predisposition is most obvious for *puerperal psychosis*; previous, subsequent and family history of mental illness are as common as in non-puerperal psychosis. Severe or psychotic puerperal depression resembles severe endogenous depression at other times with the added risk of infanticide. Manic mothers are likely to neglect their babies, and to become depressed. These disorders are best treated in psychiatric wards to which the babies can also be admitted. Medical treatment is that appropriate to the disorder. Breast-feeding is not discouraged unless benzodiazepines or lithium are prescribed. The ability to cope is reinforced. Early discharge with close follow-up and support is recommended. The short-term prognosis is excellent but there is at least a one-in-seven risk of relapse after a subsequent birth.

Neurotic depression follows at least one in ten births, is troublesome, hard to predict, often overlooked and may last longer than a year. Anxiety states may also present at this time. Questioning at the postnatal interview is likely to elicit the diagnosis. The main prevention is secondary. Treatment involves explanation, reassurance and support until the depression is relieved. The husband should be involved. Medication may be needed, and occasionally referral to a psychiatrist. Even brief postnatal depression may affect the child.

The '*blues*' is a transient emotional and cognitive disturbance in the early puerperium, of interest as a possible model for puerperal psychosis, being, as it were, writ small. It may be organically determined, but proof is lacking.

Other puerperal problems include delay in bonding, to which some obstetric practices may contribute; difficulties in readjustment to life with a new baby and establishing a routine, which may indicate that puerperal mothers are undersupported; and sexual dysfunction, which is common and warrants counselling.

Note

A useful address is: Association for Postnatal Illness, 7 Gowan Avenue, London SW6.

REFERENCES

Braverman, J. and Roux, J. F. (1978). Screening for the patient at risk for post-partum depression. *Obstet. Gynaecol.* **52**, 73.

Brewer, C. (1978). Post abortion psychosis. In *Mental illness in pregnancy and the puerperium*. (ed. M. Sandler). Oxford University Press, Oxford.

Clarke, M. and Williams, A. J. (1979). Depression in women after peri-natal death. *Lancet* **1**, 916.

Cox, J. L. (1979). Psychiatric morbidity and pregnancy: a controlled study of 263 semi rural Ugandan women. *Br. J. Psychiatr.* **134**, 401.

Cox, J. L., Connor, Y., and Kendell, R. E. (1982). Prospective study of the psychiatric disorders of childbirth. *Br. J. Psychiatr.* **140**, 111.

Dalton, K. (1971). A prospective study into puerperal depression. *Br. J. Psychiatr.* **118**, 689.

Dean, C. and Kendell, R. E. (1981). The symptomatology of puerperal illness. *Br. J. Psychiatr.* **139**, 128.

Foundeur, J., Fixsen, C., Triebel, W.A., and White, M. A. (1957). Post-partum mental illness. *Arch. Neurol. Psychiatry* **77**, 503.

Frommer, E. and O'Shea, R. (1973). Antenatal identification of women liable to have problems in managing their infants. *Br. J. Psychiatr.* **123**, 49.

Hamilton, J. A. (1962). *Post partum psychiatric problems.* C. V. Mosby, St Louis.

Hawton, K. (1982). Sexual problems in the general hospital. In *Liaison psychiatry.* (eds. F. Creed and J. Pfeffer). Pitman, London and Massachusetts.

Kane, F. J., Harman, W. J., Keeler, M. H., and Ewing, J. A. (1968). Emotional and cognitive disturbance in the early puerperium. *Br. J. Psychiat.,* **114,** 99.

Kendell, R. E., Wainwright, S., Hailey, A. and Shannon, N. (1976). The influence of childbirth on psychiatric morbidity. *Psychol. Med.* **11,** 341.

Kendell, R. E., Rennie, D., Clarke, J. A., and Dean, C. (1981). The social and obstetric correlates of psychiatric admission in the puerperium. *Psychol. Med.* **11,** 341.

Kitzinger, S. (1979). *The good birth guide.* Fontana Paperbacks, William Collins, Glasgow.

Klaus, M. H. and Kennell, J. A. (1976). *Maternal infant bonding.* C. V. Mosby, St Louis.

Kumar, R. and Robson, K. (1978). Neurotic disturbance during pregnancy and the puerperium: preliminary report of a prospective study of 119 primigravida. In *Mental illness in pregnancy and the puerperium.* (ed. M. Sandler) Oxford University Press, Oxford.

Kumar, R. (1982). Neurotic disorders in childbearing women. In *Motherhood and mental illness.* (ed. I. F. Brockington and R. Kumar). Academic Press, London; Grune and Stratton, New York.

Liedloff, J. (1975). *The continuum concept.* Gerald Duckworth, London.

Margison, F. and Brockington, I. F. (1982). Psychiatric mother and baby units. In *Motherhood and mental illness.* (ed. I. F. Brockington and R. Kumar). Academic Press, London; Grune and Stratton, New York.

Martin, D. (1968). *Adventure in psychiatry.* 2nd ed. Cassirer, Oxford.

Martin, M. (1958). Puerperal mental illness—a follow up study of 75 cases. *Br. Med. J.* **2,** 773.

Masters, W. H. and Johnson, V. E. (1966). *Human sexual response.* Little Brown, Boston.

Meares, R., Grimwade, J., and Wood, C. (1976). A possible relationship between anxiety in pregnancy and puerperal depression. *J. Psychosom. Med.* **18,** 605.

Neugebauer, R. (1983). Incidence of depression in a post-partum population: 11 per cent of 20 per cent? *Br. J. Psychiatr.* **143,** 421.

Nilsson, A. and Almgren, P. E. (1970). Paranatal emotional adjustment. A prospective investigation of 165 women. *Acta Psychiatri. Scand.* Suppl. 220.

Nott, P. N., Franklin, M., Armitage, C., and Gelder, M. G. (1976). Hormonal changes and mood in the puerperium. *Br. J. Psychiatr.* **128,** 379.

Paykel, E. S., Emms, E. M., Fletcher, J., and Rassaby, E. S. (1980). Life events and social support in puerperal depression. *Br. J. Psychiatr.* **136,** 339.

Pitt, B. (1965). *A study of emotional disturbance associated with childbearing, with particular reference to depression arising in the puerperium.* University of London, MD thesis.

Pitt, B. (1968). A typical depression following childbirth. *Br. J. Psychiatr.* **114,** 1325.

Pitt, B. (1973). Maternity blues. *Br. J. Psychiatr.* **122,** 421.

Pitt, B. (1975). Psychological reactions to childbirth. *Proc. Roy. Soc. Med.* **68,** 223.

Protheroe, C. (1969). Puerperal psychoses: a long-term study. 1927–1961. *Br. J. Psvchiatr.* **68.** 223.

Pugh, J. F., Jerath, B. K., Schmidt, W. M., and Reed, R. B. (1963). Rates of mental disease related to childbirth. *N. Eng. J. Med.* **268,** 1224.

Rees, D. and Lutkins, S. G. (1971). Parental depression before and after childbirth. *J. Roy. Coll. Gen. Practit.* **21,** 26.

Robson, K. M. and Kumar, R. (1980). Delayed onset of maternal affection after childbirth. *Br. J. Psychiatr.* **136**, 347.

Robson, K. M. and Powell, E. (1982). Early maternal attachment. In *Motherhood and mental illness.* (eds. I. F. Brockington and R. Kumar). Academic Press, London; Grune and Stratton, New York.

Ryle, A. (1964). Puerperal depression. *Lancet* **2**, 1394.

Stein, G. (1982). The maternity blues. In *Motherhood and mental illness.* (eds. I. F. Brockington and R. Kumar) Academic Press, London and Grune Stratton, New York.

Stern, G. and Kruckman, L. (1983). Multidisciplinary perspectives on postpartum depression: an anthropological critique. *Soc. Sci. Med.* **17**, 1027.

Tod, E. D. M. (1964). Puerperal depression: a prospective epidemiological study. *Lancet* **2**, 1264.

Weeks, D., Freeman, C. L. L., and Kendell, R. E. (1980). Enduring cognitive deficits following E. C. T. in depression. *Br. J. Psychiatr.* **137**, 26.

Wrath, R. M., Rooney, A., Thomas, P., and Cox, J. L. (1983). Postnatal depression and later child behaviour. *Abstracts of 7th World Congress of Psychiatry,* **S 571**, p. 136.

Yalom, I. D., Lunde, D. T., Moss, R. H., and Hamburg, R. A. (1968). Post partum blues syndrome. *Arch. Gen. Psychiatry* **18**, 16.

Section E
'New style' general practitioner obstetric care

30 The training and continuing education of the general practitioner in maternity care

M. McKendrick

INTRODUCTION

There is general agreement that despite the teaching of undergraduates in obstetrics and gynaecology and the inclusion of these subjects in their quali-fying examination there is a need for any intending general practitioner to undertake postgraduate training in obstetrics and gynaecology. Also, the established doctor cannot place reliance entirely on day-to-day clinical work to maintain the knowledge and skills needed to provide the highest stan-dards of care which are demanded particularly in the care of pregnant women, to ensure a happy and successful process and outcome. The content of training has been debated and reported on by obstetricians and general practitioners (RCOG and RCGP 1982) and the recommendations have met with widespread acceptance. Changes have occurred in the content of the work experience of the young doctor.

However, there is a need for further consideration of this phase and to the continuing professional development of the established doctor whether participating in shared care or managing full care.

BASIC MEDICAL EDUCATION

Experience and teaching in obstetrics and gynaecology is a small but im-portant component of undergraduate education. The objectives are clearly stated by the General Medical Council and include attendance at a mini-mum number of confinements. However, the experience is gained entirely in the hospital setting and is designed to enable the graduate to fulfil certain basic obligations towards the recognition and management of obstetric emergencies, including unexpected confinement. There is no argument that postgraduate training will eventually be necessary for intending general practitioners as well as specialists in obstetrics and gynaecology. Nonethe-less, there are good grounds for suggesting that attention be given to provid-ing the opportunity for undergraduates to learn about maternity services in the general practice setting. Shared antenatal care is the norm and many practices could provide good teaching in this area. In addition, contraception, preconception and postnatal care can also be demonstrated as they fall easily into the continuity of care which is the essence of general practice.

THE CONTENT OF VOCATIONAL TRAINING

It is a reasonable assumption that a large measure of hospital-based experience and teaching is appropriate; childbirth usually takes place in a hospital setting and it is there that the specialty has its main base. Six-month senior house officer appointments are the rule and fit neatly into rotational programmes. The RCOG in recent years has revised the content of the young doctor's experience to include substantial components of gynaecology including outpatient experience, counselling and family planning as well as the more traditional responsibilities of obstetric practice. Of course, there is variability from place to place. The larger, teaching hospital environment does not always enable the senior house officer to have the same first-hand experience as in the district general hospital where because of the different staffing structures there may be more direct contact with consultants in charge and more emphasis on the practical side of the service. In the latter situations the young doctor may also have greater opportunity of contact with general practitioner colleagues who may be involved in intranatal care. Registrar rotations in obstetric specialty training often bridge the two circumstances but this does not happen with senior house officers. However, the RCOG in its recognition of hospital posts is aware of these differences and recently has attempted to categorize senior house officer posts in three ways:

(i) first 6-month posts for novices to the subject;
(ii) second posts for those wishing to gain further experience perhaps with a view to pursuing a career in the subject;
(iii) senior posts for those with previous experience who should be able to take on a greater degree of responsibility in the service (RCOG and RCGP 1982).

A helpful method of joint visiting in which the RCOG inspecting team is accompanied by a representative from the RCGP enables the structure and content of the hospital posts to be viewed and debated, mainly with an eye to the needs of those who will become general practitioners, as well as the broader educational and service characteristics. Of the total number of senior house officer posts in the United Kingdom a tiny minority are needed to train intending specialists (Maternity Services Advisory Committee, 1982) so that there should be ample opportunity for general practice trainees to have at least one 6-month post in obstetrics and gynaecology.

The objectives of such training are carefully listed in the Report of the Joint Working Party. (RCOG and RCGP 1982). It has been argued that for doctors wishing ultimately to provide only antenatal and postnatal care the training needs are different. However sound this theoretical educational argument might be it is unlikely to prevail: the logistical demands cause difficulties for it is not always possible to provide experiences of varying length in rotational programmes within vocational training schemes and there is a feeling that 6 months in the discipline of obstetrics and gynaecology is little enough time to become reasonably competent in the whole care of the pregnant woman and baby. Experience in childbirth is fundamental to the full understanding of maternity care, and the 6 months which includes periods of study leave and holiday, is the minimum in which to achieve a suitable level of expertise. Also, it is easier and more convenient for a young doctor to complete a full period of training at this stage in a career rather than having to add to it at a later date when preparing to join a practice which contributes to full maternity care. The marketplace value of an obstetric post leading to eligibility to take the Diploma examination of the RCOG is not lost to these arguments.

HOW MAY VOCATIONAL TRAINING BE IMPROVED?

Young doctors do not express a great dissatisfaction with their hospital experience; they may grumble about the demands made on them in a busy unit but overall the experience, supervision and teaching are satisfactory. Nonetheless, when questioned many graduates from training are not enthusiastic about taking on the responsibility of full care in general practice and may express doubts about their competence to fulfil the role of general practitioner obstetrician. There are several reasons why this may be so: the erratic demands of clinical practice may simply be unacceptable but another possibility is that they have not seen at first-hand how rewarding maternity care in general practice can be for the family, the midwife and the doctor. They will have had scant contact with general practitioners who are enthusiastic about maternity care and more often than not will only have become involved when complications have arisen thereby gaining a distorted view about the competence of such management. The happy pregnancy with the highly satisfactory outcome managed by a skilful and interested general practitioner may not have come readily to their notice. The pursuit of 'high technology' obstetrics however important in its own right, is off-putting.

Models of training for obstetrics and gynaecology based in general practice with time spent in hospital have been proposed, notably by Ross Munro (personal communication). It is suggested that a programme be devised with a basis in a suitable general practice with a coordinated experience in hospital, antenatal clinics and other relevant situations. Such radical rethinking has inevitably not been well received although the theoretical educational basis is a sound one if the doctor intends only to provide antenatal and postnatal care. However, an alternative option of providing the opportunity for a senior house officer whether pursuing a specialist or generalist career to learn about maternity care in general practice could be both easy to arrange and have mutual learning advantages. Of course, the laudable arrangements made at Sighthill (McKee, 1983) and other projects have brought hospital and community closer together and the outcome whether measured by cold statistical analysis, the satisfaction of the families and the better working relationships between professionals is entirely satisfactory. It is tempting to extrapolate these concepts to the encouragement of junior doctors to visit practices where antenatal care is provided, and, importantly, that general practitioners should participate actively in the teaching as well as the practice, in hospital. Selected general practices, which may not necessarily be approved postgraduate teaching practices, could be involved by mutual discussion between the Regional Education Committees in the two subjects. Maternity Service Liaison Committees (Maternity Services Advisory Committee 1982) would be suitable bodies to monitor such arrangements and it is hard to believe that maternity care would not be enhanced should such arrangements be made generally available.

General practice is a major provider of contraceptive care which increasingly will include preconception counselling and also it is to the general practitioner that most women requiring confirmation of pregnancy and subsequent management first turn. Requests for termination of pregnancy are seen at the earliest stage.

However, the most powerful argument for providing an educational bridge between hospital and general practice is to link the woman's pregnancy with her home environment and with it the relationships and information which are the general practitioner's privilege. Midwives attached to practices are in no doubt of the advantages and look to colleagues in general practice to help them pursue their aims.

THE NEEDS OF THE ESTABLISHED GENERAL PRACTITIONER

It is self-evident that the maintenance of skills and updating where this is required for the established doctor should be based on day-to-day clinical work including responsibility on a regular basis for pregnant women. It is difficult to quantify this in number of pregnancies or childbirth for which the doctor may be responsible; the service demands vary and many practitioners have to provide maternity services in geographically isolated situations for there is no other alternative. Other colleagues, often practising in partnership develop special interests amongst them perhaps being obstetrics and one or two partners may accept the responsibility for a whole practice's obstetric commitment. The educational needs of these doctors must vary and a whole range of possibilities exist from short courses largely lecture-based which are ideal for a quick refreshment or updating knowledge to a week or two's clinical attachment in a consultant unit which gives time and opportunity for practical work as well as theoretical learning. It is easy to overplay such formal provisions and to underestimate the extent to which doctors seek self-improvement through their own individual learning methods. Such personal and continuing professional development is an intrinsic requirement of independent practice and deserves every encouragement. Teaching aids which include video-recording are commonplace and should enable a doctor to see new techniques in his home.

For most of us, however strongly motivated, encouragement and sometimes skilled help is needed to manage our own continuing education. We need to be able to see our own practice in the context of others and to know how to make advances. Of prime importance among the methods to achieve these aims must come small group work based on actual clinical material for which good data are available. Peer review has a strong controlling and regulating aura and this is a powerful disincentive to clinicians with a strong sense of autonomy in their practice. The discipline of obstetrics has led the way in the audit of practice through the confidential inquiry into maternal deaths and perinatal mortality studies and much has been learnt from these rigorously critical activities. However, the process of care, the way in which it is actually delivered has escaped such attention until recently when the Maternity Services Advisory Committee (1982) in *Maternity care in action* has focused sharply on the provision of antenatal and intranatal care; also the Royal College of Obstetricians and Gynaecologists has published its report on these two aspects (RCOG 1982). These developments are to be welcomed and it is of vital importance that good working links are created and fostered between service and educational authorities. Again, maternity service liaison committees should be able to provide these facilities.

TOWARDS AN INTEGRATED SERVICE

There is no place in clinical practice and in maternity care in particular, to perpetuate the division between hospital doctor and general practitioner, between hospital and the family's home environment. The educational processes outlined in this chapter maintain a theme of understanding and cooperation between pregnant women, their families and the professional responsible for their care. There need to be further forays into interdisciplinary education and the new forum within the Royal Society of Medicine is a highly praiseworthy attack in this area. Of course, in the heart-searching which is currently taking place in each professional group there is a seeking after professional identity and there is nothing innately wrong in this. However, in parallel there must be at local level, say district or hospital, a positive approach to interdisciplinary education to allow the free expression and discussion of professional aspirations in order through better understanding to provide new standards of care and to demonstrate a new responsiveness to the demands of women. These are difficult and time-consuming tasks but the rewards will be enormous. The general practitioner can play a strong if not leading part in bringing such groups together and advice and financial support should be available through regional postgraduate medical organizations.

REFERENCES

Maternity Services Advisory Committee (1982). *Maternity care in action.*

McKee, I. (1983). The Sighthill Community Antenatal Care Scheme. *In Pregnancy and its management.* Macmillan, London.

Royal College of Obstetricians and Gynaecologists and Royal College of General Practitioners (1982). Report by a Joint Working Party: *Training for obstetrics and gynaecology for general practitioners.* RCOG and RCGP, London.

RCOG (1982). Report of the Working Party: *Antenatal and intrapartum care.*

31 'New style' obstetric care

G. N. Marsh

INTRODUCTION

I have found the editing of this book a fascinating experience and I have
learned a great deal. There cannot be many texts that contain contributions
from noted feminists, distinguished professors of obstetrics, general practitioners, and practising midwives. The first group tend to express radical
views, the second more conventional ones, and the latter two groups are
pragmatic. In this final chapter I want to draw together the threads of the
various ideas in these diverse chapters. Sometimes I will be leaning more on
a quoted reference than on a text in the book and occasionally on my own
25 years obstetric experience. There will be no further references, however;
there are probably too many already! In particular I shall indicate how I will
apply what I have learned in the setting of my own practice. I hope other
general practitioners will be able to do likewise. I shall be using, incident-
ally, not just expertise from specialists in the obstetric field, which has been
the customary source of knowledge for obstetric students, but also perhaps
more importantly expertise from associated disciplines and perhaps most
importantly 'expertise' from women themselves.

Throughout the book I have tried to get authors to write cohesively and
not contradict each other, nor write anything with which I fundamentally
disagreed. But where they have, and they have stuck to their view despite
my editorial remonstrances, this final chapter provides me with an opportunity to respond. I still do not expect them to agree and readers must make
their own selection from contrary opinions. I do not regret differences,
rather do I feel that progress flows from them.

As I wrote in the introduction, the antenatal and postnatal period of a
woman's life is very central to the role of the family doctor. The
psychological rapport that can develop during those periods is of enormous
significance to the family doctor–patient relationship. Hence the importance of this book to all general practitioners. There is currently a
reawakened interest in 'holistic medicine'; but in fact where the population
is reasonably stable, general practitioners have been doing this for many
years. It can be well exemplified in good obstetric care.

COMMUNICATION, CONTINUITY, AND CONVENIENCE

Throughout this book and spelled out particularly by the non-medical contributors is a plea for better communication and more humanity in obstetric care. Better communication does not mean talking to mothers; I shall try to listen more to them and particularly ask for 'any questions' at the end of an explanation, and again at the end of a further explanation. As a splendid example Dr Burne (Chapter 28) emphasizes that parents should be told 'what you are doing and why' during the examination of their newborn. They should be given time to ask questions. Occasionally, however, there may be findings apparent only to me, that make me anxious, but I also know that they may well prove groundless; I think I should keep these to myself until the problem is confirmed or definitive action is needed. There is potential danger in overcommunicating and causing unnecessary worry which parents cannot put into the context of a broad medical knowledge. Fortunately, where doctor and patient have known each other for some time—often years—the time taken for such exchanges is not long since communication levels have been established over a long period of time.

There is strong evidence that general practitioners meet women's requirements very well and are considered the best source of information during pregnancy. Nevertheless, I shall have to give much thought to and increasingly respect the attitudes outlined by Catherine Boyd (Chapter 3). Notable amongst these are that mothers do not expect to have unwanted babies and want limited numbers; there will be very few grand multiparae. I must try and provide very effective contraception and they will expect (and have) terminations of pregnancy; this will possibly help my perinatal mortality rate. Women expect respect for single-parent status which is sometimes even voluntary and they expect respect for cohabitation as a trial for future happy marriage. I must understand that many mothers want to work, before, during and after having children. They want emotional and psychological satisfaction in pregnancy and labour and not a catalogue of medical interventions and events. This is strongly supported by Hilary Cashman (Chapter 1): 'the alternatives that women have been seeking for childbirth—home births, the Pithivier method, and so on—have two common features: they shun unnecessary interference, and they cherish the personal and emotional side of birth (both of which factors are now admitted to have medical advantages). In general practitioner care both features have been preserved.' I must ensure that that is totally true in my own work.

It seems that many general practitioners do treat women as 'total women' and that they meet their wider needs, not just their medical ones. Again this is relevant to the 'holistic' medicine currently in favour. Certainly in obstetrics where women are not ill there is a strong indication for using a more 'holistic' approach.

Hilary Cashman 'found continuity of care to be a morale booster in pregnancy' and 'it was good to see a familiar face [her general practitioner] when I was so close to delivering having seen no-one but the hospital staff for several hours'. Such comments about continuity of care are heartening to a general practitioner who year in, year out looks after the same people in the same place. The very monotony which seems implicit proves, as far as women are concerned, to be a virtue. To have all the facilities under one roof and of easy geographical and operational access is a great advantage. I must increase the facilities and oil the machinery of access frequently. More important than convenience, however, is enthusiasm and interest from the general practitioner; these two qualities are highly prized: I must manifest them more often.

Hilary Cashman writes 'there is a quality of enchantment about a first pregnancy and labour which should be left intact if at all possible: it is part of the rite of passage which turns a couple (or single woman) into a family and obstetricians should think hard and long before violating it.' The emotions underlying that sentence appeal to me; I must do everything I can to preserve 'the enchantment'.

THE PRIMARY HEALTH CARE TEAM

As I have written the chapter on the team, my enthusiasm for it is apparent and the details do not need repeating. I believe that this community-based multidisciplinary approach is the best method of providing comprehensive antenatal care to all patients whether booked for general practitioner or consultant unit delivery; fortunately such teams are increasingly common.

If you belong to a team which is incomplete then probably rereading Chapter 12 will give you ideas as to how matters can be improved. Currently my own team, for example, lacks a breast-feeding counsellor and I must do something about it. In many places the teams do exist, but their function is poor: merely a number of professionals under the same roof, but not collaborating.

Evidence of better care from the effective team is provided by two statements from consultants in this book. Dr Hall (Chapter 6) writes 'very young girls rarely present in early pregnancy unless they are seeking termination'. With our team which has been functioning effectively for approximately 15 years—that is, the whole life time of the majority of the 'very young girls'—late presentation, whether for termination or not, is extremely rare. Similarly Mr Godfrey (Chapter 11) writes 'over 25 per cent of obstetric patients do not present a reliable menstrual history'—the percentage is much smaller with us, the result of continuing educational efforts by health visitor, family planning nurse, midwife, and doctor.

Repeatedly in this book occurs evidence that low social-class women have a bad time in pregnancy and a relatively poor obstetric outcome. The comprehensive team approach can go some way to improving this. Attention to diet, grants, housing, fostering etc. can be as important in antenatal care to low social-class groups as can any medical involvement. Dr Pitt (Chapter 7) in his contribution on psychiatric care in pregnancy agrees the need for support of the deprived communities by primary health care teams.

With the presence of doctor and midwife both able to do routine antenatal care duplication of care must be guarded against. On the other hand when one or other professional is absent there is still someone to continue the care. I find my midwives are most conscientious and dependable deputies. Overall, though, in primary health care teams the midwives could be used more and given greater responsibility. By the same token there is an important role for the health visitor, not only in the postnatal period, but also antenatally. Again she should orientate her work more on the deprived and lower social classes. Increasingly I accept that she is an expert in her own right. When asked, for example, about a feeding problem I try to remember not to deal with it myself, but refer to my health visitor; she knows more about it than I do. Many general practitioners reading Chapter 26 will feel it is an account of what they themselves are doing. I must implement more the expertise of my health visitor since that chapter was written by one. The doctor's role postnatally can be found in Chapter 28.

PRE-CONCEPTION COUNSELLING

Now that the perinatal mortality rate is so low I am beginning to find it difficult to improve that measure of outcome even more. Pre-conception counselling, however, does seem to offer some possibilities. It has the added advantage of being good health advice whether women are pregnant or not. This particularly applies to advice regarding smoking and alcohol. It is obvious from my own Chapter 4 that it can be done within the setting of the primary health care team and that it can be done by nurses working to an approved protocol. Next month (or next year!) I must establish a preconception counselling clinic probably by sitting down with my family planning nurse and hammering out a simple, recordable protocol as part of the normal record system. This she can check off as patients present *en passant* during routine family planning consultations.

THE NEW-STYLE ANTENATAL PROGRAMME

I found it extremely interesting that Dr Hall (Chapter 6) begins her account of the antenatal programme with 'education for labour and parenthood'. Thus she stresses the educative component rather than the medical one. She itemizes utilization of National Childbirth Trust self-help groups and of groups at practices who can attend classes and look at videos and films etc. I must increase this in my own practice—it is rather threadbare and gets minimal 'doctor enthusiasm' at the present time. Dr Hall believes that a competent midwife can give most of the antenatal care to normal women. I think she would agree, however, that the general practitioner knowing his mothers more comprehensively should probably ordain the programme for each individual. Indeed it is this concept of an individual programme for each woman that I shall aim for in the future. In recent years too much antenatal and postnatal care has been carried out by general practitioners according to protocols which were designed during the 1940s and 1950s for a population far less affluent and less healthy than now exists. In the future I believe there should be a minimum schedule to which additions should be made rather than an extravagant all-embracing 'featherbed' system which is for most women totally unnecessary.

Using this principle and by a careful reading of Chapter 6 I have produced a new style antenatal programme for primigravidae (Tables 31.1 and 31.2) and multiparae (Tables 31.3 and 31.4). It is eminently suitable in general practice particularly in the setting of a primary health care team. As well as medical needs it concerns itself with psychological and social needs too. Hence it is a little more elaborate than the minimal care described by Dr Hall who is hospital based. The numbers of attendances and especially doctor consultations is small and the decrease as compared with currently recommended practice is shown in Table 31.5. For primigravidae it is reduced

Table 31.1 *'New style' obstetric programme for primigravidae 8–32 weeks*

Gestation in weeks	Done by	Major reasons
8	Midwife and doctor	See Table 31.6
12	Midwife	Going along OK? Any questions . . .? Any more questions?
16	—	Scan at hospital
22	Midwife	Baseline weight, blood pressure, twins Literature package (late pregnancy and labour) Arrangements for classes, films, NCT etc.
26	Midwife	Weight, blood pressure, reiterate literature, classes etc.
30	Midwife and doctor	Assess fetal size Blood pressure, weight (predictive IUGR, pre-eclampsia) Customary blood tests

Table 31.2 'New style' obstetric programme for primigravidae 34–42 weeks

Gestation in weeks	Done by	Major reasons
34	Midwife and doctor	Presentation
		Pelvic assessment, blood pressure, urine
36	Midwife and doctor	Blood pressure, urine and presentation
	Family planning nurse	Build up rapport, confidence
		Discuss labour plan
		Literature package (infant care)
		Discuss contraception
38	Midwife and doctor	As for 36 weeks (excluding literature & contraception)
		Engagement of presenting part
40	Midwife and doctor	As for 38 weeks
41	Midwife and doctor	As for 38 weeks
		Confirm normality
42	Midwife and doctor	As for 41 weeks
		Double-check dates

Table 31.3 'New style' obstetric programme for multiparae 8–32 weeks

Gestation in weeks	Done by	Major reasons
8–12	Midwife and doctor	See Table 31.6
16	Family planning	Scan at hospital
22	Midwife	Baseline weight, blood pressure, twins
		Literature package (late pregnancy and labour)
		Arrangements for classes, films, NCT etc.
30	Midwife and doctor	Assess fetal size
		Blood pressure, weight (predictive IUGR, pre-eclampsia)
		Customary blood tests

by almost 50 per cent and for multiparous women even more. When I implement this programme I shall have to explain that the antenatal clinic offers, in addition to the formal protocol, casual access to women who have a problem. In other words, patient-initiated consultations. These consultations can be with any member of the team, not just the doctor. I will have to inform the other members of the team of the programme and reassure, them and particularly the midwife, that the present good results will con-

Table 31.4 *'New style' obstetric programme for multiparae 34–42 weeks*

Gestation in weeks	Done by	Major reasons
36	Midwife and doctor	Blood pressure, and presentation Build up rapport, confidence Discuss labour plan Literature package (infant care) Discuss contraception
40	Midwife and doctor	As for 36 weeks (excluding literature and contraception) Engagement of presenting part
41	Midwife and doctor	As for 40 weeks Confirm normality
42	Midwife and doctor	As for 41 weeks Double-check dates

Table 31.5 *Number of doctor consultations in 'new and old style' antenatal care*

Period of gestation	Primigravidae		Multiparae	
	'Old style'	'New style	'Old style	'New style'
8–32 weeks	7	2	7	2
34–42 weeks	8	6	8	4
Total	15	8	15	6

tinue. It will be important to stress that each consultation will probably be longer and more leisurely, and the table describes the major reasons for each consultation. The all-important first formal antenatal attendance—as distinct from the notification of pregnancy which often takes place at a normal surgery during normal surgery hours—is described in Table 31.6. Also on Tables 31.1 to 31.5 is specified which member of the primary health care team will carry out which consultation. Although the implementation and coordination of new programmes such as this will be an effort in themselves I feel that the time saved from the current wasteful system will be more than adequate recompense. Some of it, of course, will be spent giving more care to those at greatest risk.

The programme described relates to women booked for general practitioner delivery and receiving sole care from their primary health care team. Where women are to deliver in hospital, either because of high-risk problems, or because no general practitioner facilities are available, the hospital attendances will be over and above this programme. I respectfully suggest that the principles of a caring, cost-effective system need careful institution in the current hospital programmes too.

Table 31.6 *Major reasons for first antenatal consultation*

Introduction to midwife (doctor usually known)
Assess general condition and previous significant illnesses
Obstetric history, family history
Assign to 'risk' group
Specify appropriate individual programme
Customary blood tests (including rubella)
Urine culture
Literature package for early pregnancy

SOME IMPORTANT DETAILS IN 'NEW STYLE' ANTENATAL CARE

Dr Pitt (Chapter 7) believes that childbirth puts mental health at risk, but that all the risk is post partum. He does not see abortion being associated with many psychiatric problems and feels that psychiatrically there are few problems in the antenatal period. It is interesting to find that there are fewer psychiatric admissions during pregnancy than there are for a comparable non-pregnant group. The lay view much supported by my own findings is that many women are 'never better' than when pregnant and this probably relates to the feeling of psychological wellbeing that so many women experience. Only those women who have had an earlier pregnancy terminated require a little more careful watching for depressive symptoms.

Urine culture in early pregnancy seems a valuable test and I must be a little more strict with women who are asked to bring a urine sample in a sterile bottle the day following the antenatal clinic to the surgery. Not all do and the test seems eminently worthwhile. If positive the bacteriuria should be treated. Another worthwhile test seems to be a rubella titre in every pregnancy since the level falls the further the woman is away from her antigen exposure (infection or injection).

There is no doubt that ultrasound has been the most useful development in the last decade in obstetric practice and it is fortunately totally harmless. Its precision will no doubt improve in the future, but even at the present time it has great value on a routine basis. All pregnancies should have ultrasound examination around 16–18 weeks in order to estimate gestational age by the biparietal diameter. It is heartening to find that the accuracy is plus or minus 7 days for 95 per cent of women who are screened at that time. At that stage too it can also pick up neural tube defects. There seems some evidence that it will be worth while repeating the ultrasound examination at 30 weeks for accurate determination of intrauterine growth retardation. Whether this needs to be carried out in every pregnancy may be decided by a further evaluation in the not too distant future. Ultrasound is also useful after early vaginal bleeding to determine rapidly whether the pregnancy is continuing.

Protein and calories may benefit small light women and certainly supplementation showed minor benefits to poor ill-nourished Aberdonian women, the main tangible outcome being bigger babies. Strict dieting of obese women in pregnancy is inadvisable, but they could restrict their total weight gain to 8 kg since this gives optimal perinatal mortality rate and no adverse effects on birth weight and neonatal outcome.

No woman should receive routine iron during pregnancy, but it should be reserved to treat those who are anaemic. Anaemia should be determined from the mean corpuscular volume and not the haemoglobin level. By the same token vitamins do not benefit pregnancy, but I shall keep my eye open for the large-scale trial on the prevention of neural tube defects (such as spina bifida) by giving vitamins preconceptually and in the first 8 weeks of pregnancy.

With regard to other technology used in pregnancy with great enthusiasm in the last decade, the majority of it seems to be being abandoned rather than used increasingly. However, routine amniocentesis after a maternal age of 40 for Down's syndrome and the proffering of this procedure to women between 37 and 40 years will reduce the number of mongol babies significantly. I must always remember to mention this to my older women and it must also be part of the nurses preconception counselling protocol. Premature labour is still one of the life-threatening events in pregnancy and it is important to admit all women in suspected premature labour to a hospital where if by chance the baby is born special care facilities exist for it. The diagnosis of premature labour is vital since it does seem that a small proportion of these women can have their labours delayed, allowing further intrauterine fetal growth. Fetal heart rate monitoring, fetal body and breathing movements seem unlikely to be of any use and I get the feeling that they will probably be superceded by other more accurate methods of measurement. Currently they have little to offer and the stress tests with oxytocics associated with them can be positively harmful.

Strict evaluation of fetal kick charts seems to suggest that they are little more than of psychological value.

Since epiphyseal calcification is unreliable radiology at terms seems of little use. It has helped me over the years to allow so called 'postmature' patients to become more 'postmature', but with the decreasing importance of postmaturity in otherwise normal pregnancies I think I shall abandon this. I shall also have greater confirmation of date accuracy following the routine ultrasound programme recommended above.

Plasma oestriols even serially are frequently unhelpful and their greatest use is in the high-risk fetus where if oestriol is normal the pregnancy can be allowed to continue. Such deliberations, however, are beyond the general practitioner's competence.

ARE GENERAL PRACTITIONER DELIVERIES SAFE?

Professor Stirrat (Chapter 2) states 'however, most studies on place of delivery and perinatal outcome have failed to show the clear association between general practitioner deliveries and adverse outcome that has been implicitly accepted by the profession and successive governments'. There is no evidence anywhere in this book that statistically general practitioner deliveries are unsafe. The reputation and credence of the obstetric specialist contributors is such that if there had been evidence they would have referred to it. Indeed, Marjorie Tew (Chapter 14) has amassed an enormous battering ram of statistics to show that general practitioners need not be daunted and that in the care of normal women who stay normal general practitioner care gives a lower perinatal mortality rate than specialist care. Hence there is a sound statistically based case for general practitioner and midwife looking after the majority of women. Indeed Mrs Tew goes further and suggests cogently that in normal cases intervention can do more harm than good. Thus if all women were booked into a consultant unit the results in terms of perinatal mortality and morbidity would be much worse. Normal women receiving general practitioner care—even for a home delivery—would feel very reassured by Mrs Tew's statistics. Her findings conflict with Dr Michael Bull's conventional theoretical argument for delivering all women in a large unit with general practitioner care integrated within it (Chapter 16).

Nevertheless, despite the comforting statistics it is incumbent upon at least some general practitioners doing deliveries to audit their results. Dr Bull (Chapter 15) has given an excellent account of various methods of doing this. For simple analyses concerned mostly with basic perinatal mortality rate all the partners in my practice merely need to carry out their usual antenatal, intranatal, and postnatal recording on the RCGP obstetric record card. To this has been added a few simple additional boxes about type of labour, attendance in labour, perineal repair, duration of breast feeding etc. in order to complete a logbook which can then be computed, and thus realize a significant amount of interesting practice data (Chapter 13).

ALTERNATIVE SETTINGS FOR LABOUR

Freedom of choice has always been a democratic British concept and applies not only to health, but also to other fundamental processes such as education. A lack of freedom of choice generates pressure groups for alternatives. In California 15 per cent of deliveries now take place at home because of a medical *diktat* that this should not be the case. I find that if multiple hospital alternatives are offered (a full 7 day stay, 48-hour stay, immediate discharge after labour) then home delivery is very rarely requested. I can remember one occasion in the last 5 years and 250 deliveries. In this chapter

I shall comment briefly on the four types of delivery setting and I hope make some reasonable suggestions.

Integrated unit

Dr Bull (Chapter 16) is deeply committed to his 'integrated unit' style of care. It is difficult for him to appreciate the especial qualities found in the isolated general practitioner maternity unit, or alongside unit where autonomy is virtually absolute and responsibility intense. Nevertheless his system is extremely acceptable to consultants and to his general practitioner colleagues and is being recommended as the major method of involving general practitioners in intranatal care. Accordingly what he writes is extremely worthy of study and to his credit he has preserved as much normality as he can and provided a happy atmosphere in which his general practitioner colleagues can work. It is interesting to see how even in his unit autonomy has been safeguarded. He writes 'it will be clear from the foregoing account that in the circumstances of this particular integrated general practitioner unit both doctors and community midwives have a very considerable degree of autonomy in the management of their patients in labour which is a logical extension of their roles in antenatal care'. On the fourteen-person management committee there are six general practitioners and only three consultants of whom one is a paediatrician. Nevertheless I see the potential danger of the care of normal women being affected by the consultant-style care and protocols used for abnormal women. In Dr Bull's unit consultant 'normals' had more technology than their general practitioner equivalents even though both were delivered in the same setting. I cannot help wondering, however, whether in absolute terms even the general practitioner 'normals' had more technology than general practitioner normal cases in an isolated or an alongside unit. Such comparison would be a further interesting research project. Nevertheless Dr Bull makes it apparent that general practitioners need not be daunted by the technology all around them when they work in an integrated unit. Their special role of managing normal cases in normal labour can still survive. Whether Jean Towler's (Chapter 20) beautiful description of the setting of normal obstetrics would be possible in an integrated unit must be a little in doubt. The starkly sterile laboratory-like rooms built in the modern obstetric hospitals in the 1960s and 1970s are hardly conducive to the modern normal obstetrics that she practises.

The alongside unit

In the alongside unit there is no technology present, but it is readily available 'next door' and rapid transfer is automatic. I was delighted to read that Mr Godfrey (Chapter 23) believes that there is absolutely no reason to monitor normal labour and that the general consensus of opinion is that this leads to an escalation of interventions doing more harm than good. There seems little reason why exactly similar types of booking could not be arranged for both the integrated and the alongside unit. In both units it seems there should be more flexibility of arrangements whereby women who apparently have a risk problem at the beginning of pregnancy, which does not manifest later in the pregnancy, or whose significance has disappeared, could be returned for care in labour in either an integrated or an alongside unit. In the alongside unit it should be easier to achieve the delights of Jean Towler's care to the great satisfaction of the women involved more easily than in an integrated unit. I have expressed all the pros and cons of my own alongside unit in Chapter 17.

Isolated unit

There obviously have to be more rigorous booking arrangements for an isolated unit than an integrated, or alongside one. I do not believe, however, that primigravidae should not be booked for an isolated unit so long as transfer arrangements are reasonably speedy. Delay in the first stage can be tolerated in an ambulance just as well by the woman as it can in an obstetric unit. It is more than likely that the parameters for so-called 'delay' will change and probably be lengthened as more evaluation and audit is carried out on longer labours. In the isolated unit, if the resort to rupturing membranes is delayed until labour is extremely well-established rather than carried out somewhat prematurely, as it frequently is at present, then fewer so-called 'delays' would occur. It is the potential dangers of infection and the commitment to a very much more active management of labour following too-early rupture of the membranes that causes problems in the isolated unit.

Home deliveries

Dr Sides (Chapter 19) estimates that the perinatal mortality rate at home for low-risk normal women possibly rises by one per 1000 births—say from five or six deaths per 1000 to six or seven per 1000. Some women believe that the advantages of home confinement 'outweigh the slight increase in risk'. Obstetricians argue that anything can happen even to the most normal women in labour. Indeed they say that of the low-risk normals in hospital 10 per cent developed abnormalities in labour. This is not as horrendous as it sounds. Many of the problems that do occur are in the first stage and are not all that urgent; so if they were at home they could be transferred to hospital.

Furthermore, many of the so-called abnormalities are not serious, nor in any way life-threatening, but merely reflect variations from strict hospital norms. For example a first stage longer than 12 hours, or a second stage longer than 1 hour, would be defined as 'abnormal'—the fact that the

Apgar score of the baby exposed to either of those situations could be 10/10 would be irrelevant: the labour was still 'abnormal'. Similarly a postpartum haemorrhage of 600 ml would be described as 'abnormal' even though the haemoglobin was normal 3 days later—and the matter patently of little import to mother or baby. Slow delivery of the placenta or maternal blood pressure of 150/95 during labour do not really matter much although defined as abnormalities.

Many mothers believe that even these minor abnormalities would not arise if they were happily at home instead of in strange hospital surroundings attended by people whom they may never have met and do not know. Finally, some women believe that some of the abnormalities are a sequel to 'interference' in their labour (for example, being put to bed when they would rather walk about). I find it hard to argue with this mixture of statistics and emotion and even harder to deny freedom of choice at the end of any discussion. If a woman who has had one, two, or three babies perfectly normally, and has had a normal pregnancy this time, asks me if she can have her baby at home I will happily look after her there. I will explain the risks—such as they are—I will tell her that *I* would be happier with her under a hospital roof—but if at the end of the day she wants her baby to be born at home I shall care for her meticulously—and try to enjoy the event with her.

DETERMINATION OF 'RISK'

Determination of 'risk' is still very important, but it is difficult to know where the cutoff comes for consultant care as opposed to general practitioner care in labour. Some of the factors affecting perinatal mortality rate indentifiable by history and examination do not necessarily all preclude general practitioner booking—some disappear in importance, for example illegitimacy; some wane, for example bleeding at 6 weeks; but several factors together increase anxiety. It is important to remember that screening later in the pregnancy can show that risks have gone and care in labour can be returned to the general practitioner. Dr Newcombe's tables (Chapter 8) help to highlight bad risks; as an example, previous perinatal death is more than twice as likely to repeat itself. Women under 16 are at very high risk of perinatal death and social class V women have a high perinatal death rate and also a high incidence of low birth weight at term. Similarly women under 45 kg have a bad perinatal mortality rate and also a high incidence of low birth weight at term. Heavier patients seem to be relatively low risk. Mothers smoking 20 or more cigarettes a day have a high incidence of low birth weight at term, but a very low abnormal delivery rate. Rather surprisingly grand multiparity only seems to be very much greater risk after five or more previous deliveries and not three or four as has been previously thought. I see no reason why I should not book all my gravida 4 para 3 mothers. Dr Hall (Chapter 6) considers there is no greater risk of complication after having a previous termination of pregnancy and with the high prevalence of this procedure I would certainly have more patients by being able to overlook this as a 'previous complication'. More important Dr Hall also finds, and I would very much agree, that women's experiences in labour can determine the setting of their next booking. A mother who has had inadequate pain relief in her first labour may well ask for an epidural in the second and specialist care, whereas another mother who feels she has had too much 'interference' in her first labour may well ask for general practitioner care in an attempt to avoid this subsequently. These are extremely cogent and relevant reasons and I acquiesce to them.

THE 'NEW STYLE' LABOUR PROGRAMME

It has been customary for a midwife—often with a pupil midwife—to carry out general practitioner unit, or even home deliveries on her own and call the general practitioner if and when necessary. Often enough this has been merely for the repair of the perineum. This must change. I believe and I feel most people (lay and professional) would agree that every baby 'lives dangerously' in the first 10 minutes of life. Accordingly skilled pairs of trained hands, one of which belongs to a doctor, should be present at the delivery. The general practitioner obstetrician today should attend each labour in the first stage (usually a fairly leisurely appearance), in the second stage, and stay with the woman and her midwife until the third stage is complete and the baby in a stable condition with a good Apgar score. The major reasons for these attendances are listed in Table 31.7. Thereafter care can largely be undertaken by the midwife whether it be in hospital or in the home until the health visitor enters the programme, at around 10–14 days. The general practitioner needs to visit once at home—as opposed to the ritualistic alternate-day routine practised heretofore—ideally around the 6th day to assess the family setting and check the baby comprehensively with a full physical examination. Table 31.7 shows the programme up to the 6-week postnatal examination. Such a programme can only be justified, however, if midwife, health visitor, and doctor are truly working as a team, know of each other's role and function and meet almost daily (Chapter 12).

'NEW STYLE' LABOUR

In this era of high technology labours I am considerably heartened by Professor Stirrat (Chapter 2) when he writes 'in women who are already at low risk there is little room for improvement. Indeed intervention can do more harm than good.' The more so when Mr Godfrey, another specialist

Table 31.7 *'New style' obstetric programme from labour–six weeks post partum*

'New style'	Done by	Major reasons
First stage	Doctor and midwife	Doctor provides continuity and confirms normality; instils confidence into woman and companion; supports midwife, deals with minor abnormalities; decides on referral
Second stage	Doctor and midwife	As above; provides second pair skilled hands
Third stage	Doctor and midwife	As above scores bonding; checks baby
Day 1	Doctor and midwife	Checks baby
Day 2–10 (at home)	Midwife	Daily care
Day 6	Doctor and midwife	Comprehensive baby check
10 days to 6 weeks	Health visitor	
6 weeks	Doctor and midwife	Pelvic history and examination; cervical cytology; preconception
	family planning nurse	counselling; contraception; baby check, immunization programme

obstetrician writes (Chapter 23) 'fetal heart monitoring of low-risk cases produced no significant improvement in perinatal mortality rate, or importantly in *morbidity*' (my italics). Furthermore most studies show an increase in forceps and ventouse deliveries and caesarean sections in association with an increase in monitoring. Accordingly it is vitally important to determine 'low risk' and this needs to be coupled with listening to what the woman herself would like.

Against that background it is not surprising that Professor Stirrat goes on to suggest that a strong theoretical case can be made for the majority of women, who are after all normal, being looked after by general practitioner and midwife. So many of the physical problems and social shortcomings and psychological overlays with which general practitioner and midwife frequently coped in earlier decades have all diminished. Obstetrics should increasingly become more normal. Jean Towler's account of normal physiological labour (Chapter 20) is so sensitively and beautifully written that it requires little comment. Her table describing 'the birth process' and comparing 'unnatural' labour/birth with 'natural' labour/birth (Table 20.1) summarizes cogently what she thinks and certainly stimulates me to evaluate most carefully everything that she writes. The importance of a plan being made for labour, including normal labours with which I am concerned, and including contingency plans in the event of complications, along the lines of the 'what if . . .' questions suggested by Dr Zander (Chapter 13) seems to be vital. I have always felt that the later antenatal attendances were of great significance and I feel the more so now. Tables 31.2 and 31.4 show what a high proportion of consultations the doctor does at the end of the pregnancy compared with the small number in early pregnancy (see Tables 31.1 and 31.3).

I like Dr Bull's suggestion that general practitioners should physically carry out occasional normal deliveries in order to keep in practice. Having not done any for quite a long time I shall lean heavily initially on the expertise of the midwife who will be supervising me!

Because of the potential normality of women in general practitioner obstetrics, I shall try not to over-react with drugs, drips, machines, and other interventions to minor abnormalities or minor delays in potentially very normal cases. I shall merely observe more acutely whether the normal process will see my patient through. Thus I may be able to avoid exposing a significant number of normal mothers and children to the risk of unnecessary medical intervention, the sort of thing which might be ordained on a 'routine' basis in a specialist unit. I appreciate this will put a greater burden on the midwives, but I think they will be happy to respond to this when they see that it gives them greater responsibility and leaves them more in charge.

Increasingly I shall try to avoid the use of drugs and use people instead. The more I read about drugs and their deleterious effects, and the more I see them changing from decade to decade the more suspicious of them I become. This applies to their use for pathological conditions just as much as it does for the use in a physiological process like labour. With the father present to give encouragement, a good midwife giving reassurance, and importantly a general practitioner paying an occasional visit to confirm that all is well in the various stages of labour, the resort to drugs can be minimal.

In early labour, especially if the woman has been admitted too soon, two tablets of dichloralphenazone (Welldorm) if requested give a reasonably tranquil night. Barbiturates and diazepam have no use in labour and should be abandoned, the more especially if one thinks of the health of the fetus. I shall carefully appraise women who have been in *established* labour for 8 hours, and where I anticipate that the labour is going to continue for several more hours it may be necessary to resort to intravenous fluids. However, their value must be balanced against the dilatation of the cervix, whether the woman is walking about, whether she wishes to continue to do so, her general condition etc. I cannot agree with Lim and Hawkins (Chapter 21) that 'any woman in established labour for 8 hours needs intravenous fluids'. This smacks of the sort of 'routine' or *diktat* that has provoked so much criticism of the hospital specialist management of normal labours in recent years.

Lim and Hawkins feel that gas and air is a harmless and reasonably successful analgesic and I shall try to use this first before I resort to pethidine. This the more so if there seems some possibility that the second stage is rapidly approaching. When narcotics are given 50 per cent of women develop nausea and vomiting and then need further drugs to control the side-effects, not to mention intravenous fluids to counteract any resultant dehydration. Hence the use of narcotics is always debatable and should never be 'routine'. Furthermore, Lim and Hawkins write that only 40 per cent of women in labour found 50–100 mg of pethidine helped them, and that even 150 mg of pethidine gave 'useful but incomplete relief to 50–60 per cent of mothers'. There are also deleterious effects on the baby. This gives me a wider perspective on the 'value' of routine pethidine which has been a mainstay of my obstetric practice for many years. I think I shall be using pethidine less and less in the future.

There seem to be increasingly differing views about the routine use of oxytocics in the third stage. Double-bind trials did not exist when these drugs were first evaluated, and have never been done. There is no doubt that increasing amounts of oxytocics seem to result in decreasing amounts of bleeding. I shall watch the literature, but I anticipate a decline in the routine use of oxytocics in the third stage of normal labours. I no longer fret if my midwife forgets, or does not give, Syntometrine with the anterior shoulder since I have seen many perfectly normal physiological expulsions of the placenta, albeit a little more slowly.

SOME DETAILS OF 'NEW STYLE' LABOUR ACCORDING TO STAGE

Stage 1

A companion should be present and ideally it should be the father; he should be involved and cared for throughout labour, and armchairs, light refreshments etc. should be provided. From time to time he should be asked how he feels! The woman herself should not have a perineal shave—perhaps a trim of long hair instead—an enema should be optional and she should use the vertical position, and walk about if she feels able, until ideally 7 or 8 cm dilatation. In future I shall look upon lying down as being ever so slightly dangerous! Standing-up labour pains are stronger and less painful and women currently spend too much time in or on a bed. Anything that prevents ambulation should have its value carefully assessed and be disregarded if the need is for cervical dilatation.

Longer labours could be permitted more frequently if there was less resort to rupturing membranes too early in the first stage. I must realize that once I have ruptured the membranes I have committed myself to possibly an interfering style of labour. I shall leave membranes unruptured until labour is extremely well established and thus perhaps prevent recourse to so many accelerations.

Much of the first stage of labour could take place at home, more especially if midwives visited the home at the onset of labour. This currently takes place for women who are booked by domiciliary midwives for early discharge schemes and it is rare for these women to be admitted 'too early'. If midwives visited all women in early labour then this would prevent too early admission, or even avoid admission for so called 'false labour'.

Inductions for uncomplicated postmaturity are usually ill-advised. They probably mean that the dates are wrong. If all the parameters of normality are satisfactory I shall leave my apparently 'postmature' women well alone, certainly until about 17 days 'post-mature'. That protocol should certainly ensure a chance of a normal labour for the great majority of normal women.

It is of great importance to keep the mother calm in labour and this means keeping oneself and all other attendants tranquil too. The deleterious effects of fear and anxiety are increasingly being substantiated by greater scientific knowledge of catecholamine studies.

Stage 2

The father should of course be present throughout the second stage and help to encourage and calm the mother. He should also be present at minor 'abnormal' events such as forceps delivery and perineal repair.

Masks and headwear are not needed for normal delivery; scrupulous cleanliness, but not (unattainable) sterility, should be the aim.

I shall use a permissive attitude in the second stage especially with regard to the woman's delivery position. I see no reason why a woman should not have her baby kneeling, sitting, standing, or lying down according to her personal preference and according to the way in which she can use her contractions best. Overall, squatting is probably the best position.

I shall no longer shout 'push'; I shall try to avoid even saying it! Maternal relaxation gives better control and easier stretching of the perineum. If the perineum stretches more easily there should be fewer tears.

With this approach to the second stage and realizing that the desire to bear down does not necessarily coincide immediately with full dilatation a normal second stage can last 2 hours. This may play havoc with my day (or night) but such interruptions are uncommon and must be taken as part of the routine of good general practitioner obstetrics. There is patently conflict between the physiological function and the busy (or sleepy) doctor!

Stage 3

Fathers too can bond with their babies so presence immediately after delivery—if not actually at it—should be positively encouraged.

I find that using Rhiannon Walters' word (Chapter 24) 'cut' or 'wound' instead of episiotomy or incision makes me a little more sensitive to what I am doing. I shall discuss episiotomies in late pregnancy and only do one if it is definitely indicated. I must ensure that the woman's perineum is well anaesthetized before the episiotomy is done and also during the repair. I shall remember from now on that one in five women had 'painful or very painful stitching' (Chapter 24). I shall be doing fewer episiotomies in the future and particularly trying to avoid them in primigravidae so that further episiotomy or repairs in subsequent pregnancies are avoided.

The above management of the three stages of labour are very different from Dr Bull's account (Chapter 23) of 'active management'. This he bases on a better physiological understanding of labour and he uses a prospective approach to anticipating or averting problems. The difficulty of course is that the physiology of labour is still not at all that well understood. In particular, physiological norms for each individual woman cannot be precisely determined. Hence 'errors' in management creep in as a result of lack of precise knowledge of what is normal for any particular individual. Once intervention has begun there can follow the side-effects of that intervention which in turn can set off further intervention and further side-effects. Ultimately whether the mother is any longer giving birth, or rather 'having birth done to her' becomes doubtful. Associated with intervention comes a greater need for drugs and machines. Ultimately the staff feel they cannot manage without them. I subscribe to the consensus view that the escalation of the number of caesarean sections, forceps, and ventouse deliveries in the United Kingdom in recent decades is largely due to a more 'active' approach to labour. At times that approach is patently life-saving. But as a general practitioner managing low-risk cases I shall try as far as possible to avoid too much intervention and aim to achieve all the creditable components that characterize a home delivery, yet under a hospital roof.

THE 'NEW STYLE' PUERPERIUM

Skin-to-skin contact and other methods of bonding between mother and baby and father should be encouraged. I like to score the bonding in my mind using the following 'measures' of the parents when baby is 'handed over': How do they look, what do they say, what do they do, how do they relate to each other? After the bonding comes fairly immediate breast-feeding. Then mother, father, and baby should be left alone for half an hour or so to commune as they wish.

I shall try to persuade the midwifery hierarchy in my own district that women should be discharged according to their individual needs. This will vary from an hour or two after delivery to 10 days when social circumstances at home are fairly desperate. On the whole earlier and earlier discharge should be ordained. Most primiparae could return home after 48 hours given adequate community midwife support. Lying-in wards could contract significantly.

Having read the chapters by Chloe Fisher and Sandy Tinson (Chapters 25 and 26) I am all the more convinced of the importance of the midwife and health visitor in the puerperium and thereafter, and the relatively small role of the general practitioner. I am even more prepared to let them get on with it.

Dr Pitt's excellent description (Chapter 29) of neurotic depression is one that any general practitioner would recognize: the gradual onset, the lingering symptoms, usually better by the baby's first birthday; 10 per cent of mothers have this type of depression in the puerperium.

For mothers who have had a severe psychotic depression in the puerperium I found it helpful from the point of view of advice to know that one in six will have a recurrence in a subsequent pregnancy.

Professor Morrell (Chapter 27) convinces me that I should change my postnatal examination at 6 weeks. The question 'knowing what you know now, how do you want matters changing next time?' seems to be a good starting point, followed by 'how does your husband (partner) want matters changing?' and then on to preconception counselling. I shall only do haemoglobins for those women under 50 kg, those with a low mean corpuscular volume in pregnancy, those of low social class and those who have had a postpartum haemorrhage or caesarean section. Effectively this means I shall stop doing the majority of haemoglobins that I currently do. I shall only do a cervical smear if none has been done for 3 years, but I shall ask two sensitive questions with regard to the genitourinary system. First I shall enquire whether sex has restarted and if so is it satisfactory. If it has not restarted I shall intimate that tolerance of discomfort should not be long term, certainly not more than 2 or 3 weeks. I shall tell them to report if all is not well by that time. Secondly I shall enquire about their urinary function and advise women with either frequency or incontinence what to do, and to report back if matters do not rectify within a few weeks. I shall emphasize the importance of exercise—pram pushing is a good one to start with—as a means of promoting healthy family activities.

FINALE

As the reader goes to his surgery tomorrow I hope he will have several ideas for immediate change in his obstetric care, several more for a few months time, and finally some as distant pipedreams. I hope he implements many of them.

Index